ANTIBIOTIC AND ANTIMICROBIAL USE IN DENTAL PRACTICE

Second Edition

ANTIBIOTIC AND ANTIMICROBIAL USE IN DENTAL PRACTICE

Second Edition

Edited by

Michael G. Newman, DDS
Adjunct Professor of Periodontics
School of Dentistry
University of California at Los Angeles
Los Angeles, California

Arie J. van Winkelhoff, PhD
Professor of Oral Microbiology
Academic Centre for Dentistry Amsterdam
Amsterdam, The Netherlands

Quintessence Publishing Co, Inc

Chicago, Berlin, London, Tokyo, Paris, Barcelona, São Paulo, Moscow, Prague, and Warsaw

Library of Congress Cataloging-in-Publication Data

Antibiotic and antimicrobial use in dental practice / edited by Michael G. Newman, A.J. van Winkelhoff. — 2nd ed.
  p. ; cm.
  Rev. ed. of: Antibiotic/antimicrobial use in dental practice. c1990.
  Includes bibliographical references and index.
  ISBN 0-86715-397-0
  1. Antibiotics. 2. Material medica, Dental. I. Newman, Michael G. II. Winkelhoff, A.J. van III. Antibiotic/antimicrobial use in dental practice.
  [DNLM: 1. Antibiotics—adverse effects. 2. Antibiotics—therapeutic use. 3. Mouth Diseases—drug therapy. 4. Tooth Diseases—drug therapy. WU 166 A629 2000]
  RK715.A58 G85 2000
  617.6'061—dc21

                                                                00-045822

quintessence
books

© 2001 Quintessence Publishing Co, Inc

Quintessence Publishing Co, Inc
551 Kimberly Drive
Carol Stream, Illinois 60188
www.quintpub.com

Editor: Lisa C. Bywaters
Assistant Editor: Katie Funk
Production: Susan Robinson
Design: Michael Shanahan

Printed in the USA

DEDICATION

We dedicate this book to our families, our patients, and our colleagues, whose support and encouragement have been sincerely appreciated.

CONTENTS

CONTRIBUTORS

J. Craig Baumgartner, DDS, MS, PhD
Chairman
Department of Endodontology
Oregon Health Sciences University
Portland, Oregon

Thomas Beikler, Dr med
Assistant Professor
Clinic of Periodontology
Center for Dentistry and Oral Medicine
Westfalian-Wilhelms University
Muenster, Germany

Sebastian G. Ciancio, DDS
Professor and Chair
Department of Periodontics
Director, Center for Dental Studies
School of Dental Medicine
State University of New York
Buffalo, New York

Jacob Fleischmann, MD
Professor
Section of Oral Biology and Medicine
School of Dentistry
University of California at Los Angeles
Los Angeles, California

Thomas F. Flemmig, Prof Dr med dent
Chairman
Clinic of Periodontology
Center for Dentistry and Oral Medicine
Westfalian-Wilhelms University
Muenster, Germany

Larry Peterson, DDS, MS
Clinical Professor
Department of Oral and Maxillofacial
  Surgery
Ohio State University
Columbus, Ohio

Douglas Harrington, DDS
Private Practice
Pediatric Dentistry and Orthodontics
San Diego, California

David Herrera, DDS, Dr Odont
Associate Professor
Faculty of Odontology
Complutense University of Madrid
Madrid, Spain

Stefan A. Hienz, PhD, DMD
Section of Periodontics
School of Dentistry
University of California at Los Angeles
Los Angeles, California

Perry R. Klokkevold, DDS, MS
Associate Professor and Clinical Director
Postgraduate Periodontics and Implant
  Surgery
School of Dentistry
University of California at Los Angeles
Los Angeles, California

Robert Lindemann, DDS, MEd, MS
Professor and Associate Dean
School of Dentistry
University of California at Los Angeles
Los Angeles, California

Andrea Mombelli, DDS, PhD
Professor and Chair
Department of Periodontology and Oral
  Pathophysiology
School of Dental Medicine
University of Geneva
Geneva, Switzerland

Sushma Nachnani, MS
Director
University Health Resources Group
Culver City, California

Joan Otomo-Corgel, DDS, MPH
Chair of Research
Dental Service
Veterans Administration Greater Los Angeles
  Healthcare System
Los Angeles, California

Adjunct Assistant Professor
Section of Periodontics
School of Dentistry
University of California at Los Angeles
Los Angeles, California

Mark Redd, DDS
Private Practice
Periodontics and Dental Implants
Laguna Hill, California

Mariano Sanz, MD, DDS
Vice-Dean
Faculty of Odontology
Complutense University of Madrid
Madrid, Spain

Stephen T. Sonis, DMD, DMSc
Professor and Chair
Department of Oral Medicine and
  Diagnostic Sciences
Harvard School of Dental Medicine
Boston, Massachusetts

Chief
Division of Oral Medicine, Oral and
  Maxillofacial Surgery and Dentistry
Dana-Farber Cancer Institute
Boston, Massachusetts

Senior Surgeon
Brigham and Women's Hospital
Boston, Massachusetts

Maurizio S. Tonetti, DMD, PhD, MMSc
Professor and Chair
Department of Periodontology
Eastman Dental Institute and Hospital
University College London
London, United Kingdom

**Christina M.J.E. Vandenbroucke-Grauls,
  MD, PhD**
Professor
Medical Microbiology and Infection
  Prevention
Academic Hospital Vrije University Amsterdam
Amsterdam, The Netherlands

Arie J. van Winkelhoff, PhD
Professor
Department of Oral Microbiology
Academic Centre for Dentistry Amsterdam
Amsterdam, The Netherlands

Edwin J. Zinman, DDS, JD
Attorney at Law
San Francisco, California

Former Lecturer
Department of Periodontology
University of California at San Francisco
San Francisco, California

PREFACE

Antibiotics and antimicrobials have become a critical and integral part of dental practice. Accordingly, there is a growing need for precise strategies and guidelines governing their use. The new and updated information contained in this completely revised second edition is essential for every practitioner. Although modernized in appearance and updated in content, the book remains the same important reference and resource that has become one of the most popular books in its field.

This second edition of *Antibiotic and Antimicrobial Use in Dental Practice* integrates basic facts and principles with concepts that have emerged during the last 6 years. As in the previous edition, a group of internationally recognized experts has been assembled to provide the most direct and pertinent information for application to clinical practice.

Above all, this book is user-friendly. Useful and informative tables, charts, algorithms, and information boxes support concise discussions of relevant information. In addition, icons have been generously dispersed throughout each chapter to alert the reader to important facts and principles.

A new chapter on general principles describes the infections and bacteriologically associated complications that can arise in the oral cavity. These conditions, diseases, and complications are among the most common situations dealt with in clinical practice. This background serves as the foundation for many of the systemic and topical agents described in the rest of the book.

Completely new or expanded chapters on viral and fungal infections, oral malodor, systemic disease complications, and special considerations for female patients, as well as a revised chapter on topical agents, offer a comprehensive view of the proper prescription and use of the bewildering array of agents currently available. Essential information about new therapies, including a form of periodontal therapy involving devices that deliver local controlled release of antimicrobials in the periodontal pocket, are discussed in a straightforward, practical manner.

Recognizing the integral role implants play in dental practice, specific guidelines are provided to assist the practitioner in the use of antimicrobials for the treatment of peri-implant infections as well as in the maintenance and treatment of plaque-associated conditions. Another chapter addresses the growing need for awareness of legal issues associated with the use of antibiotics and antimicrobials in clinical practice. This chapter illustrates the pertinent medicolegal and ethical issues through real-life examples drawn from cases, trials, and verdicts.

The chapter on restorative dentistry considerations discusses the mutual relationship between restorative dentistry and periodontics. This chapter also provides up-to-date information and suggestions for diagnosing, treating, and preventing infections in patients with removable prostheses.

Finally, this new edition consolidates the most significant information discussed in detail in the text in a series of highly useful quick-access tables, boxes, and charts. A listing of the most useful tables, boxes, and charts and where they can be found is provided in the Quick Cross-Reference Guide starting on page xiii.

The editors would like to thank the contributors for their excellent work and their dedication to improving the lives of patients, who depend on clinicians to have the most useful and accurate information possible. They also would like to thank the staff at Quintessence Publishing, whose collaboration and hard work helped to make this edition a truly comprehensive revision.

Quick Cross-Reference Guide

The Quick Cross-Reference Guide lists the pages in this book where information on a given topic has been conveniently summarized for easy access. To use this Guide, simply look for a description of the information you need within one of the following five categories: General Principles, Drug Selection, Pharmacokinetics, Drug Interactions and Adverse Effects, and Prophylaxis and Prevention. For example, to find out which antibiotics should be used to treat an oral *Candida* infection, look for this topic under the category "Drug Selection." Once you find the correct entry, you can go to the page(s) listed to find the information you need in an easy-to-read table, box, or figure format.

General Principles	
Antimicrobial failures and errors	Page 11, Boxes 1-6 and 1-7
Antimicrobial dosing and minimum inhibitory concentrations	Page 8, Box 1-3; page 49, Box 3-2; page 276, Appendix 2; page 277, Appendix 3
Considerations for antibiotic treatment	Page 19, Box 1-9
Endodontic indications for adjunctive antimicrobials	Page 147, Table 10-2
Errors in antimicrobial chemotherapy	Page 11, Box 1-7
Infection management	Page 167, Table 11-4; page 49, Box 3-2; page 17, Figure 1-3; page 275, Appendix 1
Legal—standard of care	Page 259, Box 19-1
Major drugs and agents used in odontogenic infections	Page 166, Table 11-3
Oral malodor	Page 128, Box 9-1; page 135, Box 9-3
Principles of diagnosis	Page 22, Box 2-1
Rules for bacterial sampling	Page 23, Box 2-2
Types of bacteria from odontogenic infections	Page 34, Table 3-1

QUICK CROSS-REFERENCE GUIDE

QUICK CROSS-REFERENCE GUIDE

Section

1

General Principles

Arie J. van Winkelhoff, PhD
Christina M.J.E. Vandenbroucke-Grauls, MD, PhD

1

PRINCIPLES OF ANTIMICROBIAL CHEMOTHERAPY IN DENTAL AND OROFACIAL INFECTIONS

A Brief History

Humans share the world with a large and diverse population of microorganisms, the majority of which are necessary for human survival. Microorganisms decompose much of our waste, process our food, provide essential nutrients, and give us substances—namely antibiotics—with which to treat infectious diseases. A small number of the many thousands of microbial species are potentially hazardous for humans; these are considered human pathogens.

Control of microorganisms is not a twentieth-century invention. Salting, smoking, pickling, and drying are methods of preserving food that date back to early civilizations. People have used herbs, strong perfumes, oils, and vinegar to protect themselves from infectious diseases such as the plague. The Greeks and Romans burned clothing and corpses during epidemics.

Today, much time, effort, and money are spent to control microorganisms. Most of our food and drinking water is sanitized, and we clean our bodies and our environment to prevent microbial contamination. In daily life we use various physical methods (filtration, heat, radiation, and ultraviolet rays), gas (ethylene oxide), and chemicals to control "bugs" (microorganisms) and to treat infectious diseases. This chapter deals with the principles of antimicrobial chemotherapy.

3

Microbial Control Terminology

Agents that kill microorganisms are called *cides*, which is a word often used in combination with the target organism. Thus, a *bactericide* kills bacteria (not the endospore); a *fungicide* kills fungal spores, hyphae, and yeasts; a *virucide* deactivates viruses; a *sporocide* kills bacterial endospores; a *germicide* kills pathogenic microorganisms; and a biocide kills not only microorganisms but all living organisms.

Agents that primarily prevent the multiplication of microorganisms are called *static* (from the Greek *stasis*, to stand still). A *bacteriostatic* antimicrobial agent prevents the multiplication of susceptible bacteria, thereby supporting the host defense system's efforts to eliminate the pathogen. *Fungistatic* agents inhibit fungal growth.

A *disinfectant* is a group of germicidal agents that kills bacteria but does not kill endospores. At effective concentrations, many disinfectants are toxic for human tissues and are therefore used only on inanimate surfaces. Any disinfectant used on human body sites must show a selective toxicity for microorganisms.

Antiseptic agents are chemicals that kill vegetative pathogens. Used to prevent sepsis (growth of microorganisms in blood and other tissues), they are applied directly to tissues (surgical incisions, wounds, and body surfaces). Examples of antiseptic measures include the application of iodine compounds prior to a surgical incision and the use of hydrogen peroxide in a prepared root canal.

Any substance used in the treatment or prophylaxis of disease is called a *chemotherapeutic* agent. Chemotherapeutic drugs used to treat infectious disorders are called *antimicrobial chemotherapeutics* and are capable of killing or halting the multiplication of pathogens at human body sites. Historically the term *antibiotic* referred to antimicrobial drugs produced by living microorganisms (bacteria or fungi) as a result of their natural metabolism, whereas *chemotherapeutic* referred only to artificially prepared antimicrobial agents. Today all natural antibiotics are chemically modified (semisynthetic) to improve their pharmacokinetic properties, making the distinction between antibiotics and chemotherapeutic agents obsolete. The current trend is to use the words *antibiotic* and *antimicrobial agent* for all antimicrobial drugs, regardless of their origin.

Drugs Against Bugs

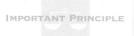

The use of antimicrobial agents is based on selective toxicity, a principle introduced by Ehrlich, who thought that selective staining might be used to target and kill microorganisms. Antimicrobial agents have selective toxicity, which means that they severely damage microorganisms but, ideally, have no effect on eukaryotic cells.

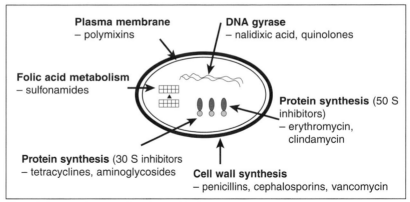

Fig 1-1 Mode of action of major antibiotics.

Table 1-1 The antimicrobial activity of various antimicrobial agents

Activity	Agent
Antimetabolic	Sulfonamides, trimethoprim
Cell wall inhibitor	Penicillins, cephalosporins, vancomycin
Bacterial protein synthesis inhibitor	Tetracyclines, clindamycin, aminoglycosides
DNA gyrase inhibitor	Naladixic acid, ciprofloxacin, ofloxacin

Types of Antibiotics

Some antimicrobial agents interrupt microbial metabolic pathways, which are not found in the host cell. These antimicrobial agents, known as antimetabolites, can be competitive inhibitors of microbial enzymes or false substrates that lead to the production of compounds that are toxic for the microorganism. Examples of antimetabolites are sulfonamides and trimethoprim.

A major structural component of the bacterial cell wall is peptidoglycan, and chains of peptidoglycans are linked by peptide side-chains (Fig 1-1). This amine linkage is the target for β-lactam antibiotics (penicillins, cephalosporins, monobactams, and penems). Other cell wall inhibitors prevent peptidoglycan synthesis (vancomycin, teicoplanin), acting mainly against gram-positive bacteria.

Another group of antibiotics (naladixic acid, ofloxacin, ciprofloxacin) interferes with DNA gyrase, an enzyme that supercoils bacterial DNA. Several antibiotics inhibit bacterial protein synthesis (aminoglycosides, tetracyclines, and chloramphenicol). Thus, different groups of antibiotics have different modes of action (Fig 1-1; Table 1-1). By nature, some antibiotics are active against a small range of bacteria and are called narrow-spectrum antibiotics; others damage or kill a wide range of microorganisms and are called broad-spectrum antibiotics.

5

> **Box 1-1** Characteristics of the ideal antibiotic
>
> Is selectively toxic to the microbe but nontoxic to eukaryotic cells
>
> Is bactericidal rather than bacteriostatic
>
> Remains relatively soluble and active even when highly diluted in body fluids
>
> Remains active long enough to be effective
>
> Does not easily induce antimicrobial resistance
>
> Complements and assists the activities of the host's defense
>
> Does not induce allergies in the host
>
> Does not affect the commensal microflora to a notable extent
>
> Has minimal to no drug interactions or adverse effects

The Ideal Antimicrobial Agent

All clinically active agents have advantages and disadvantages; however, the ideal antimicrobial agent has the characteristics listed in Box 1-1 and described below.

Activity

KEY FACTS

The activity of the ideal antimicrobial agent would damage pathogenic organisms while having minimal effect on the commensal microorganisms. The antibiotic should preferably be rapidly bactericidal. Activity can be diminished by the presence of resistant organisms that inactivate the antimicrobial agent.

Toxicity

KEY FACTS

Low toxicity for the host is an essential criterion for any antibiotic. Although minor adverse effects are common, severe adverse effects can lead to permanent damage (eg, loss of hearing after gentamicin therapy) and even threaten life. One example is an infection caused by a commensal colon bacterium *(Clostridium difficile)* that may be resistant to an antimicrobial medication and, as a result, can lead to the development of pseudomembranous colitis.

An antimicrobial agent may act as a sensitizing agent; for instance, approximately 15% of the North American population is hypersensitive to all penicillins. Photosensitivity may occur after use of chlortetracycline or naladixic acid. Topically applied antimicrobial agents may act as primary irritants. Several antibiotics can affect the nervous system; for example, aminoglycoside antibiotics have a specific action on the cochlear and vestibular nerves, and other antibiotics (polymyxin) can affect the optic nerve. Liver damage can be caused by erythromycin estolates, while aminoglycosides are nephrotoxic. Some antibiotics, such as metronida-

SPECIAL IMPORTANCE
FOR WOMEN

> **Box 1-2** Pharmacokinetic variables in antimicrobial therapy
>
> 1. **Diffusion** of the drug into the infected site: Depends on the lipid solubility, acid dissociation constant, and pH of the surrounding tissue.
>
> 2. Plasma **protein binding:** Only free antimicrobial agents can diffuse into tissues. Protein binding varies from 80-96% for doxycycline, clindamycin, and some penicillins to less than 25% for ciprofloxacin, amoxicillin, and metronidazole.
>
> 3. **Inoculum effect:** Loss of optimal effect of the antimicrobial agent due to dense microbial population. Reduction of the microbial mass (scaling and root planing in periodontitis, drainage in case of an abscess) may reduce the inoculum effect.
>
> 4. **Renal or liver impairment:** May limit the metabolism and excretion of the antimicrobial agent.

zole, are indirectly toxic and have teratogenetic (harmful to the fetus) effects when used during pregnancy. When administered to the mother during pregnancy, tetracyclines may have undesirable effects on the developing bone and dental tissues of the fetus.

Pharmacology

KEY FACTS

Effective treatment of an infection depends on knowledge of all infecting organisms and their susceptibility to the antimicrobial agent. The site of the infection, the spectrum of action, and the dosage are additional factors that contribute to the outcome of the therapy.

The absorption, distribution in body tissues and fluids, metabolism, and excretion of an antimicrobial drug should be such that an adequate concentration can be rapidly reached in the environment of the infecting organism and maintained there for an adequate length of time. An antibiotic that is excreted quickly needs frequent or continuous administration. The antibiotic blood level attained should exceed the in vitro minimal inhibitory concentration by a factor of 2 to 8 depending on the site of infection, among other factors. All antibiotics are bound to blood and tissue proteins to some extent, reducing the direct availability of the drug (Box 1-2).

Dosing

CLINICAL INSIGHT

The optimal dose of an antimicrobial agent is the amount that results in the maximum clinical effect with the least harm to the host and to the host's natural microbial flora. One strategy used in antimicrobial chemotherapy is to apply a high dosage for a short time as the clinical situation permits. Such a regimen rapidly provides a high concentration of the antimicrobial agent. A major factor in the success of many antimicrobial agents is the height of serum concentration and the level of the agent within the infected tissue. A shorter therapy reduces the chance for toxic and allergic adverse effects.[1]

> **Box 1-3** Principles of antibiotic dosing for orofacial infections
>
> 1. Employ high doses for a short time; this is more critical for concentration-dependent antibiotics such as metronidazole and quinolones than for β-lactam antibiotics.
> 2. Use a loading dose where indicated; this is especially important for tetracyclines.
> 3. Achieve a blood level of the antimicrobial agent of 2-8 times the minimal inhibitory concentration; this compensates for tissue barriers.
> 4. Use frequent dosing intervals for half-life times of penicillins and cephalosporins in order to maintain effective blood levels.

In acute infections, determination of the sensitivity (minimal inhibitory concentration [MIC]) of the pathogen(s) often is not possible, allowing for an initial loading dose higher than the maintenance dose. A loading dose may be justified when more than 10 to 12 hours is required to achieve the maximum blood concentration of an antibiotic or when the serum half-life (number of hours required for serum level to fall to half the maximum level) is longer than 3 hours. The half-life for tetracyclines, for example, varies from 5 (chlortetracycline) to 15 hours (doxycycline) (Box 1-3).

Time- and concentration-dependent antibiotics

Unlike bactericidal antibiotics, bacteriostatic antimicrobial agents such as erythromycin, tetracyclines, and clindamycin affect microorganisms at any reasonable concentration above the minimal inhibitory concentration. The effect of these antibiotics is either concentration-dependent or time-dependent.

Concentration-dependent antibiotics The activity of concentration-dependent antibiotics depends on the ratio between the peak drug concentration in the blood and the in vitro minimal inhibitory concentration of the pathogen. Examples of concentration-dependent antibiotics are metronidazole and the fluoroquinolones (ciprofloxacin, ofloxacin). For concentration-dependent drugs, a single dose resulting in a peak concentration 8 to 10 times greater than the in vitro minimal inhibitory concentration of the pathogen may be the optimum dosing strategy. This is because the killing rate is proportional to the drug concentration. Doubling the concentration of a concentration-dependent drug in vitro will kill the same number of organisms in half the time.

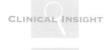

Time-dependent antibiotics Time-dependent antimicrobial agents kill microorganisms during time periods when the concentration of unbound drug exceeds the in vitro minimal inhibitory concentration for the pathogen. β-Lactam antibiotics (penicillins and cephalosporins) are examples of time-dependent and concentration-independent antimicrobial agents. Once a threshold concentration has been achieved (4 to 5 times greater than the minimal inhibitory concentration), increasing the drug concentration will not prolong or increase the bacterial killing. Cell wall inhibitors (β-lactams, vancomycin) are effective only against multiplying microorganisms because cell wall inhibition can be achieved only during cell wall formation. The goal of dosing with β-lactam drugs is to maximize the time of exposure to active drug levels and to maintain drug levels above the minimal inhibitory concentration for as long a period as possible.

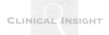

Post-antibiotic effect

The post-antibiotic effect of a drug refers to the period after the drug concentration has fallen below the minimal inhibitory concentration of a pathogen when bacterial growth is inhibited. This effect varies considerably depending on the type of antibiotic, the concentration of the drug, the length of the therapy, and the type of microorganism involved, and it differs for gram-positive and gram-negative bacteria. Post-antibiotic effects tend to last longer for antimicrobial agents that inhibit protein synthesis (eg, macrolides, clindamycin, and tetracyclines) than for β-lactam antibiotics.

Antibiotic Combinations

In some infections a single antibiotic therapy may not be sufficient to control the disease, requiring the combining of two antimicrobial agents. However, one must recognize that two antibiotic agents do not always kill a pathogen better than one agent alone (Box 1-4).

The guidelines in Box 1-5 should govern the simultaneous administration of more than one antimicrobial agent. Two antimicrobial agents may have synergistic effects on a bacterial pathogen by interfering in a bacterial metabolic pathway at different points. One example of such an effect involves sulfonamides and trimethoprim, two antimicrobial agents that interfere with the bacterial metabolism of para-aminobenzoic acid (PABA). These two drugs are combined in one medication in the treatment of gram-negative bacterial infections. Metronidazole with amoxicillin and metronidazole with ciprofloxacin display synergistic actions against the periodontal pathogen *Actinobacillus actinomycetemcomitans*. The minimal inhibitory concentrations of each of these two antimicrobial agents are significantly reduced in a synergistic interaction between the two drugs. This means that in vivo even low concentrations of both drugs are bactericidal at the infected site. Especially in infected sites that are difficult for antimicrobial agents to penetrate, synergy between two antibiotics may be the only way to resolve the infection. In *Helicobacter pylori* gastritis, two antibiotics are always necessary to eradicate the infectious agent.

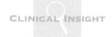

Box 1-4 Interactions between two antimicrobial agents

- Bacteriostatic + bacteriostatic: usually results in additive effects (1 + 1 = 2)
- Bactericidal + bacteriostatic: often results in antagonistic effects (1 + 1 < 1)
- Bactericidal + bactericidal: may result in synergistic effects (1 + 1 > 2)

Box 1-5 Guidelines for administering more than one antimicrobial agent

1. To broaden the antimicrobial range of the therapeutic regimen beyond that of a single antibiotic. This is often needed in the treatment of mixed infections (more than one pathogen with different antimicrobial susceptibility profiles).
2. To prevent or delay the emergence of bacterial resistance by using agents with overlapping antimicrobial spectra.
3. To lower the required dose of a potentially toxic drug.
4. To exploit synergistic interactions between two drugs.

Antibiotic Choice

A number of factors should be considered before choosing an antibiotic to treat a bacterial infection. In addition to considering the characteristics of the infectious agent, pharmacology, and toxicity, the cost of the drug should also be taken into account (Table 1-2).

Failure of Antimicrobial Therapy

An antimicrobial therapy can fail for a number of reasons (Box 1-6). The clinician may have selected the wrong antibiotic. The dose may have been too small, or a correct dose may have been given for too short a period (Box 1-7). The antibiotic may not be able to sufficiently penetrate into the infected area (eg, β-lactam antibiotic in an abscess). The presence of foreign bodies (heart implants, orthopedic devices, and dental implants) may decrease the effect of an antibiotic. Poor vascularization and poor blood flow can result in local concentrations that may be too low for controlling the infection.

Toxicity, hypersensitivity, and other adverse effects may require cessation of the therapy. The patient may fail to take the antibiotics properly. When the host defense system does not function optimally (previous disease, age, immunological disorder), it is significantly more difficult to overcome an infection even when potent antibiotics are used. A competent host defense system is essential when bacteriostatic antimicrobial

Table 1-2 Factors influencing antibiotic choice

Factor	Notes
Activity	Can be different in vitro and in vivo; is the pathogen known?
Concentration at site of infection	Poor in abscesses
Pharmacokinetics	The local antibiotic concentration should be significantly higher than the in vitro minimal inhibitory concentration; high dose is important for metronidazole and quinolones; prolonged dose is essential for penicillins and cephalosporins
Adverse effects	Hepato- and nephrotoxicity, allergy (ampicillin rash), superinfection (thrush, pseudomembranous colitis)
Costs	Availability of cheaper alternatives; duration of therapy

Box 1-6 Causes of failure in antimicrobial therapy

1. The organism is not susceptible to the prescribed antimicrobial agent
2. The pathogen(s) may have become resistant
3. Wrong diagnosis
4. Wrong antibiotic or combination of incompatible antibiotics
5. Incorrect dose
6. Mixed infection present with insufficient antibiotic coverage
7. Side effects and drug withdrawal
8. Superinfection
9. Inadequate surgery (debridement, drainage)
10. Inadequate host defense system

Box 1-7 Common errors in antimicrobial chemotherapy

1. Viral infections do not respond to antibiotics
2. Ineffective dose of the appropriate antibiotic is administered
3. Toxic agents are used when less toxic medication is available
4. Expensive drugs are prescribed when equally effective but less expensive drugs are available
5. Susceptibility profile of the pathogen is not known
6. Patient's progress is not monitored

Table 1-3 Some factors that influence the clinical efficacy of an antimicrobial drug

Factor	Description
1. Binding of the drug to tissues	Tetracycline binds to dentin and is released over an extended period of time.
2. Protection of key organisms	In a mixed microbial population, some bacteria may inactivate an antibiotic, thereby protecting target organisms. Metronidazole can be inactivated by *Enterococcus*, which protects *Bacteroides fragilis*, a penicillinase-producing commensal bacterium that can protect a penicillin-sensitive target organism.
3. Total bacterial load	The total number of bacteria at the infected site may be too high to be controlled by an antimicrobial agent (inoculum effect). Reducing the total number of bacteria, eg, by drainage of pus, facilitates the effectiveness of the agent.
4. Bacteriostatic (tetracyclines)	Use of bacteriostatic antibiotics may not result in elimination of the infection, especially in neutropenic patients.
5. Degrading enzymes	Penicillins and cephalosporins can be degraded by penicillinases and cephalosporinases.
6. Biofilm effects	Bacteria in biofilms need a higher antibiotic concentration to be killed in comparison to planctonic bacteria. Minimal inhibitory and bactericidal concentrations may exceed breakpoint concentrations.

agents are used. An antibiotic therapy may not be effective against all the organisms present. Orofacial infections are often caused by multiple bacterial pathogens (odontogenic abscesses, periodontitis, and endodontic infections). Bacteriological examination of exudate is therefore essential for selection of the correct antibiotic or antibiotics. Some factors that influence the clinical efficacy of antimicrobial drugs are summarized in Table 1-3.

The Drug-Bug-Host Triangle

IMPORTANT PRINCIPLE

The concept of anti-infective therapy involves three components: the drug, the bug, and the infected host. A systemic antimicrobial agent supports the infected host to overcome the infection by killing or halting the growth of the invading microorganisms. In addition, the host defense system eliminates the microorganisms. Figure 1-2 shows the interactions between the host, the drug, and the infecting organisms. The antimicrobial agent is selected on the basis of its activity against the organism. The antimicrobial agent can be bactericidal or bacteriostatic *(1)*. The influence of the microorganism on the drug is "consumption" and possible production of enzymes that degrade the antibiotic and creates microbial drug resistance *(2)*. The microorganism affects the host and causes disease. The virulence and pathogenicity of the microorganism are determining factors for the course and outcome of the disease *(3)*. In response to the growth of the infecting organism, the host defense system tries to eliminate the pathogen through cellular and humoral immune responses

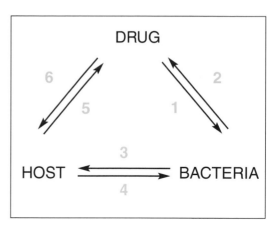

Fig 1-2 Interactions between the drug, the bug and the host. There is antimicrobial activity of the drug against the pathogenic microorganisms *(1)*. The microorganisms consume the drug and may be capable of degrading the antimicrobial agent through enzymatic action *(2)*. The pathogen with a certain virulence and pathogenicity affects the host *(3)*. In return, the host defense system tries to eliminate the infectious agent *(4)*. The host will bind the drug to plasma proteins and digest the drug *(5)*. The drug can adversely affect the host and the commensal microflora of the host *(6)*.

(4). The host binds the drug to plasma proteins, "digests" the antimicrobial agent through metabolic processes, and excretes the metabolic end products in urine and feces *(5)*. Some antibiotics are active through metabolic products that are formed in the host. These metabolic products can display greater in vivo antimicrobial activity than the original compound. The host is also capable of developing an immunological reaction toward an antimicrobial agent. The antimicrobial agent can cause adverse effects in the host *(6)*. Antimicrobial therapy may result in superinfection, that is, the outgrowth of commensal microorganisms that are relatively resistant to the drug and cause an inflammatory response. An example is *Candida albicans*, a yeast present in the mouth and vagina that can cause oral or vaginal candidiasis.

Antimicrobial drugs assist the patient in overcoming an infectious disorder. However, one should always bear in mind that antibiotics have adverse side effects and should therefore be used with great caution and based on defined criteria.

Adverse Effects of Antibiotics

Chemotherapy, by its very nature, involves contact with foreign chemicals that can potentially harm human tissues. It is estimated that approximately 5% of the individuals taking an antibiotic drug develop some form of serious adverse reaction. Box 1-8 lists the three basic types of adverse effects that can be distinguished.

> **Box 1-8** Three basic types of adverse antibiotic effects
>
> 1. Direct tissue damage through toxicity
> 2. Allergic reactions
> 3. Disruption of the balance of the commensal microbial flora

Toxicity

The organs and tissues most subject to toxicity are the liver (hepatotoxic), kidneys (nephrotoxic), gastrointestinal tract, cardiovascular system, blood-forming tissue, nervous system (neurotoxic), skin, teeth, and bone.

The liver metabolizes and detoxifies foreign chemicals. A chemotherapeutic or its metabolite may lead to hepatitis, while enzymatic abnormalities may damage liver cells. The kidneys act as blood filters and excrete drug metabolites that may damage kidney tissue. Antibiotics such as chloramphenicol can interfere with the blood-forming cells in the bone marrow, possibly resulting in reversible or irreversible (fatal) anemia. Some drugs hemolyze red blood cells, others can cause leukopenia, and still others can damage platelets, thereby interfering with blood clotting. Certain antimicrobial drugs can affect the brain and cause seizures; others, such as aminoglycosides, can damage nerves (commonly the eighth cranial nerve) and cause dizziness, vertigo, and deafness. When drugs block the transmission of impulses to the diaphragm, respiratory failure can be the result. The skin is a frequent target of antibiotic adverse effects. Skin disorders can be a symptom of an allergic reaction or a sign of direct toxic effects. Some antibiotics (tetracyclines) may interact with sunlight and cause photodermatitis. Tetracyclines are contraindicated for children under the age of 8 years because they bind to enamel of the teeth and cause discoloration. Pregnant women should avoid tetracyclines because they can cross the placenta and affect the development of bones and teeth in the fetus.

Allergic responses to antibiotics

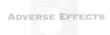

A frequent adverse effect of antibiotics is the development of allergy. Allergy is an immunological reaction toward a foreign molecule. Antimicrobial drugs or metabolites of the drug can act as antigens against which antibodies are produced. Penicillin, for example, is converted in the body to a molecule that may combine with large serum protein carrier molecules to form an antigenic hapten-carrier complex. Approximately 2.5% of individuals produce antibodies in response to these complexes, leading to allergic reactions. Allergic reactions have been described for all major types of antibiotics, but penicillins account for the greatest number of antibiotic-induced allergies.

Suppression and alteration of the commensal microflora

The normal microbial flora of the skin, the mouth, the outer openings of the urogenital tract, and the large intestine comprise a wide variety of bacteria that colonize the healthy human body. These resident bacteria are normally harmless and maintain an ecological balance. Broad-spectrum antibiotics may disturb this balance and cause outgrowth of specific species, which may in turn lead to superinfection. For example, when a cephalosporin is used to treat an *Escherichia coli* urinary tract infection, a large number of lactobacilli in the vagina may also be killed. These lactobacilli maintain a low pH in the vagina by producing large amounts of lactic acid. The low pH is a defense mechanism against outgrowth of *Candida albicans*. Reduction of lactobacilli during antibiotic therapy may lead to increased pH outgrowth of *C albicans* and vaginitis. The same phenomenon can occur in the oropharynx and cause thrush.

Another example of a superinfection following an antibiotic therapy is antibiotic-associated colitis or pseudomembranous colitis, sometimes seen after oral therapy with several antimicrobial agents. This superinfection is caused by selective outgrowth in the bowel of *Clostridium difficile*, a spore-forming anaerobic bacterial species. This organism can produce toxins that cause severe diarrhea, fever, and abdominal pain. Superinfections have become a serious problem in hospital patients.

Drug Interactions

When given simultaneously, two drugs may interact and influence each other's effect or cause unexpected side effects. (For possible interactions between antimicrobial agents, see "Antibiotic Combinations" above). Antimicrobial agents can also interact with other drugs. Table 1-4 summarizes the most important factors to consider when choosing an antimicrobial agent. One of the factors listed is the importance of taking a medical history to find out about any other drugs the patient might be using.

Interaction between two drugs may occur before absorption of the drugs. An example is the diminished absorption of tetracycline when taken with metallic ions, which tend to chelate the tetracycline. This effect may be such that the achieved concentration of the drug is insufficient for a therapeutic effect. After absorption, competition for protein binding sites may lead to increased effective activity of the displaced drug. Sulfonamides are especially well known for their competition for albumin binding sites with drugs like warfarin (an anticoagulant) or methotrexate (a cytostatic agent). This results in increased anticoagulant activity or cytotoxicity, and then the dosage of the other drugs needs to be adjusted. Conversely, sulfonamides may be displaced from their binding sites by salicylates, indomethacin, and phenylbutazone, leading to increased sulfonamide activity.

Table 1-4 Examples of interactions of antimicrobial agents with other drugs

Antimicrobial drug	Interacting drug	Effect of interaction
Aminoglycosides	Furosemide	Increased oto- and nephrotoxicity
	Cephalosporins and vancomycin	Increased nephrotoxicity
	Muscle relaxants	Neuromuscular blockade
Tetracyclines	Antacids and iron	Diminished absorption of tetracycline
	Carbamazepine, diphenylhydantoine, and barbiturates	Decreased half-life of tetracycline
	Oral contraceptives	Decreased oral contraceptive effect
	Oral anticoagulants	Potentiating effect on anticoagulation
Rifampin	Many compounds*	Reduction in oral bioavailability and decreased serum half-life
Metronidazole	Alcohol	Disulfiram effect (nausea)
	Oral (coumarin-type) anticoagulants	Inhibition
Macrolides	Several compounds	Increased levels of the drugs
Clindamycin	Neuromuscular blocking agents	Enhanced effect
Sulfonamides	Anticoagulants	Enhanced effect
	Chlorpropamide, tolbutamide	Increased hypoglycemic effect
	Diuretics, phenytoin, uricosuric agents	Potentiating effect
Trimethoprim-sulphamethoxazole (cotrimoxazole)	Phenytoin methotrexate	Increased levels
	Cyclosporine	Inhibition of renal creatinine excretion
Quinolones	Antacids	Reduced oral bioavailability of quinolone
	Theophylline, caffeine	Impaired elimination
	Nonsteroidal anti-inflammatory drugs	Seizures
	Morphine	Decreased serum concentration of quinolone

*At least 50 different drugs.

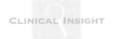
CLINICAL INSIGHT

An important mechanism of interaction is the induction or inhibition of hepatic enzymes responsible for drug inactivation. One of the most potent inducing agents for hepatic enzymes is rifampin, which leads to a decreased serum half-life for prednisone, digitoxin, oral contraceptives, quinidine, sulfonylurea, and several other drugs. Such interaction may decrease the efficacy of oral contraceptives, cause arrhythmias during quinidine therapy, cause decompensation during digitoxin therapy, and may affect diabetes regulation.

Interaction involving the kidneys can lead to increased nephrotoxicity. The potential for such interaction must always be borne in mind

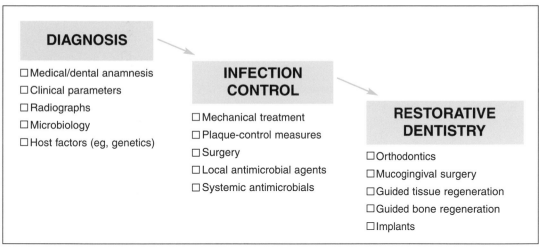

Fig 1-3 Three basic steps in dental management of infectious disorders.

when treating patients taking diuretic drugs (eg, furosemide), which tend to increase the nephrotoxicity of antimicrobial agents.

The possibility of adverse drug interactions should always be considered before prescribing an antimicrobial agent for any patient taking medication, and it is important to follow the manufacturer's instructions or to request advice from a pharmacist or physician.

IMPORTANT PRINCIPLE

Three Basic Steps in the Dental Management of Infectious Disorders

IMPORTANT PRINCIPLE

In dentistry, treatment of infectious disorders consists of three basic steps: diagnosis, infection control, and restorative measures (Fig 1-3).[2] Following this protocol is essential in obtaining a predictable treatment outcome.

Diagnosis

The diagnostic phase in the treatment of orofacial infections is of paramount importance. Since most if not all infectious disorders are multifactorial, it is crucial to obtain as much relevant diagnostic information as possible. A detailed diagnosis will enable the clinician to select the most effective anti-infective treatment. Diagnosis involves not only collecting information and clinical data from the patient but also understanding the disease process in an individual patient, estimating the prognosis of the disease progression, and identifying potential risk factors for therapy failure. Furthermore, a diagnosis should enable the clinician to make a rational choice among alternative treatments. A diagnosis requires a

1. Medical history
2. Dental history
3. Radiographic examination (upon indication)
4. Review of current medications, including recent use of antibiotics
5. Documentation of drug hypersensitivity
6. Risk assessment

The need for additional information depends on the type of orofacial infection.

In the case of a young-adult patient with severe periodontitis, for example, besides the dental, periodontal, and radiographic information, several additional factors may be of importance. Putative risk factors for chronic, aggressive, and refractory periodontitis include smoking, stress, genetic disposition, intrafamily transmission of periodontal pathogens, systemic disorders (diabetes mellitus), and medical infections (eg, HIV). Information about these factors will contribute to an optimal diagnosis and prognosis.

When a systemic antimicrobial chemotherapy is considered, microbiological diagnosis can assist in selecting the most effective drug regimen. A rational view of the treatment needed to control the infection is enabled in the diagnostic phase.

Infection control

KEY FACTS

Measures that are essential in the management of orofacial infections are drainage of pus, debridement of affected tissues, and removal of foreign bodies when present. Unless the source of the infection is eliminated, every therapy will ultimately fail.

Evacuation of pus is the first and most essential step in the treatment of odontogenic abscesses. Mechanical removal of bacterial deposits in endodontal and periodontal infections will lower the bacterial load and is a critical step in the anti-infective treatment. In periodontitis, supra- and subgingival debridement is the first and crucial phase of periodontal infection control.[3] Antimicrobial oral rinses can support mechanical treatment in controlling the microflora after, for instance, periodontal surgery. Irrigation of deepened periodontal pockets or dental root canals with an anti-infective agent can enhance the effects of mechanical debridement. A systemic antimicrobial therapy should be used when it seems likely that withholding the antibiotic therapy will result in therapy failure or will significantly lengthen the time of disease. Immunocompromised patients or individuals with a systemic disease more often

---

> **Box 1-9** Considerations for antibiotic treatment
>
> 1. Fever and/or chills within the last 24 hours
> 2. Malaise, fatigue, weakness, dizziness, rapid respiration
> 3. Trismus
> 4. Cellulitis: infection extending rapidly into adjacent spaces or tissues with abscess formation
> 5. Local or systemic infection with a history of rheumatic fever, endocarditis, heart prosthesis
> 6. Immunocompromised status (AIDS, cancer, autoimmune disease, corticosteroid therapy)
> 7. Allograph (cardiac, renal, bone marrow, liver, osseous implant)
> 8. Diabetes mellitus Type I, II, or III

IMPORTANT PRINCIPLE

need systemic antibiotics to overcome an infectious disorder. Antibiotics should definitely be considered for patients with orofacial infections when one or more of the signs, symptoms, or conditions shown in Box 1-9 is present. In many patients with one of these conditions, the dental professional will initiate therapy in collaboration with a physician to ensure optimal treatment for the patient.

Restorative measures

IMPORTANT PRINCIPLE

Following infection control measures, active repair of lost tissues and restoration of functions are integral parts of modern dentistry. It is of paramount importance to complete the infection-control phase before restorative treatment is initiated to prevent future complications. Guided bone and tissue regeneration using barrier membranes, dental implants to support crowns and bridges, and mucogingival surgery are treatments that now have predictable outcomes.

References

1. Pallash TJ. Pharmacokinetic principles of antimicrobial therapy. Periodontol 2000 1996;10:5.
2. Van Winkelhoff AJ, Winkel EG. Systemic antibiotic therapy in severe periodontitis. Cur Opin Periodontol 1997;4:35-40.
3. Van Winkelhoff AJ, Rams TE, Slots J. Systemic antibiotic therapy in periodontics. Periodontol 2000 1996;10:45-78.

Arie J. van Winkelhoff, PhD
Christina M.J.E. Vandenbroucke-Grauls, MD, PhD

Microbiological Sampling and Sensitivity Testing

The Role of Microbiological Diagnosis

An integral step in the diagnosis of an infectious disorder is the identification of the microorganisms involved. One of the services of a microbiology laboratory is to provide accurate information about the presence or absence in a specimen of microorganisms that may be involved in a disease process. In addition, it provides relevant information on the antimicrobial susceptibility profile of the pathogen(s).

The ability to achieve an optimal microbiological diagnosis depends on the interaction between the clinician and the laboratory. The clinician must be aware of the critical steps involved in collecting and transporting a specimen, while the microbiologist must appreciate the patient's condition, must be able to understand the disease process, and should assist the clinician in interpreting the test results. The goal of sample collection is to gather information to serve as a basis for the clinician to select the most effective treatment.

In acute orofacial infections, treatment will be initiated on the basis of the "most likely pathogen(s)." Sample collection in such a case should be carried out before antimicrobial therapy is started. The results of the microbiological analysis may lead to a change in the antibiotic therapy. In chronic or subacute infections, a microbiological diagnosis can precede the selection of a systemic antimicrobial chemotherapy (Box 2-1).

IMPORTANT PRINCIPLE

KEY FACTS

Mixed infections

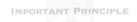

Exudates from soft and osseous orofacial tissues usually contain a mixed microflora of aerobic, facultative anaerobic, and strict anaerobic bacterial species, making interpretation of the results difficult. It is the clinician's responsibility to request either detection of a specific pathogen or analysis of the presence and proportions of all bacteria present. For instance, in a case of stomatitis a clinician may request a test on the *Candida* species, whereas in a case of an odontogenic abscess all bacteria present should be analyzed.

It is of paramount importance to inform the laboratory of the origin of the specimen. α-Hemolytic streptococci or *Actinomyces* species in a throat sample will be regarded as normal microflora of the oropharynx, whereas a large number of the same species in an exudate of an orofacial infection can be significant pathogens. It is the responsibility of the clinician to instruct the laboratory in the analysis of a specimen.

Collecting a Specimen

To obtain the most useful information from the microbiological laboratory, the clinician should comply with the rules listed in Box 2-2.

Submucosal lesions

Before exudate from a submucosal abscess or lesion is aspirated, the surface should be carefully decontaminated with an antiseptic (eg, aqueous iodine or nonphenolic compound). Skin can be decontaminated with io-

---

> **Box 2-2** Rules for bacteriologic sampling
>
> 1. Use sampling materials and guidelines recommended by the laboratory.
> 2. Select the proper device to collect a specimen. Use sterile absorbent paper points to sample a root canal or periodontal pockets. Sterile swabs can be used to collect mucosal specimens.
> 3. To avoid contamination of the specimen, carefully isolate the site of collection. Local antiseptics are helpful for disinfecting the sampling site in case of tissue penetration. Mechanically remove supragingival plaque deposits and gently air dry before sampling a deepened periodontal pocket.
> 4. Use an appropriate transport device to send the sample to the laboratory. Anaerobic bacteria must be transported rapidly in a special anaerobic transport system containing defined transport fluids.
> 5. Provide the laboratory with information relevant to the type of infection and be clear in the type of testing required.

IMPORTANT PRINCIPLE

dine and 70% alcohol. The exudate can be collected with a 20-gauge needle and syringe. If the exudate is transported in the syringe, the material should be immediately sent to the laboratory. The exudate can also be transferred to an anaerobic transport vial containing an appropriate anaerobic fluid. In all cases the material should be processed as soon as possible to keep the anaerobic bacteria viable and to prevent selective outgrowth of facultative anaerobic bacteria.

Incised lesions or abscesses can be sampled with a sterile swab, which should be placed in an anaerobic transport tube containing an appropriate transport medium. If actinomycosis is suspected, the sample of the lesion should be presented both for culture and for microscopic detection of sulfur granules. In case of an *Actinomyces* infection, gram staining will reveal gram-positive branching rods.

Mucosal lesions

Mucosal lesions can be sampled with a sterile wooden applicator after the surface has been cleaned with sterile saline. Since strict anaerobic bacteria belong to the normal flora of all oral mucosal surfaces, detection of anaerobes provides very little information.[1] Dry smears of a mucosal surface specimen can be prepared on a glass slide and stained (crystal violet or Gram stain). A wet smear of a mucosal surface specimen can be used to detect motile bacteria (motile rods and spirochetes).

Cariogenic microorganisms

To detect and enumerate cariogenic bacteria, supragingival plaque or saliva samples can be collected. Plaque can be removed from smooth and occlusal surfaces using sharp dental instruments, while interproximal sites can be sampled with dental floss.

Table 2-1 Bacterial species associated with progressive periodontitis and superinfecting microorganisms in periodontal infections

Species	Presence
Actinobacillus actinomycetemcomitans	Especially in early onset periodontitis and refractory periodontitis
Porphyromonas gingivalis	Present in severe adult periodontitis
Prevotella intermedia	Present in most forms of periodontitis
Bacteroides forsythus	Present in adult/refractory periodontitis
Fusobacterium nucleatum	Present in most forms of periodontitis
Peptostreptococcus micros	Present in most forms of periodontitis
Eubacterium	Present in adult/refractory periodontitis
Staphylococci*	Superinfecting organisms in adult periodontitis
Enteric rods*	Superinfecting organisms in adult periodontitis
Enterococcus*	Superinfecting organisms in adult periodontitis
Candida*	May multiply after systemic antimicrobial therapy
β-Hemolytic streptococci*	May cause streptococcal stomatitis/gingivitis

*Superinfecting microorganisms that may be important to detect.

Periodontal samples

CLINICAL INSIGHT

In cases of aggressive forms of periodontitis such as early onset periodontitis, refractory periodontitis, and periodontitis in immunocompromised patients, microbiological analyses of the subgingival microflora can assist in selecting adjunctive antimicrobial chemotherapy. To avoid contamination of the subgingival sample, the sampling site should be carefully isolated with cotton rolls, cleared of supragingival plaque, and air dried. Specimen collection can be performed with a sterile scaler or sterile paper points. A scaler will remove both attached and nonattached bacterial deposits. Absorbent paper points will collect nonattached microorganisms. In cases of generalized periodontitis, it is recommended to sample the deepest bleeding pocket in each quadrant of the dentition and to pool the four samples; in this way the major strict anaerobic periodontal pathogens can be collected.[2] In cases of local periodontal breakdown (localized juvenile [aggressive] periodontitis), all deepened periodontal pockets can be sampled and either pooled or analyzed separately. For clinical purposes, detection of a limited number of periodontal bacteria in subgingival plaque is performed (Table 2-1). Since most periodontal pathogens are commensal microorganisms, it is important to determine relative proportions rather than mere presence.

Peri-implantitis

When signs of infection and inflammation occur around one or more dental implants, treatment may involve antimicrobial therapy (see chapter 14). Samples may be obtained with sterile paper points or with a sterile (plastic) scaler. In the partially edentulous patient it may also be useful to sample deepened periodontal pockets when present. These periodontal sites may have been the initial reservoirs for infection of the peri-implant lesion. An integral part of the peri-implantitis treatment may thus be a (renewed) periodontal infection-control program.

Safety

It is sensible to assume that all clinical specimens are potentially infectious. This is true not only for samples containing blood but also for saliva samples. Clinical specimens should be handled with suitable precautions during transportation and in the laboratory. Specimens obtained from patients known to be positive for hepatitis B or human immunodeficiency virus (HIV) should be clearly labeled as such both on the sample device and on the request form.

Antimicrobial Susceptibility Testing of Bacteria

Many orofacial infections are treated successfully without identifying or testing the antimicrobial susceptibility of the pathogen(s). Therapy failure may occur, however, if the pathogens involved are resistant to the drugs of choice. Further, orofacial infections are usually mixed infections, and insufficient antimicrobial coverage in a mixed microflora may cause persistence of the infection. In a mixed infection, one bacterial species may produce an enzyme that destroys penicillins (penicillinases) and protects penicillin-susceptible bacteria.

Antimicrobial susceptibility testing is performed to guide the clinician in decision making. It should be borne in mind that in vitro susceptibility does not guarantee clinical efficacy. The choice of antimicrobial agent should be based on knowledge of the causing agent, its antimicrobial susceptibility, the pharmacology of the drug, possible or previous adverse and/or side effects, and other details of the medical and dental history of the patient. Consulting the patient's physician may be necessary to help in understanding the patient's current medical condition.

Susceptibility tests

Laboratory tests for antimicrobial susceptibility fall into two main categories:

- Dilution tests
- Diffusion tests

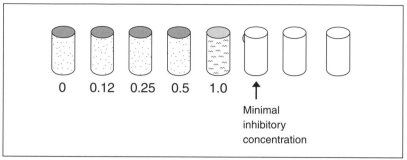

Fig 2-1 Antibiotic assay by the tube dilution method, which permits determination of the minimal inhibitory concentration (MIC). A series of increasing concentrations of an antibiotic is prepared in the culture medium. Each tube is inoculated with the same number of bacterial cells and incubated. Growth (turbidity) occurs in those tubes with an antibiotic concentration below the MIC.

Dilution tests A quantitative method for measuring the susceptibility of an antimicrobial agent is the minimal inhibitory concentration (MIC) test, which determines the lowest concentration of an antimicrobial agent that will inhibit visible growth in vitro. In an MIC test, a series of dilutions of an antimicrobial agent is prepared in broth and inoculated with the standard inoculum size of the test organism. After overnight incubation at an appropriate temperature (usually 37°C), the highest dilution in which there is no visible growth is recorded as the MIC (Fig 2-1). The MIC test can be used to determine an antimicrobial agent's minimal bactericidal concentration (MBC), which is the lowest concentration that kills the inoculated bacteria. The MBC is determined by subculturing aliquots of each dilution onto fresh medium without the antimicrobial agent and incubating overnight. The antimicrobial agent is considered bactericidal when the MBC is equal to or less than fourfold higher than the MIC. Determining the MIC or MBC of an antimicrobial agent is costly in terms of both time and money and is not always necessary. These tests play a role in the management of serious infections (eg, endocarditis) and those that fail to respond to apparently appropriate treatment.

Several other methods to test for antimicrobial susceptibility have been described and are currently in use, among them the macro- and microdilution techniques, the disk tube method, and the agar dilution method. In general, dilution tests are recommended for slow-growing organisms, including strictly anaerobic oral bacteria. Dilution tests also result in minimal inhibitory and bactericidal concentrations.

Diffusion tests Diffusion tests are performed with filter paper disks or tablets containing the antimicrobial agent. A plate is seeded over the entire surface with a bacterial isolate and disks are placed on the surface of

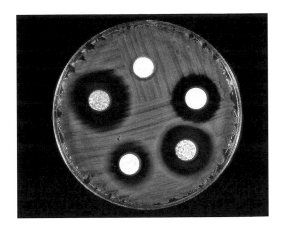

Fig 2-2 Diffusion test. The test organism shows sensitivity to some antibiotics as indicated by zones of inhibition of bacterial growth around the disks. The bacterial isolate shows resistance to one antibiotic as indicated by absence of inhibition.

the agar plate. After an appropriate period of incubation, the plate is examined for zones of growth inhibition around each antibiotic disk (Fig 2-2). The amount of antibiotic in each disk is related to achievable concentration of the drug in serum. Therefore, inhibition zones for different antibiotic disks vary. The larger the inhibition zone (expressed in millimeters), the more susceptible the isolate.

These inhibition zones are compared with the inhibition zone of a reference organism, and the test isolate's susceptibility is expressed as either susceptible (S), intermediate (I), or resistant (R). An "I" indicates that the antibiotic is less susceptible than the norm and that it may not be the first drug of choice or that the doses should be increased. The size of the inhibition zone is determined by the inoculum size of the organism, the antibiotic concentration in the disk, and the incubation time. For a number of bacterial pathogens, the relationship between inhibition zones and the MIC has been established. The MIC of an unknown isolate can be read from a regression line after the inhibition zone has been determined. This technique, called the Kirby-Bauer method, can only be used when the standard techniques are strictly followed.

The terms *susceptible* and *resistant* are laboratory parameters related to clinical outcomes after drug administration. An organism is described as sensitive or resistant depending on whether treatment with the usual recommended dose of an antibiotic is likely to result in successful therapy or failure, respectively (Box 2-3). The agar diffusion test is not suitable for accurate susceptibility testing of strict anaerobic organisms, which need a long incubation time.

KEY FACTS

> **Box 2-3** Terminology used in antimicrobial testing
>
> An organism is considered **sensitive** if treatment with an antibiotic at standard doses is likely to be successful.
>
> Treatment for a **moderately sensitive** organism is likely to be successful if an increased dose of antibiotic is used.
>
> An organism that is **resistant** is unlikely to be successfully treated with a given antibiotic, irrespective of the dosage.

Whole-plaque susceptibility testing

The subgingival microflora in periodontitis consist of large numbers of different bacterial species. Selection of an antimicrobial drug based on antimicrobial susceptibility testing of one or a few isolates may not predict clinical efficacy. Therefore, some authors have proposed a technique by which whole subgingival plaque is suspended, diluted, and streaked on a blood agar plate containing the breakpoint concentration of a given antimicrobial agent. The proportion of whole plaque that is inhibited by the antimicrobial drug in the agar plate is expressed as a percentage relative to the number of colonies growing on a blood agar plate without the drug.[3] Using this technique, it has been shown that some antibiotics (eg, amoxicillin) are able to inhibit 99% of the microorganisms of the subgingival plaque from deepened periodontal pockets.[4] However, it has also been shown that an antibiotic that is effective in vitro may not be effective in controlling a periodontal infection.[5]

Interpretation of test results

CLINICAL INSIGHT

The result of an in vitro test, an MIC value needs to be related to the clinical efficacy of the drug, and this is determined in part by peak blood and tissue concentrations. A systemic antimicrobial agent will be administered when the MIC is substantially lower (4 to 8 times, depending on the site of infection) than the achievable peak blood and tissue concentration.

Selecting the Correct Drug

CLINICAL INSIGHT

Besides sensitivity, a number of other factors influence the choice of an antimicrobial agent, including the spectrum of the drug, expected adverse and side effects, the condition of the patient, and the cost of the medication. In general it is preferable to choose the drug with the narrowest spectrum without loss of clinical efficacy, the highest selective toxicity for the infectious organism, and the lowest toxicity for the patient.

The ratio between the toxic dose and the lowest therapeutic dose of a drug is known as its therapeutic index. The smaller the ratio, the greater is the potential for toxic drug reactions.

For example, a drug with a therapeutic index of

$$\frac{12 \ \mu L/mL = \text{toxic dose}}{6 \ \mu L/mL \ (MIC)} = 1.2$$

represents a higher risk for failure than one with a therapeutic index of

$$\frac{10 \ \mu L/mL = \text{toxic dose}}{1 \ \mu L/mL \ (MIC)} = 10$$

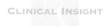

When a number of antimicrobial agents have similar MICs, the drug with the highest therapeutic index—that is, the drug with the widest margin of safety—is selected.

References

1. Van der Velden U, van Winkelhoff AJ, Abbas F, de Graaff J. The habitat of periodontopathic microorganisms. J Clin Periodontol 1986;13:243–248.

2. Mombelli A, McNabb H, Lang NP. Black-pigmented gram-negative bacteria in periodontal disease. II. Screening strategies for detection of *P. gingivalis.* J Periodontal Res 1991;26:308–313.

3. Van Winkelhoff AJ, Winkel EG, Barendregt D, et al. beta-Lactamase producing bacteria in adult periodontitis. J Clin Periodontol 1997;24:538–543.

4. Walker CB, Gordon JM, Socransky SS. Antibiotic susceptibility testing of subgingival plaque samples. J Clin Periodontol 1983;10:422–432.

5. Winkel EG, van Winkelhoff AJ, Barendregt D, et al. Clinical and microbiological effects of initial periodontal therapy in conjunction with amoxicillin and clavulanic acid in patients with adult periodontitis. A randomised double-blind, placebo-controlled study. J Clin Periodontol 1999;26:461–468.

Section

2

Drugs of Choice

Mariano Sanz, MD, DDS
David Herrera, DDS, Dr Odont

3

INDIVIDUAL DRUGS

Using antibiotics effectively in the treatment of orofacial infections (those occurring in the orofacial tissues) requires thorough understanding of the infecting microbiota. Odontogenic infections—those affecting teeth or periodontal tissues—are the most common type of orofacial infection. Most odontogenic infections involve a combination of gram-positive, gram-negative, facultative anaerobic, and strict anaerobic bacteria (usually dominated by the latter) (Table 3-1). Over the last 50 years, evolving technology has allowed for the isolation and growth of many fastidious anaerobic bacterial species.

Before 1970, when anaerobic bacteria were very difficult to grow, odontogenic infections were thought to be caused mainly by *Streptococcus* or *Staphylococcus* species and were treated with penicillin and erythromycin. Today we know that from 79% to 100% of odontogenic infections involve anaerobes and that facultative anaerobic bacteria are seldom present alone. Different antibiotics may be effective in treating odontogenic infections, either as a single regimen or in combination.

Besides the composition of the microflora, other factors that may influence the antimicrobial activity of systemic antibiotics[1] include:

1. Total bacterial mass
2. Bacterial invasion into root and periodontal tissues
3. Microorganisms in biofilms
4. Subgingival recolonization of the pocket from supragingival plaque
5. Binding of the drug to other nontarget microorganisms and tissues
6. Presence of β-lactamase–producing microorganisms

Table 3-1 Types of bacteria isolated from different odontogenic infections

Type of infection	Total flora	With anaerobes	Only anaerobes	Strict anaerobes*	References
Bacteremia secondary to tooth extraction		79%		71%	17
Orofacial odontogenic infections		95%	42%		18
Pulp necrosis—intact teeth	10^3–10^5			91%	19
Pulp necrosis—nonintact teeth	$10^{4.8}$			64%	20, 21
Periapical periodontitis	$10^{2.2}$	86–100%	14–39%	44–45%	22, 23
Periodontal abscess	>10^6	100%	0%	45–60%	24–27
Periodontitis		100%	0%		1

*Percentage of strains isolated.

Table 3-2 Pharmacokinetic characteristics of frequently used systemic antimicrobial agents

Antimicrobial agent	Route*	Excretion†	Serum-binding protein (%)	Peak serum level (µg/mL)	Time (h) for peak concentration	Half-life (h)
Penicillins						
Penicillin G	O	R	60		.75	1
Ampicillin	O/IM/IV	R	20	4	1	1.5
Amoxicillin	O/IM/IV	R	20	6,15	1.5	1–1.2
Amoxicillin/clavulanate	O/IM/IV	R	17/22	7.1/3.1	1	1–1.1
Cephalosporins						
Cephalexin	O	R	5–15	17		0.67
Tetracyclines						
Tetracycline	O	R/B	20–25	3	2	6–10
Doxycycline	O	R/B	75	1–6	2	12–22
Minocycline	O	R/B	90	0.7–4.5	3	11–20
Macrolides						
Erythromycin (base)	O	H/R	70	1	1.5	1.5
Erythromycin (ester)	O	H		1		1.5
Azithromycin	O	B	7	2–3	2	68
Spyramicin	O	H		1.1–1.8	2	5
Lincomycins						
Lincomycin	O	H			4	4–5
Clindamycin	O	H	Very high	5	.75	2
Nitroimidazoles						
Metronidazole	O	R	<20	12	1	8
Quinolones						
Ciprofloxacin	O	R			1.5	

*O—Oral; IM—Intramuscular; IV—Intravenous.
†R—Renal; B—Biliary; H—Hepatic.

Table 3-3 Serum and crevicular fluid concentrations after standard dosages of frequently used systemic antimicrobial agents[2–4]

Antimicrobial agent	Route*	Dose†	Time (h)	Maximum levels Serum (µg/mL)	Maximum levels Crevicular (U/mL)
Penicillins					
Penicillin G	O	10^6 UI	1–2		0.045
Ampicillin	O/IM/IV	500 mg SD	1–3	2–4	nd
Amoxicillin	O/IM/IV	500 mg SD	1–8	5.5–7.5	3–4
Amoxicillin/clavulanate	O/IM/IV	500+125 mg			
Cephalosporins					
Cephalexin	O	500 mg SD	1–3	5–17	nd
Tetracyclines					
Tetracycline	O	250 mg QID	48	1.9–2.5	4.0–8.0
Doxycycline	O	100 mg OID	48–105	2.1–2.9	6
Minocycline	O	100 mg BID	168–192	2.6–3.3	8–15.5
Macrolides					
Erythromycin (base)	O	250 mg QID	1–54	0.4–4.8	0.4–0.8
Azithromycin	O	500 mg OID	12–156	0.33–0.35	3.30–6.47‡
Spyramicin	O	2 g	2	1.1–1.8	10§
Lincomycins					
Clindamycin	O	300 mg SD	1–7	1.9	1–2
Nitroimidazoles					
Metronidazole	O	250 mg TID	120	14.3	13.7
Quinolones					
Ciprofloxacin	O	500 mg SD	1.25	2.4	nd

*O—Oral; IM—Intramuscular; IV—Intravenous.
†SD—Single dose; OID—once per day; BID—twice per day; TID—three times per day; QID—four times per day.
‡Levels measured in the gingival tissues.
§Levels measured in saliva.

Approximately 20 distinct antibacterial drugs, each with a well-defined mechanism of action, pharmacology, and antimicrobial profile, are available; about half of these have been used in the treatment of oral infections. This chapter reviews these drugs, emphasizing their pharmacology (Tables 3-2 and 3-3). The different types of antibiotics are presented according to their mode of action.

Inhibition of Cell Wall Synthesis

β-Lactam antibiotics

β-Lactam antibiotics include penicillins and cephalosporins, which have similar chemical structures. Penicillins can be classified on the basis of their antibacterial activity:

1. Natural penicillin (penicillin G), derived from *Penicillium chrysogenum*, and the only natural penicillin still in use
2. Penicillinase-resistant penicillins, including the isoxazolylpenicillins (oxacillin sodium, cloxacillin sodium, dicloxacillin sodium)
3. Aminopenicillins, including ampicillin-like agents and amoxicillin
4. Expanded-spectrum penicillins, including ureidopenicillins (ticarcillin, azlocillin, mezlocillin sodium, piperacillin)
5. Carbapenems (imipenem, meropenem)
6. Monobactams (aztreonam)
7. β-Lactamase inhibitors, which have a weak antibacterial activity and are used in combination with other penicillins and cephalosporins. This group includes clavulanic acid, sulbactam, and tazobactam.

Penicillins share a 6-aminopenicillanic acid nucleus, which includes the β-lactam ring. This structure is connected by an amide linkage to an acyl side chain, in which modifications and substitutions are responsible for the different β-lactam drugs.

β-Lactam antibiotics inhibit bacterial cell wall synthesis by inhibiting cross-linking between the peptidoglycan molecules. Because β-lactam antibiotics inhibit the transpeptidation mechanism of the cross-linking process, the new peptidoglycan chains are not cross-linked and lack tensile strength, which leads to cell rupture through osmotic lysis. This mode of action is bactericidal and affects only multiplying bacterial cells.[5]

Penicillin G (benzylpenicillin) *Absorption* Oral absorption is erratic; to obtain complete absorption, the parenteral route is preferred. Penicillin V (phenoxymethyl penicillin) is similar to penicillin G except that it is relatively acid stable and is well absorbed orally.

Distribution Widely distributed throughout the body, penicillin G has a short half-life in serum (20 minutes), requiring continuous administration at high dosages to maintain adequate serum levels. It crosses the placenta but not the blood-brain barrier in healthy individuals, and it is excreted in breast milk in low concentrations.

Excretion The antibiotic is cleared by the renal system. Different formulations—penicillin G procaine and penicillin G benzathine—extend the effect of this drug.

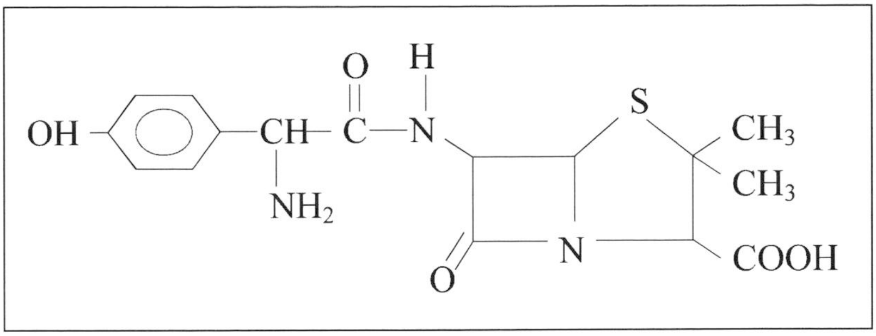

Fig 3-1 Structure of amoxicillin.

Mode of action Penicillin G inhibits cell wall synthesis.

ADVERSE EFFECTS

Adverse effects Adverse effects include hypersensitivity (0.6% to 10%), fatal anaphylaxis, diarrhea, and other gastrointestinal disturbances. At high doses, toxic effects such as hemolytic anemias, encephalitis, and nephritis may occur.

Spectrum Penicillin G is mainly active against gram-positive bacteria, including streptococci, staphylococci (excluding most *Staphylococcus aureus*), clostridia, and corynebacteria, and some gram-negative cocci, including *Neisseria meningitidis*. Among the gram-negative anaerobes, it is active against *Fusobacterium* and *Porphyromonas* species, some *Bacteroides* (not *Bacteroides fragilis*), and some anaerobic cocci.

INFORMATION ABOUT SPECIFIC DRUG

Amoxicillin *Absorption* The absorption of amoxicillin (Fig 3-1) is significantly higher than that of ampicillin; it has a bioavailability of 70% to 80%.

SPECIAL IMPORTANCE FOR WOMEN

Distribution It has good diffusion to organic fluids and infected tissues. It does not pass the blood-brain barrier in healthy patients, but adequate levels have been detected in surgical patients. Very low levels are secreted in breast milk.

Excretion Sixty percent of the amoxicillin is eliminated by urine during the first 4 hours.

Mode of action Amoxicillin has a quicker bactericidal action than ampicillin.

ADVERSE EFFECTS

Adverse effects Amoxicillin's adverse effects are similar to those of penicillin G.

Spectrum It has a broad spectrum. It is less effective than penicillin G against gram-positive cocci but more active against gram-negative cocci and gram-negative bacilli.

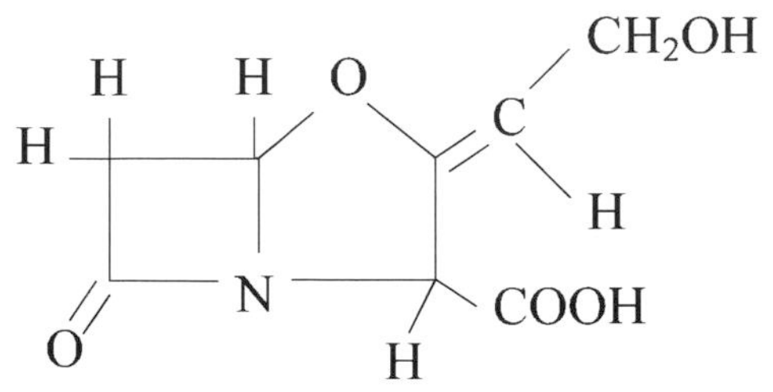

Fig 3-2 Structure of clavulanic acid.

INFORMATION ABOUT SPECIFIC DRUG

Amoxicillin/clavulanic acid The similar pharmacokinetic characteristics of these two drugs favor their combination.[6] Although clavulanic acid (Fig 3-2) has low antibacterial activity, it extends the spectrum of amoxicillin by inhibiting β-lactamase activity.

Absorption Clavulanic acid is well absorbed orally, allowing maximum serum levels to be reached in less than 1 hour, and has a bioavailability of 75%.

Distribution The combination has good diffusion to organic fluids and infected tissues.

Excretion It is excreted mainly at glomerular level. Forty percent of the clavulanic acid is eliminated by urine during the first 3 hours; it is also eliminated via feces, and it is metabolized in the liver.

ADVERSE EFFECTS

Adverse effects Gastrointestinal problems, including nausea, vomiting, diarrhea, and pain, affect 8% of those who take it. Allergic reactions and *Candida* superinfections may also occur.

INFORMATION ABOUT SPECIFIC DRUG

Cephalosporins These semisynthetic compounds, derived from cephalosporin C, share the β-lactam ring with the penicillins, the lateral chain being a six-member dihydrothiazine ring. They have been classified according to their generation (Box 3-1).

Indications Cephalosporins are indicated for nonhospital-acquired *Klebsiella* infections and as a substitute for penicillins.

Absorption Most cephalosporins are not absorbed well after oral administration and thus are only available for intramuscular or intravenous administration.

> **Box 3-1** Generational classification* of cephalosporins
>
> **First generation:** cephalothin, cephalexin, cephatrizine
> **Second generation:** cefuroxime, cefamandole, cefaclor
> **Third generation:** cefoperazone sodium, cefotaxime, moxalactam
> **Fourth generation:** cefepime, cefpirome
> *Cephamycins (cefoxitin) are structurally similar to the cephalosporins.

Distribution Cephalosporins are widely distributed throughout the body. Most of the dose is excreted unmodified via urine within 4 to 6 hours. They cross the placenta but not the blood-brain barrier (not useful in meningitis) and are excreted in breast milk in low concentrations.

Excretion Cephalosporins are cleared by renal glomerular filtration.

Mode of action Like penicillins, cephalosporins are bactericidal and inhibit cell wall synthesis.

Adverse effects Allergic reactions, including possible cross-reactivity with penicillins, are seen in approximately 10% of patients. Other possible effects are hemolysis, renal damage, oral moniliasis, local pain, tissue sloughing at the injection site, rash, urticaria, fever, gastrointestinal disorders, glossitis, neutropenia, and superinfection with *Pseudomonas* and *Enterobacter* species.

Spectrum Cephalosporins are broad-spectrum antibiotics, affecting most gram-positive bacteria as well as some gram-negative bacteria such as *Proteus mirabilis, Escherichia coli, Haemophilus influenzae, Klebsiella*, and *Enterobacter*. The third-generation cephalosporins extend their spectrum to gram-negative anaerobes.

Glycopeptides (vancomycin hydrochloride and teicoplanin)

Glycopeptides are large polar molecules that cannot penetrate the outer membrane of gram-negative bacteria. Vancomycin hydrochloride is a glycopeptide first isolated from *Streptomyces orientalis.*

Indications Vancomycin hydrochloride is mainly used in gram-positive infections unresponsive to β-lactam antibiotics or in patients who are sensitive to β-lactam antibiotics.

Mode of action Vancomycin hydrochloride, a bactericidal agent, inhibits peptidoglycan synthesis by interfering with chain lengthening.

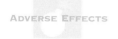

Fig 3-3 Structure of tetracycline.

Adverse effects Vancomycin hydrochloride and teicoplanin may cause severe side effects.

Spectrum Vancomycin hydrochloride is effective against all gram-positive bacteria. Bacterial resistance to the agent is extremely uncommon but has been reported in strains of enterococci.

Drug form and use In most cases, vancomycin hydrochloride and teicoplanin are administered intravenously; however, oral therapy with vancomycin hydrochloride is used to treat pseudomembranous colitis.

Cyclic peptides (bacitracin)

Bacitracin is bactericidal against some gram-positive bacteria and *Neisseria*. Because of its toxicity, bacitracin is used only as a topical agent in the treatment of superficial infections.

Inhibition of Protein Synthesis

Tetracyclines

A group of antibiotics with a common tetracyclic structure of four fused rings (Fig 3-3), tetracyclines are classified according to their pharmacologic action: short action—chlortetracycline, oxytetracycline, and tetracycline; intermediate action—demeclocycline; and long action—doxycycline and minocycline.

Indications The use of tetracyclines has declined because of an increase in bacterial resistance to these drugs. They are useful for treating acne and a variety of rarely occurring infections. In the oral cavity, they have been used systematically and locally as an adjunct in the treatment of periodontitis, acute necrotizing ulcerative gingivitis (ANUG), and periodontal abscesses and in the prophylaxis of bacterial endocarditis.

Absorption Tetracycline hydrochloride is absorbed approximately 70% orally; however, since tetracycline binds to calcium, antacids and dairy products may inhibit its absorption. Doxycycline and minocycline are absorbed approximately 100% and 95%, respectively.

Distribution Tetracyclines are widely distributed throughout the body; however, they may concentrate in gingival crevicular fluid at higher levels than in plasma. They cross the placenta barrier and are present in breast milk in low concentrations.

Excretion Tetracyclines are excreted via the renal system by glomerular filtration.

Mode of action These drugs, which are bacteriostatic at common concentrations, bind to the 30 S ribosomal subunit and specifically inhibit the binding of aminoacyl-t-RNA synthetases to the ribosomal acceptor site. Apart from their antibacterial properties, several nonantimicrobial benefits have been reported, including inhibition of host collagenase and enhancement of periodontal reattachment and bone formation.

Adverse effects Side effects of tetracyclines include gastrointestinal problems (diarrhea) and monililial infections (gastrointestinal, vaginal, oral). Tooth staining (permanent discoloration of dentin during tooth formation) may also occur, which contraindicates the use of tetracyclines during pregnancy and early childhood. Photosensitivity reactions also are common, and hepatotoxicity and nephrotoxicity may occur at high doses. The incidence of allergic reactions is uncommon. Vestibular alterations (vertigo, tinnitus) are common with the use of minocycline.

Spectrum Tetracyclines are broad-spectrum antibiotics effective against gram-positive and gram-negative bacteria, treponemas, mycoplasmas, chlamydiae, rickettsiae, and protozoa. Minocycline may be active against staphylococci.

Drug variations Tetracyclines have been evaluated in different formulations as locally delivered agents for the adjunctive treatment of periodontitis (see chapter 4). These formulations include ointments, irrigating solutions, acrylic strips, dialysis tubing, gels for root conditioning, resorbable controlled-release devices, and different types of fibers.

Macrolides

Macrolides are antibiotics with a common structure of macrocyclic lactam rings linked with amino sugars. The 40 different compounds in the macrolide group can be categorized according to the number of carbon atoms. The group with 14 atoms includes erythromycin, roxithromycin, clarithromycin, and dirithromycin. The group with 16 atoms includes spiramycin, josamycin, and diacetilmidecamycin. A new class of macrolides, the azalides (15 atoms), have improved pharmacokinetic properties, tissue distribution, and half-life and are active against gram-negative anaerobes. Azithromycin is the best known drug in this group.

Mode of action Macrolides, which are bacteriostatic drugs, interfere with bacterial protein synthesis by binding to the 50 S ribosomal subunit, it is thought by binding to the donor site during the translocation step.

Erythromycin *Indications* Erythromycin often is indicated in the treatment of diphtheria, atypical pneumonia including legionellosis and pertussis, and *Mycoplasma pneumoniae* infection and as an alternative for penicillin in penicillin-sensitive patients. It is also the drug of choice in neonatal chlamydial infection. However, it is not the drug of choice for anaerobic odontogenic infections.

Absorption One limitation of erythromycin is poor tissue concentration. Erythromycin base has a low solubility and is destroyed by gastric acid. To protect the drug, enteric-coated capsules may be used, but this may be counterproductive, resulting ultimately in incomplete absorption. Esters of erythromycin with stearate, estolate, and succinate improve absorption.

Distribution Erythromycin is distributed to most body tissues, with peak blood levels occurring 1 to 4 hours after oral administration. The stearate and succinate esters reach similar serum levels while the estolate compounds reach 3 to 4 times higher concentrations. Low levels are reached in the gingival crevicular fluid. It is secreted in breast milk, passes the placenta barrier, and reaches the cerebrospinal fluid in meningitis.

Excretion Erythromycin is excreted via bile, urine, and feces. Nonrenal mechanisms are more important.

Mode of action Erythromycin inhibits protein synthesis via an unknown action against ribosomal function.

Adverse effects It is well tolerated by most patients, although gastrointestinal symptoms such as vomiting, nausea, and diarrhea have been reported. Cholestatic jaundice (associated with the estolate form) and theophylline toxicity have also been described.

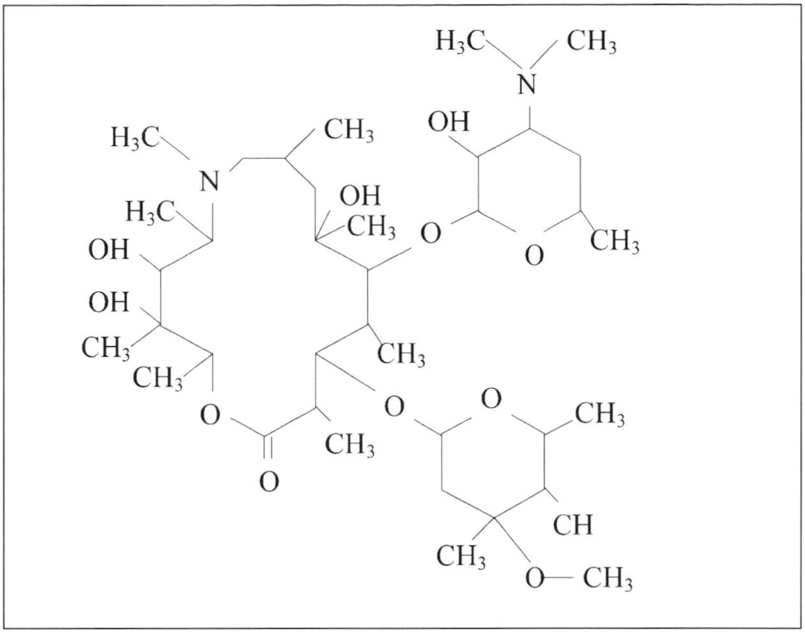

Fig 3-4 Structure of azithromycin.

Spectrum Erythromycin is active against gram-positive facultative anaerobic and strict anaerobic bacteria. Because erythromycin is unable to penetrate the lypopolysaccharide–cell wall complex, most gram-negative bacteria are not affected by the agent.

INFORMATION ABOUT SPECIFIC DRUG

Azithromycin *Indications* Azithromycin (Fig 3-4) is used to treat upper and lower respiratory tract infections, skin and soft tissue infections, sexually transmitted diseases, persistent chlamydial infections, and, in some cases, oral infections such as periodontitis,[7] periodontal abscesses,[8] and other acute oral infections.[9]

Absorption Azithromycin has better oral absorption than erythromycin because it has a higher resistance to gastric acids. The bioavailability is approximately 37%.

Distribution This drug is characterized by a unique pharmacokinetic profile.[10] Although blood levels are low (0.4 μg/mL 2 to 3 hours after a single 500 mg oral dose), the tissue levels are high (approximately 10 times higher than blood levels and up to 100 times higher than serum concentrations), with high levels in saliva, bone, and gingival tissues.[2] Azithromycin also reaches very high intracellular concentrations. It is secreted in breast milk.

Excretion Excretion is very slow; levels of the unmodified drug have been detected in the urine 14 days after administration. The principal route of excretion is hepatic bile.

Mode of action It has been shown that an active intake by phagocytes can transport the drug to the infected site.[11]

Adverse effects Azithromycin is associated with a low incidence of side effects; those that do manifest are mainly gastrointestinal problems. The drug is well tolerated in most individuals, including the elderly and children.

Spectrum It is effective against a wide range of microorganisms, including gram-positive aerobes, gram-negative aerobes, and strict anaerobes such as *Bacteroides fragilis, Fusobacterium* species, or *Peptostreptococcus* species. Azithromycin also has shown activity against *Actinobacillus actinomycetemcomitans*[12] and *Porphyromonas gingivalis*.[13]

Clindamycin Clindamycin is a semisynthetic derivative of lincomycin that usually is presented as a salt, such as clindamycin hydrochloride (Fig 3-5).

Absorption The absorption of clindamycin is almost total after oral administration and is better than lincomycin.

Distribution It passes readily into most tissues, with special relevance for its active transport to the interior of macrophages and leukocytes (high concentration in abscesses) and into bone tissues. It crosses the placenta barrier but does not pass through inflamed meninges.

Excretion Clindamycin is metabolized in the liver and excreted mainly in bile, but also through urine and feces.

Mode of action This bacteriostatic antibiotic binds to the 50 S ribosomal subunit and interferes with protein synthesis.

Adverse effects Diarrhea is reported to occur in 10% to 20% of patients using clindamycin, and morbiliform eruption appears in 3% to 5% of individuals. An uncommon but potentially serious side effect of clindamycin is the development of pseudomembranous colitis, an intestinal disease caused by overgrowth of *Clostridium difficile* (see chapter 7).

Spectrum Like erythromycin, clindamycin is active against most gram-positive facultative or strict anaerobic bacteria. It is particularly effective

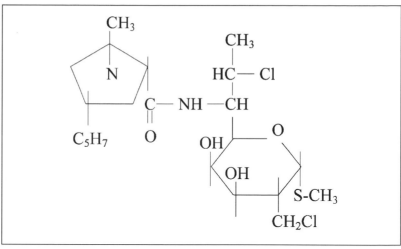

Fig 3-5 Structure of clindamycin hydrochloride.

against gram-negative strict anaerobic bacteria but not against most gram-negative strict aerobic bacteria.

Drug variations A formulation of clindamycin hydrochloride in a gel has been evaluated for local use in the adjunctive treatment of periodontitis.

Aminoglycosides Aminoglycosides include streptomycin, gentamicin, tobamycin, sisomicin, kanamycin, amikacin, paromomycin, framycetin, and neomycin.

Mode of action They inhibit protein synthesis by binding to the 30 S ribosomal subunit.

Adverse effects Ototoxicity and nephrotoxicity occur in 2% to 10% of patients using aminoglycosides. Effective doses are close to toxic levels.

Spectrum They are active against aerobic and facultative anaerobic gram-negative bacilli but not against strict anaerobic bacteria.

Drug form and use Because aminoglycosides are not absorbed from the gastrointestinal tract, they must be administered parenterally or topically. They are available in creams and ointments for topical use.

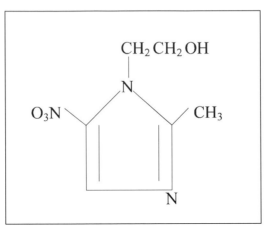

Fig 3-6 Structure of metronidazole.

Interference with Nucleic Acid Synthesis

Nitroimidazoles

The most important member of this group is metronidazole (Fig 3-6), but other agents also exist, including nimorazole, ornidazole, tinidazole, caridazole, and secidazole. Nitroimidazoles are bactericidal drugs. They act as an electron-acceptor at low redox potential, allowing the formation of toxic metabolites that are lethal to the organism.

Metronidazole *Indications* Metronidazole was first used to treat trichomonal vaginitis. It is the drug of choice in treating giardiasis; amebic dysentery; amebic abscess; anaerobic bacterial infections such as abdominal sepsis, brain abscess, and lung abscess; and oral infections such as periodontitis.

Absorption Metronidazole is well absorbed orally.

Distribution It passes readily into most tissues and saliva. Metronidazole also crosses the placenta barrier, is secreted in breast milk, and may cause mutagenic effects; therefore, it should not be prescribed to pregnant or nursing women.

Excretion Metronidazole is excreted via the renal system.

Mode of action Metronidazole, a bactericidal drug, can diffuse into both aerobic and anaerobic bacteria. Inside the cell, it is reduced at the 5-nitro position through a process involving anaerobic metabolic pathways. Due to the decrease in intracellular metronidazole, a promotion of further intake seems to occur. Inside the cell, the metronidazole metabolites react with DNA and other macromolecules, resulting in cell death.

Adverse effects A disulfiram (antabuse) reaction, caused by the accumulation of acetaldehyde in the blood, can develop in patients who drink alcohol while taking metronidazole. It also potentiates the effects of anticoagulants and may leave a metallic taste in the mouth. Nausea occurs in 12% of patients, sometimes with headache, anorexia, and vomiting. Convulsive seizures have also been associated with metronidazole use, and large doses may cause peripheral neuropathy. Other possible side effects include drowsiness, headache, depression, skin rashes, and vaginal and urethral burning.

Spectrum Metronidazole is effective against strict anaerobic gram-positive and gram-negative bacteria, *Trichomonas vaginalis, Giardia lamblia,* and *Entamoeba histolytica.*

Drug variations Metronidazole has been evaluated as an agent for subgingival topical application in irrigation solutions, gels, dialysis tubing, acrylic strips, and surgical cements, and it is commercially available (see chapter 4).

Quinolones

Nalidixic acid was the first member and prototype of the quinolones, a synthetic group of drugs. The fluoroquinolones, which improved upon the spectrum of nalidixic acid, include norfloxacin (the first fluoroquinolone), enoxacin, ofloxacin, pefloxacin, amifloxacin, sparfloxacin, and ciprofloxacin. When DNA is transcribed, the supercoiled molecule must be unwound in order to allow the process of transcription. Quinolones interfere with the action of DNA topoisomerase (ATP hydrolyzing), the bacterial enzyme responsible for this process.

Ciprofloxacin *Indications* Ciprofloxacin (Fig 3-7) is used to treat *Pseudomonas aeruginosa* infections, chlamydial infections, hospital-acquired gram-negative pneumonia, and cystic fibrosis (recurrent *Pseudomonas* infection) in children.

Absorption After oral administration of ciprofloxacin, absorption is 50% to 98%.

Distribution Ciprofloxacin passes into most body fluids. It also crosses the placenta barrier and is secreted in breast milk.

Excretion Ciprofloxacin is excreted via the renal system, mainly tubular secretion.

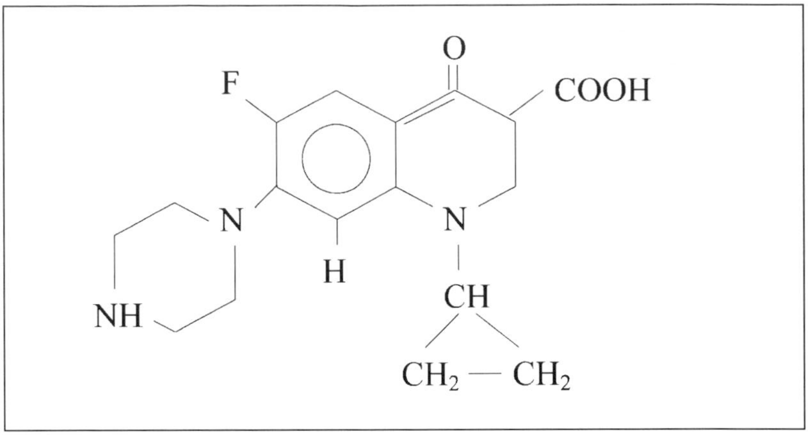

Fig 3-7 Structure of ciprofloxacin.

Mode of action It is generally bactericidal; however, it is bacteriostatic at low concentrations. Quinolones penetrate cells, including macrophages and polymorphonuclear leukocytes.

ADVERSE EFFECTS

Adverse effects Ciprofloxacin is well tolerated but may be associated with nausea, vomiting, diarrhea, abdominal pain, photosensitivity, xerostomia, insomnia, headache, dizziness, and drowsiness. White blood cell and blood glucose disorders also have been reported in patients using ciprofloxacin. Allergic reactions are rare and mainly manifest in the form of skin rashes.

Spectrum It is effective against facultative gram-negative and gram-positive bacteria but not against most strict anaerobic bacteria.

INFORMATION ABOUT SPECIFIC DRUG

Cotrimoxazole

Cotrimoxazole is a combination of sulfamethoxazole (a sulfamide) and trimethoprim (derived from folic acid), both synthetic drugs that interfere with enzymes responsible for the folate biosynthetic pathway. Individually, the drugs are bacteriostatic against a broad spectrum of bacteria, including mycobacterium, chlamydia, and *Pneumocystis carinii*. In combination, the drugs have synergistic effects, resulting in bactericidal activity. This combination is used frequently in the treatment of urinary infections and in the prevention and treatment of *P carinii* pneumonia in patients with AIDS, but not for treatment of orofacial infections.

> **Box 3-2** General principles for antimicrobial dosing in orofacial infections[15]
>
> - Employ high doses for a short duration
> - Use the oral route
> - Aim to achieve blood levels of the antibiotic 2 to 8 times higher than the minimal inhibitory concentration of the pathogen
> - Use frequent dosing intervals
> - Determine the duration of therapy by the remission of disease

Sulfonamides

Indications Sulfonamides have been used for prophylaxis and treatment of meningococcal disease; however, resistance to the agents develops quickly.

Mode of action Sulfonamides are synthetic bacteriostatic antimicrobial agents that affect the synthesis of folic acid by interfacing with the bacterial uptake of para-aminobenzoic acid (PABA) because they are structurally similar.

Spectrum Sulfonamides primarily affect gram-positive bacteria.

Summary of Recommendations

Different systemic antibiotics and dosages are used in various situations in dentistry. The following section summarizes general guidelines for the use of systemic antimicrobial therapies in dentistry.[14]

Treatment of acute orofacial infections

CLINICAL INSIGHT

It is imperative to treat directly the source of infection by incision and drainage (depending upon indication). These procedures will facilitate access of the antibiotic to the infected site. Evidence-based information related to the proper dosages, dosing intervals, and dose duration is limited. The selection of an antimicrobial drug is usually empirical, but pharmacokinetic properties such as diffusion of the drug in abscesses and infected tissues should be taken into account. Box 3-2 lists the general principles that should be applied when determining antimicrobial dosing for orofacial infections. Common dosages for antibiotics are shown in Table 3-4.

Table 3-4 Usual dosages for adults and children for frequently used systemic antimicrobial agents

Antimicrobial agent	Usual adult dosages*			Usual child dosages*		
	Route	Dose	Interval	Route	Dose	Interval
Penicillins						
Penicillin G	IM	10^6 IU	6 h	IV	20000 IU/kg (<10 y)	4 h
Ampicillin	O	500–1000 mg	6–8 h	O	50–100 mg/kg (lactating)	24 h
					250 mg (<2 y)	8 h
Amoxicillin	O	500–750 mg	8 h	O	40–80 mg/kg (<2 y)	24 h
					125 mg (2 to 7 y)	8 h
					250 mg (7 y)	8 h
Amoxicillin/clavulanate	O	500–875/125 mg	8 h	O	40–80 mg/kg (<2 y)	24 h
					125 mg (2 to 7 y)	8 h
					250 mg (7 y)	8 h
Cephalosporins						
Cephalexin	O	250–1000 mg	6 h	O	125 mg (<1 y)	6 h
					125–250 mg (1 to 6 y)	6 h
					250–500 mg (>6 y)	6 h
Tetracyclines						
Tetracycline	O	250–500 mg	6 h		Contraindicated	
Doxycycline	O	100 mg	12–24 h		Contraindicated	
Minocycline	O	100 mg	24 h		Contraindicated	
Macrolides						
Erythromycin (base)	O	250–500 mg	6–8 h	O	10–20 mg/kg	8 h
Azithromycin	O	500 mg	24 h	O	10 mg/kg for 3 days (loading dose); then 5 mg/kg for 5 days	24 h
Lincomycins						
Lincomycin	O	500 mg	6–8 h	IM	10 mg/kg	12–24 h
Clindamycin	O	150–450 mg	6 h	O	2–6 mg/kg	6 h
Nitroimidazole						
Metronidazole	O	500 mg	8 h	O	7.5 mg/kg	8 h
Quinolones						
Ciprofloxacin	O	500–750 mg	12 h		Contraindicated	

*O—Oral; IM—Intramuscular; Kg—Kg of body weight.

Adjunctive treatment in certain types of periodontitis

Treatment history and the clinical form of aggressive periodontitis (refractory patients, early onset periodontitis, periodontitis in immunocompromised patients) play a role in the decision to use an adjunctive systemic antimicrobial therapy. Determination of the microbiological composition of the subgingival plaque may assist in selecting the most appropriate drug. Tetracyclines, metronidazole, amoxicillin/clavulanate, clindamycin, ciprofloxacin, and amoxicillin with metronidazole are the most frequently selected drugs.[16] Various dosages and regimens have been used in the adjunctive treatment of adult periodontitis (see chapter 8).[1]

Prophylaxis of infections/traumatic sequelae of oral surgery

There is no evidence in the literature to prove that the use of antibiotics concomitant with surgical procedures improves treatment outcome. However, an infection control regimen, usually involving antibiotic use, is recommended when implants or other devices (such as membranes) are surgically placed.

Prophylaxis of bacteremia-related infections

Various antibiotic protocols are recommended by health agencies for prevention of bacteremia-related infections in high-risk patients (see chapter 15).

References

1. Slots J, van Winkelhoff AJ. Antimicrobial therapy in periodontics. J Calif Dent Assoc 1993;21(11):51–56.
2. Malizia T, Tejada MR, Ghelardi E, Senesi S, Gabriele M, Giuca MR, et al. Periodontal tissue disposition of azithromycin. J Periodontol 1997;68:1206–1209.
3. Slots J, Rams TE. Antibiotics in periodontal therapy: Advantages and disadvantages. J Clin Periodontol 1990;17:479–493.
4. Goodson JM. Antimicrobial strategies for treatment of periodontal diseases. Periodontol 2000 1994;5:142–168.
5. Walker CB. Selected antimicrobial agents: Mechanism of action, side effects and drug interactions. Periodontol 2000 1996;10:12–28.
6. Brogden RN, Carmine A, Heel RC, Morley PA, Speight TM, Avery GS. Amoxycillin/clavulanic acid: A review of its antibacterial activity, pharmacokinetics and therapeutic use in urinary tract infections. Drugs 1981;22:337–362.
7. Pajukanta R, Asikainen S, Saarela M, Alaluusua S, Jousimies-Somer H. In vitro activity of azithromycin compared with that of erythromycin against *Actinobacillus actinomycetemcomitans*. Antimicrob Agents Chemother 1992;36:1241–1243.
8. Pajukanta R. In vitro antimicrobial susceptibility of *Porphyromonas gingivalis* to azithromycin, a novel macrolide. Oral Microbiol Immunol 1993;8:325–326.

9. Sefton AM, Maskell JP, Beignton D, Whiley A, Shain H, Foyle D, et al. Azithromycin in the treatment of periodontal disease. Effect on microbial flora. J Clin Periodontol 1996;23:998–1003.

10. Lode H. The pharmacokinetics of azithromycin and their clinical significance. Eur J Clin Microbiol Infect Dis 1991;10:807–812.

11. McDonald PJ, Pruul H. Phagocyte uptake and transport of azithromycin. Eur J Clin Microbiol Infect Dis 1991;10:828–833.

12. Herrera D, Roldán S, O'Connor A, Sanz M. The periodontal abscess (II). Short-term clinical and microbiological efficacy of two systemic antibiotics regimes. J Clin Periodontol 2000;27:395–404.

13. Lo Bue AM, Sammartino R, Chisari G, Gismondo MR, Nicoletti G. Efficacy of azithromycin compared with spiramycin in the treatment of odontogenic infections. J Antimicrob Chemother 1993;31(suppl E):119–127.

14. Slots J, Pallasch TJ. Dentists' role in halting antimicrobial resistance. J Dent Res 1996; 75:1338–1341.

15. Pallasch TJ. Pharmacokinetic principles of antimicrobial therapy. Periodontol 2000 1996;10:5–11.

16. American Academy of Periodontology. Systemic antibiotics in periodontics. J Periodontol 1996;67:831–838.

17. Okabe K, Nakagawa K, Yamamoto E. Factors affecting the occurrence of bacteremia associated with tooth extraction. Int J Oral Maxillofac Surg 1995;24:239–242.

18. Chow AW, Roser SM, Brady FA. Orofacial odontogenic infections. Ann Intern Med 1978;88:392–402.

19. Sundqvist G, Johansson E, Sjogren U. Prevalence of black-pigmented *Bacteroides* species in root canal infections. J Endod 1989;15:13–19.

20. Gomes BP, Lilley JD, Drucker DB. Clinical significance of dental root canal microflora. J Dent 1996;24:47–55.

21. Orstavik D, Kerekes K, Molven O. Effects of extensive apical reaming and calcium hydroxide dressing on bacterial infection during treatment of apical periodontitis: A pilot study. Int Endod J 1991;24:1–7.

22. Iwu C, MacFarlane TW, MacKenzie D, Stenhouse D. The microbiology of periapical granulomas. Oral Surg Oral Med Oral Pathol 1990;69:502–505.

23. Matusow RJ, Goodall LB. Anaerobic isolates in primary pulpal-alveolar cellulitis cases: Endodontic resolutions and drug therapy considerations. J Endod 1983;9:535–543.

24. Topoll HH, Lange DE, Müller RF. Multiple periodontal abscesses after systemic antibiotic therapy. J Clin Periodontol 1990;17:268–272.

25. Newman MG, Sims TN. The predominant cultivable microbiota of the periodontal abscess. J Periodontol 1979;50:350–354.

26. Hafström CA, Wikström MB, Renvert SN, Dahlén GG. Effect of treatment on some periodontopathogens and their antibody levels in periodontal abscesses. J Periodontol 1994;65:1022–1028.

27. Herrera D, Roldán S, González I, Sanz M. The periodontal abscess (I). Clinical and microbiological findings. J Clin Periodontol 2000;27:387–394.

Andrea Mombelli, DDS, PhD
Maurizio S. Tonetti, DMD, PhD, MMSc

4

TOPICAL ANTIMICROBIAL AGENTS:
General Principles and Individual Drugs

The Rationale for Local Antimicrobial Therapy

Longitudinal studies have shown that periodontal disease can usually be treated successfully through a combination of mechanical therapies, including systematic scaling and planing of the root surfaces, meticulous daily oral hygiene, and regular removal of newly formed subgingival deposits. In some patients with periodontitis, however, this nonspecific mechanical approach can cause irreversible hard tissue damage (loss of tooth substance) and gingival recession. In fact, conventional periodontal therapy and maintenance often involve repeated treatment of sites that are locally unresponsive or have recurrent disease, resulting in occasional hard tissue trauma.

Microbiological studies have shown that mechanical treatment may not predictably eliminate putative pathogens, such as *Actinobacillus actinomycetemcomitans,* from the subgingival area.[1,2] Although mechanical periodontal therapy may be clinically successful for those patients in whom all putative pathogens are not completely eradicated, the persistence or regrowth of microorganisms in treated sites should be considered an unsatisfactory treatment outcome. Pathogens may be unreachable because they reside in sites inaccessible for periodontal instruments—for example, in deep vertical defects or furcation areas—or because of their ability to invade periodontal soft tissues or dentin tubules.

IMPORTANT PRINCIPLE

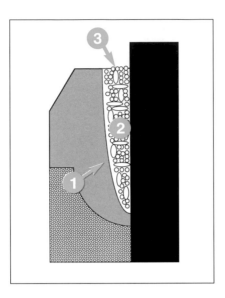

Fig 4-1 Specific conditions for the use of antimicrobial agents in periodontal therapy: (1) The agent must be available at a sufficiently high concentration not only within but also outside the periodontal tissues in the subgingival environment. (2) The subgingival bacteria are protected from antimicrobial agents in a biofilm. (3) The periodontal pocket as an open site is subject to recolonization after therapy.

Subgingival microorganisms accumulate on the root surface to form a structured, adherent layer of plaque. This phenomenon, known as biofilm formation, effectively protects them from antimicrobial agents (Fig 4-1).[3,4] Concentrations of antimicrobial agents necessary to kill the bacteria embedded in biofilms may not be reached in the subgingival environment if they are administered systemically at commonly recommended dosages. Moreover, adverse systemic reactions are more common at elevated doses, and this can severely decrease patient compliance. Local concentrations high enough to affect microorganisms even in mechanically undisturbed biofilms may be achieved by direct placement of agents into periodontal pockets. This approach to therapy appears particularly promising if pathogenic microorganisms are confined to areas difficult to reach by mechanical instrumentation.

Principles for Local Antibiotic Therapy

For the treatment of periodontal disease, antimicrobials can be delivered locally by means of pocket irrigation or placement of drug-containing ointments and gels or by using sophisticated devices for prolonged release of antibacterial agents. To be effective, the drug should reach the entire area affected by the disease, including the base of the pocket, and should be maintained at a sufficiently high local concentration for a prescribed period of time.[5]

A mouthrinse, or *supragingival* irrigation, will not predictably deliver an agent to the deeper parts of a periodontal defect.[6,7] Agents brought into periodontal pockets by *subgingival* irrigation may be washed out rapidly by the gingival fluid. Based on an assumed pocket volume of 0.5 µL and a gingival fluid flow rate of 20 µL/h, it has been estimated that the half-life of a nonbinding drug placed into a pocket is about 1 minute.[5] Thus, within minutes, even a highly concentrated, highly potent agent would be diluted below a minimal inhibitory concentration for oral microorganisms.

Some medications have an intrinsic ability to bind to surfaces of soft and/or hard tissues and thus establish a drug reservoir. The bound drug is gradually released in biologically active form, thereby prolonging the half-life of elimination of the drug. This ability to bind to oral structures, form an equilibrium with free drug, and be released in active form is known as *substantivity,* and it was first described in dentistry for chlorhexidine used as a mouthrinse.[8] Although there are indications that this effect may also occur to some extent within the periodontal pocket— for instance, after prolonged subgingival irrigation with tetracycline[9]— the potential to create a drug reservoir of significant size on the small surface area available in a periodontal pocket is limited. To maintain a high concentration over a prolonged period of time, the flushing action of the crevicular fluid flow must be counteracted by a steady release of the drug from a larger reservoir.

Local Delivery Devices

The purpose of local delivery devices is to establish a drug reservoir in the periodontal pocket that can maintain effective concentrations at the site of action for prolonged periods of time despite loss from crevicular fluid clearance. Conceptually, a local delivery device consists of a drug reservoir and an element to limit the rate of drug release. The rate-limiting mechanism could be:

- Pure diffusion (a diffusion-controlled system)
- Chemical reaction at the continuously depleted interface between the polymer and the dissolution medium (a chemically controlled system)
- Countercurrent diffusion of the dissolution medium at constant penetration velocity in the polymer (a swelling-controlled system).[10]

A variety of local delivery devices have been designed specifically for use in the periodontal pocket (Table 4-1). Some of these devices are not resorbable; most, however, are biodegradable. Table 4-1 shows that a limited number of antimicrobials have been considered in the creation of most delivery devices. Although all of these antimicrobials have demonstrated an effect against periodontitis-associated bacteria, they differ in terms of their mode of action and their spectrum of susceptible microorganisms. Also, some of the proposed drugs have additional nonantibiotic effects such as the anticollagenase effect of some modified tetracyclines.[11] To establish a drug reservoir large enough to replace the drug continuously cleared by the flushing action of crevicular fluid over a

Table 4-1 Devices tested for local delivery of antimicrobials in the periodontal pocket

Author	Antimicrobial agent	Concentration in carrier (%)	Composition of delivery system
Goodson et al[55]	Tetracycline	20	Dialysis tubing
Coventry and Newman[56]	Chlorhexidine	20	Dialysis tubing
Addy et al[57]	Chlorhexidine	10–50	Polyethylmethacrylate
	Tetracycline	40	Polyethylmethacrylate
	Metronidazole	40	Polyethylmethacrylate
Friedman and Golomb[58]	Chlorhexidine	30	Ethylcellulose + polyethylenglycol
Goodson et al[23]	Tetracycline	25	Ethylene-vinyl acetate
Golomb et al[59]	Metronidazole	30	Ethylcellulose + polyethylenglycol
Noguchi et al[60]	Tetracycline	1	Hydroxypropylcellulose
	Chlorhexidine	5	Hydroxypropylcellulose
Satomi et al[61]	Minocycline	2	OH-ethylcellulose + aminoalkyl-methacrylate + triacetine + glycerinum + $MgCl_2$
Minabe et al[62]	Tetracycline	50	Cross-linked collagen
Deasy et al[63]	Tetracycline	10–25	Polyhydroxybutyric acid
	Metronidazole	25	Polyhydroxybutyric acid
Passler and Nossek[64]	Metronidazole	8	Polyvinylalcohol
Eckles et al[65]	Tetracycline	40	White petrolatum (USP)
Steinberg et al[66]	Chlorhexidine	10–50	Byco protein + glycerol
Higashi et al[67]	Ofloxacin	10	Methacrylic acid + hydroxypropyl-cellulose
Higashi et al[68]	Clindamycin	5	Eudragit + plasticizers
Norling et al[69]	Metronidazole benzoate	25	Glycerylmono-oleate + sesame oil
Sauvêtre et al[70]	Clindamycin	1	Carbopol + EDTA + TEA
Jones et al[71]	Minocycline	–	Poly(glycolide-co-DL-lactide)
Jeong et al[72]	Tetracycline	5	Poloxamer + ethanol + citric acid + carbopol
Gates et al[73]	Metronidazole	–	Cellulose acetate phtalate + polyoxy (ethylene + propylene) + pluronicL101
Roskos et al[74]	Tetracycline	10	Poly(ortho) esthers + Mg(OH)$_2$
Polson et al[75]	Doxycycline	10	Poly(DL-lactide) + N-methyl-2-pyrrolidone

specified period, a delivery device should be able to expand the volume of the periodontal pocket. Moreover, it should remain dimensionally stable for a specified period of time to avoid premature removal by the tissue tonus of the pocket wall (such as occurs, for example, following subgingival application of a fluorescein gel by irrigation, wherein a large portion of the gel is immediately squeezed out of the pocket).[12]

> **Box 4-1** Functional requirements for an antimicrobial drug to be of use in periodontal therapy
>
> - Shows in vitro activity against the organisms considered most important in the etiology of the disease
> - Demonstrates that a sufficient dose can be reached and maintained within the subgingival environment for a sufficiently prolonged period to kill the target organisms
> - Causes no major local or systemic adverse effects
> - Demonstrates a favorable clinical outcome of chemical therapy in periodontal patients through well-controlled longitudinal studies
> - Demonstrates a practical advantage over conventional treatment alternatives (eg, better outcome, fewer adverse effects, easier to deliver)

The few published papers that have addressed the availability of drugs in periodontal pockets after local delivery indicate exponential kinetics of decay for viscous and/or biodegradable carriers, leading to a depletion of the drug reservoir within hours of placement. To improve the antimicrobial effect, repeated applications have been recommended. Controlled delivery of an antimicrobial agent over several days has been shown for tetracycline released from nondegradable monolithic ethylene vinyl acetate fibers.[9]

Evaluation of Antimicrobial Agents for Local Periodontal Therapy: General Issues

A number of study protocols have been used to test the efficacy of local antimicrobial therapy (Box 4-1). Trials vary not only in the type of treatment provided but also in sample size, selection of subjects, range of parameters, duration of study, and controls. Unfortunately, many studies are difficult to interpret due to the unclear baseline status of patients, insufficient or nonstandardized maintenance after therapy, brevity of observation periods, or lack of randomization and controls. Comparison of various forms of therapy is complicated because only a single form of local drug delivery is usually included in one study.

Most of the evidence for a therapeutic effect of local delivery devices comes from trials involving patients with previously untreated adult periodontitis. Some protocols compare local drug delivery to a negative control such as the application of carrier without the drug. These studies may be able to show the drug's net effect, but they are not able to demonstrate a benefit over the most obvious alternative: scaling and root planing. Even if a study can demonstrate that local drug delivery is as effective as scaling and root planing on untreated periodontitis, the question remains as to how much value the procedure has when combined with standard mechanical treatment. Few studies have addressed the use of local drug delivery in recurrent or persistent periodontal lesions, potentially the most valuable area for application.

Among the broad range of antimicrobial agents available, a limited number have been tested thoroughly for use in periodontal therapy, including:

• Minocycline
• Doxycycline
• Metronidazole
• Tetracycline
• Chlorhexidine

Evaluation of Antimicrobial Agents for Local Periodontal Therapy

Two-percent minocycline ointment

The efficacy of a 2% minocycline ointment (Dentomycin; Cyanamid, Lederle Division, Wayne, NJ) has been assessed in a series of clinical trials mainly conducted in adult patients in Japan. The safety and efficacy of subgingivally applied 2% minocycline ointment was tested at four Belgian universities in a randomized, double-blind study of 103 adults with moderate to severe periodontitis.[13] Repeated subgingival administration of minocycline ointment yielded an adjunctive improvement after subgingival instrumentation in both clinical and microbiological variables over a 15-month period.[14]

Subgingival delivery of different forms of minocycline—for example, in bioabsorbable 10% minocycline–loaded microcapsules—is also being investigated. Proof of principal studies involving relatively small numbers of patients with chronic periodontitis indicate that, compared to scaling and root planing, such local subgingival delivery systems may better reduce bleeding on probing and may induce a microbial response more favorable for periodontal health.[15]

Doxycycline hyclate in a biodegradable polymer

The clinical efficacy and safety of doxycycline hyclate, delivered subgingivally in a biodegradable polymer (poly[DL-lactide] dissolved in N-methyl-2-pyrrolidone) (Atridox, Block Drug, Jersey City, NJ), was compared to placebo control, oral hygiene, and scaling and root planing in two multicenter studies, each involving 411 patients who demonstrated moderate to severe adult periodontitis. Comparisons showed the treatment to be statistically superior to placebo control and oral hygiene and as effective as scaling and root planing in reducing the clinical signs of adult periodontitis over a 9-month period.[16] Clinical changes resulting

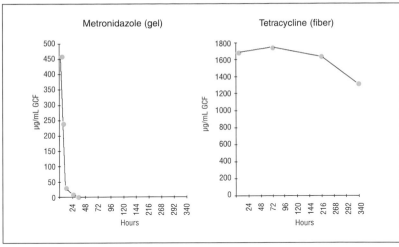

Fig 4-2 Concentrations of metronidazole after application of 25% metronidazole dental gel[76] and of tetracycline in gingival crevicular fluid (GCF) during tetracycline fiber treatment.[9]

from local delivery of doxycycline hyclate or traditional scaling and root planing were evaluated in a group of patients undergoing supportive periodontal therapy. Attachment level gains and probing depth reductions were similar at 9 months after therapy.[17]

Metronidazole gel

Dialysis tubing, acrylic strips, and poly-OH-butyric acid strips have been tested as solid devices for delivery of metronidazole. At present the only commercially distributed and most extensively used device for metronidazole application is a gel consisting of a semisolid suspension of 25% metronidazole benzoate in a mixture of glyceryl mono-oleate and sesame oil (Elyzol Dental Gel, Dumex, Copenhagen, Denmark). Applied with a syringe inserted into the pocket, the gel is expected to increase in viscosity after placement. It has been reported that 40% of the applied gel remained in place while 60% was immediately lost and probably swallowed.[18] After treating an average of 18 teeth in 14 patients, a mean peak metronidazole plasma concentration of 0.6 μg/mL was reached within 2 to 8 hours. The estimated mean dose of metronidazole per treated tooth was 3 mg. The drug concentration in crevicular fluid was determined to be below 1 μg/mL in 50% of the sampled sites after 1 day and in 92% of the sites after 36 hours (Fig 4-2). The clinical response to subgingival application of the metronidazole gel was compared to the effect of subgingival scaling in a large multicenter study of 206 patients with untreated adult periodontitis.[19] Differences between the effects of gel application and scaling were considered clinically insignificant by the authors. Using a similar design, the microbiological outcome of two gel applications was compared to scaling in 24 subjects during a 6-month observation period.[20] The total bacterial cultivable count and the proportions of anaerobic bacteria were comparably affected in the two groups, and both treatments reduced probing depth and bleeding on probing equally well. Although in theory the antimicrobial action of metronidazole is bactericidal and independent of time, in practice a sufficient period of drug presence is important regardless of whether a substance has demonstrated bactericidal or bacteriostatic properties in the laboratory.

A subsequent controlled, randomized, blind study extended the previous observations to include clinical attachment level measurements. A study of 164 subjects detected no significant difference between metronidazole gel application and scaling and root planing.[21] This raises the question of equivalence between the two treatment modalities. From a practical standpoint, one form of a treatment may be preferred over another of equal efficacy if it offers greater tolerability, lower costs, and so forth. Equivalence between scaling and root planing and metronidazole gel therapy has been evaluated using the lower bounds of confidence intervals in a parallel arm, multicenter, controlled clinical trial that included 84 subjects.[22] The estimates provided by this study indicate that metronidazole gel therapy is 82% as good as mechanical debridement at the 95% confidence level.

INFORMATION ABOUT
SPECIFIC DRUG

Tetracycline in a nonresorbable plastic copolymer

Hollow devices such as dialysis tubing and solid devices such as acrylic strips, collagen, and poly-OH-butyric acid strips have been tested for tetracycline delivery. Semisolid viscous media include white petrolatum and poloxamer or carbopol gels. The most extensively tested tetracycline-releasing device that has been approved in both the United States and Europe for the treatment of adult periodontitis is the Actisite periodontal fiber (Alza, Palo Alto, CA; Solco, Birsfelden, Switzerland). Actisite is a biologically inert, nonresorbable plastic copolymer (ethylene and vinyl acetate) containing 25% tetracycline hydrochloride powder. Manufactured as a monolithic 0.5-mm-diameter thread, it is packed into the periodontal pocket, secured with a thin layer of cyanoacrylate adhesive, and left in place for 7 to 12 days.[23,24] Through continuous delivery of tetracycline, local concentration of the active drug in excess of 1,000 mg/L can be maintained throughout that period (see Fig 4-2).[9] The drug also is deposited on the root surface and penetrates into the soft periodontal tissues. Salivary tetracycline concentrations ranging from 8 to 51 mg/L have been measured when treating multiple sites while serum concentrations remained below detection level.[25,26]

Several clinical studies have been performed with these devices[27]; however, only three large multicenter trials will be discussed here. The safety and efficacy of tetracycline fiber therapy was investigated in a 60-

day multicenter study conducted in 107 periodontitis patients already treated with supragingival scaling and prophylaxis. The fiber therapy significantly increased attachment levels and decreased pocket depth and bleeding to a greater extent than the control procedures.[28] A second multicenter study is of particular interest for two reasons: it was conducted in periodontal maintenance patients needing treatment of localized recurrent periodontitis, and it evaluated the effect of fiber therapy as an adjunct to scaling and root planing.[29] After 6 months, sites that received the combined treatment showed a significantly higher attachment level, a significantly greater reduction in pocket depth, and less bleeding on probing than those treated with scaling and root planing alone. A third large-scale multicenter study demonstrated that results obtained within 3 months of therapy were maintained over 1 year and that combined treatment resulted in a significantly lower incidence of disease recurrence than achieved with any of the other tested treatment modalities.[30]

Chlorhexidine gluconate in a gelatin chip

While acrylic strips and ethylcellulose compounds have been used for chlorhexidine application, resorbable gelatin chips are the most extensively tested chlorhexidine delivery devices. The safety and efficacy of PerioChip (Perio Products, Jerusalem, Israel), a degradable, subgingivally placed drug delivery system containing 2.5 mg chlorhexidine, were evaluated in a multicenter study of 118 patients with moderate periodontitis.[31] A split-mouth design was used to compare the treatment outcomes of scaling and root planing alone with the combined use of scaling and root planing and PerioChip in pockets with probing depths of 5 to 8 mm. The average reduction in pocket depth in the sites treated with the chip was significantly greater than in the sites that received mechanical treatment only (mean difference of 0.42 mm at 6 months). The efficacy of the chlorhexidine chip when used as an adjunct to scaling and root planing in adult periodontitis was evaluated in two double-blind, randomized, placebo-controlled, multicenter clinical trials. At 9 months the chlorhexidine chip showed significantly better results with regard to reducing probing depth and improving clinical attachment level from baseline compared with mechanical control treatments.[32]

Adverse Reactions

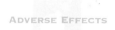

Local delivery of antimicrobial agents requires the same degree of caution as one would observe with systemic delivery. In particular, local delivery devices should not be used:

- In subjects with known allergy to the active drug
- In subjects with known allergy to components of the drug delivery device (or its breakdown products).

In general, the ability to minimize the incidence of adverse effects, especially those frequently associated with delivery via the systemic route, is one advantage of local delivery of antimicrobials.[33] For the most part, only minor adverse effects, such as transient discomfort or sensitivity related to the physical placement of the device, have been associated with local delivery.[32]

However, local delivery does not preclude the selection of resistant bacterial strains or the overgrowth of intrinsically resistant organisms either at the site of administration or at other body sites. So far no data are available on the possible effects that local delivery within the oral cavity may have on the microflora of the gastrointestinal tract. This lack of hard data has spurred speculation as well as concern about the possible spread of bacterial resistance to the antimicrobials used and even of possible increase in the risk of transfer of multidrug resistance.

In terms of effects on the oral microflora, only a few studies have addressed the issue of the increase in bacterial resistance following local delivery of tetracycline and minocycline. These studies show a significant increase in the proportions of resistant strains immediately after local delivery, albeit in a very limited number of cases. Baseline levels of resistant organisms were observed 3 to 6 months following therapy, indicating that the phenomenon was transient in nature.[34–36]

Given the increasing problems associated with bacterial resistance, antibiotics should be used very selectively in the treatment of periodontal disease. Narrow indications should replace the indiscriminate, repeated use advocated by some manufacturers.

Comparison of Treatment Methods and Strategies

Few studies have focused on understanding how local delivery devices could be incorporated into an overall treatment strategy. The evidence in this area is scant and most has not been independently confirmed. More research is needed to precisely determine the relative usefulness of various treatment options and to identify clinical situations in which a systemic or local chemotherapy or one particular local delivery device may be more beneficial than another.

Comparison of Local Delivery Systems

Most studies have tested a single form of local drug delivery instead of comparing various forms of therapy. In one recent study, however, the efficacy of three commercially available local delivery systems as adjuncts to scaling and root planing was tested in patients with persistent periodontal lesions.[37,38] Treatment modalities included scaling and root planing alone and in conjunction with the application of 25% tetracycline fibers, with 2% minocycline gel, and with 25% metronidazole gel. Although all three locally applied antimicrobial systems seemed to offer some benefit over scaling and root planing alone, a treatment regimen of scaling and root planing plus tetracycline fiber placement gave the greatest reduction in probing depth over the 6 months after treatment. Suppuration was most effectively reduced in the scaling plus tetracycline fiber group followed by the minocycline group.

Comparison of Local and Systemic Antibiotics

Clarification is needed in the process of selecting local or systemic delivery when the use of an antibiotic is indicated. One investigation addressed this question in patients with rapidly progressing periodontitis.[39] Overall, no significant differences were noted between systemic administration of amoxicillin–clavulanic acid and the use of tetracycline fibers as an adjunct to mechanical therapy. For patients with adult periodontitis, two studies reported better results from scaling and root planing supplemented with locally applied metronidazole rather than with adjunctive systemic metronidazole.[40,41]

Recolonization

Different oral distribution patterns for microorganisms such as *Porphyromonas gingivalis* can be recognized in periodontitis patients.[42,43] Local therapy may be less successful in patients where these organisms are widespread than when confined to isolated areas. This hypothesis was tested in a study comparing two extreme forms of local therapy. In one group of patients, full-mouth scaling and root planing, application of tetracycline fibers, and chlorhexidine rinse were combined. In the other group, only two teeth were treated locally and no attempt was made to interfere with the overall conditions of the oral environment. The recolonization kinetics indicated that disinfected pockets in disinfected dentitions (full-mouth treatment) did not display significant recolonization. Disinfected pockets in infected dentitions, however, demonstrated significant rates of recolonization.[44] Moreover, major clinical differences were found in the local healing response depending on whether the rest of the dentition was left untreated or also subjected to therapy.[45]

These findings concur with earlier studies that showed the importance of plaque control as a key component of mechanical periodontal therapy.[46–48] A more recent study underscored the importance of oral hygiene by showing differences in outcomes attributable to the level of postoperative oral hygiene after a combination of mechanical debridement and administration of various systemic antibiotics.[49] Current evidence suggests that local delivery may be most beneficial in the control

KEY FACTS

KEY FACTS

of ongoing localized disease in otherwise stable patients. Maintenance patients with a few nonresponding sites may therefore benefit most from local antimicrobial therapy, a concept corroborated in a multicenter study.[29]

Oral chlorhexidine rinses were able to suppress recolonization with putative pathogens after application of tetracycline fibers and scaling and root planing.[50,51] While the local delivery device suppresses the established subgingival microflora, chlorhexidine mouth rinsing serves to prevent the early recolonization of treated sites.

CLINICAL INSIGHT

Local Delivery Devices and Specific Clinical Situations

An investigation to evaluate the effectiveness of local delivery (tetracycline fibers) combined with scaling and root planing and chlorhexidine mouth rinsing in altering the distribution of infected sites in generalized *P gingivalis*–infected periodontitis sites found that *P gingivalis* was most likely to persist in second molars.[52] This observation indicates that some sites may be difficult to access with local delivery devices.

Factors Influencing Success of Treatment

CLINICAL INSIGHT

In establishing the appropriate treatment strategy, the following local factors should be carefully considered:

- Accessibility of site
- Extent of periodontal destruction
- Unfavorable anatomy
- Difficulty in plaque control

KEY FACTS

It is important to note that most of the studies reviewed in this discussion so far explicitly excluded teeth with furcation involvement. A study by Minabe and coworkers evaluated the effect of repeated drug delivery application with or without mechanical therapy in molar furcation defects.[53] The effectiveness of adjunctive local drug delivery in the control of mandibular Class II furcations during maintenance care was evaluated in a randomized, single-blind, multicenter, controlled clinical trial.[54] One hundred twenty-seven patients presenting with Class II mandibular furcations with bleeding on probing were included in the study. Treatments consisting of scaling and root planing combined with local controlled drug delivery with tetracycline fibers yielded better outcomes than scaling and root planing alone. Differences in improvement of probing depth and bleeding on probing were significant after 3 months, but their duration did not extend to the 6-month evaluation.

Conclusion

To treat periodontal disease successfully, local delivery devices must provide therapeutic levels of antimicrobial agents in the subgingival area over prolonged periods. Clinical trials demonstrate the efficacy of topical antimicrobial therapy under these conditions. Local delivery of antimicrobial agents is most effective in the treatment of localized nonresponding or recurrent periodontal disease.

References

1. Mombelli A, Gmür R, Gobbi C, Lang NP. *Actinobacillus actinomycetemcomitans* in adult periodontitis. II. Characterization of isolated strains and effect of mechanical periodontal treatment. J Periodontol 1994;65:827–834.

2. Mombelli A, Schmid B, Rutar A, Lang NP. Persistence patterns of *Porphyromonas gingivalis*, *Prevotella intermedia/nigrescens*, and *Actinobacillus actinomycetemcomitans* after mechanical therapy of periodontal disease. J Periodontol 2000;71:14–21.

3. Anwar H, Dasgupta MK, Costerton JW. Testing the susceptibility of bacteria in biofilms to antibacterial agents. Antimicrob Agents Chemother 1990;34:2043–2046.

4. Anwar H, Strap JL, Costerton JW. Establishment of aging biofilms: Possible mechanism of bacterial resistance to antibiotic therapy. Antimicrob Agents Chemother 1992;36:1347–1351.

5. Goodson JM. Pharmacokinetic principles controlling efficacy of oral therapy. J Dent Res 1989;68(special issue):1625–1632.

6. Eakle W, Ford C, Boyd R. Depth of penetration in periodontal pockets with oral irrigation. J Clin Periodontol 1986;13:39–44.

7. Pitcher G, Newman H, Strahan J. Access to subgingival plaque by disclosing agents using mouthrinsing and direct irrigation. J Clin Periodontol 1980;7:300–308.

8. Bonesvoll P, Gjermo P. A comparison between chlorhexidine and some quaternary ammonium compounds with regard to retention, salivary concentration and plaque-inhibiting effect in the human mouth after mouth rinses. Arch Oral Biol 1978;23: 289–294.

9. Tonetti M, Cugini MA, Goodson JM. Zero-order delivery with periodontal placement of tetracycline loaded ethylene vinyl acetate fibers. J Periodont Res 1990;25: 243–249.

10. Langer R, Peppas N. Present and future applications of biomaterials in controlled drug delivery systems. Biomaterials 1981;2:201–214.

11. Golub LM, Wolff M, Lee HM, et al. Further evidence that tetracyclines inhibit collagenase activity in human crevicular fluid and other mammalian sources. J Periodont Res 1985;20:12–23.

12. Ooster Waal PJ, Mikx FH, Renggli HH. Clearance of a topically applied fluorescein gel from periodontal pockets. J Clin Periodontol 1990;17:613–615.

13. van Steenberghe D, Bercy P, Kohl J, et al. Subgingival minocycline hydrochloride ointment in moderate to severe chronic adult periodontitis: A randomized, double-blind, vehicle-controlled, multicenter study. J Periodontol 1993;64:637–644.

14. van Steenberghe D, Rosling B, Söder PO, et al. A 15-month evaluation of the effects of repeated subgingival minocycline in chronic adult periodontitis. J Periodontol 1999;70:657–667.

15. Yeom HR, Park YJ, Lee SJ, et al. Clinical and microbiological effects of minocycline-loaded microcapsules in adult periodontitis. J Periodontol 1997;68:1102–1109.

16. Garrett S, Johnson L, Drisko CH, et al. Two multi-center studies evaluating locally delivered doxycycline hyclate, placebo control, oral hygiene, and scaling and root planing in the treatment of periodontitis. J Periodontol 1999;70:490–503.

17. Garrett S, Adams DF, Bogle G, et al. The effect of locally delivered controlled-release doxycycline or scaling and root planing on periodontal maintenance patients over 9 months. J Periodontol 2000;71:22–30.

18. Stoltze K, Stellfeld M. Systemic absorbtion of metronidazole after application of a metronidazole 25% dental gel. J Clin Periodontol 1992;19:693–697.

19. Ainamo J, Lie T, Ellingsen BH, et al. Clinical responses to subgingival placement of a metronidazole 25% gel compared to the effect of subgingival scaling in adult periodontitis. J Clin Periodontol 1992;19:723–729.

20. Pedrazzoli V, Kilian M, Karring T. Comparative clinical and microbiological effects of topical subgingival application of metronidazole 25% dental gel and scaling in the treatment of adult periodontitis. J Clin Periodontol 1992;19:715–722.

21. Grossi SG, Dunford R, Genco RJ, et al. Local application of metronidazole dental gel (IADR Abstract #543). J Dent Res 1995;74(special issue):468.

22. Pihlstrom B, Michalowicz B, Aeppli D, et al. Equivalence in clinical trials (IADR Abstract #1038). J Dent Res 1995;74(special issue):530.

23. Goodson JM, Holborow D, Dunn R, Hogan P, Dunham S. Monolithic tetracycline containing fibers for controlled delivery to periodontal pockets. J Periodontol 1983;54:575–579.

24. Goodson JM, Cugini M, Kent R, et al. Multicenter evaluation of tetracycline fiber therapy: I. Experimental design, methods and baseline data. J Periodontal Res 1991;26:361–370.

25. Rapley JW, Cobb CM, Killoy WJ, Williams DR. Serum levels of tetracycline during treatment with tetracycline-containing fibers. J Periodontol 1992;63:817–820.

26. Goodson JM, Offenbacher S, Farr D, Hogan P. Periodontal disease treatment by local drug delivery. J Periodontol 1985;56:265–272.

27. Tonetti MS. The topical use of antibiotics in periodontal pockets. In: Lang NP, Karring T, Lindhe J (eds). Proceedings of the Second European Workshop on Periodontology. Berlin: Quintessenz Verlag, 1997: 78–109.

28. Goodson JM, Cugini M, Kent R, et al. Multicenter evaluation of tetracycline fiber therapy: II. Clinical response. J Periodontal Res 1991;26:371–379.

29. Newman MG, Kornman KS, Doherty FM. A 6-month multi-center evaluation of adjunctive tetracycline fiber therapy used in conjunction with scaling and root planing in maintenance patients: Clinical results. J Periodontol 1994;65:685–691.

30. Michalowicz BS, Pihlstrom BL, Drisko CL, et al. Evaluation of periodontal treatments using controlled release tetracycline fibers: Maintenance response. J Periodontol 1995;66:708–715.

31. Soskolne WA, Heasman PA, Stabholz A, et al. Sustained local delivery of chlorhexidine in the treatment of periodontitis: A multi-center study. J Periodontol 1997;68: 32–38.

32. Jeffcoat MK, Bray KS, Ciancio SG, et al. Adjunctive use of a subgingival controlled-release chlorhexidine chip reduces probing depth and improves attachment level compared with scaling and root planing alone. J Periodontol 1998;69:989–997.

33. Nord CE, Edlund C. Ecological effects of antimicrobial agents on the human intestinal microflora. Microb Ecology Health Dis 1991;4:193–207.

34. Goodson JM, Tanner A. Antibiotic resistance of the subgingival microbiota following local tetracycline therapy. Oral Microbiol Immunol 1992;7:113–117.

35. Preus H, Lassen J, Aass A, Ciancio S. Bacterial resistance following subgingival and systemic administration of minocycline. J Clin Periodontol 1995;22:380–384.

36. Larsen T. Occurrence of doxycycline resistant bacteria in the oral cavity after local administration of doxycycline in patients with periodontal disease. Scand J Infect Dis 1991;23:89–95.

37. Radvar M, Pourtaghi N, Kinane DF. Comparison of 3 periodontal local antibiotic therapies in persistent periodontal pockets. J Periodontol 1996;67:860–865.

38. Kinane DF, Radvar M. A six-month comparison of three periodontal local antimicrobial therapies in persistent periodontal pockets. J Periodontol 1999;70:1–7.

39. Bernimoulin P, Purucker H, Mertes B, Krüger B. Local versus systemic adjunctive antibiotic therapy in RPP patients [abstract #647]. J Dent Res 1995;74(special issue):481.

40. Noyan U, Yilmaz S, Kuru B, et al. A clinical and microbiological evaluation of systemic and local metronidazole delivery in adult periodontitis patients. J Clin Periodontol 1997;24:158–165.

41. Paquette D, Ling S, Fiorellini J, et al. Radiographic and BANA test analysis of locally delivered metronidazole: A phase I/II clinical trial. J Dent Res 1994;73(special issue):305.

42. Mombelli A, McNabb H, Lang NP. Black-pigmenting gram-negative bacteria in periodontal disease. II. Screening strategies for *P. gingivalis.* J Periodontal Res 1991; 26:308–313.

43. Mombelli A, McNabb H, Lang NP. Black-pigmenting gram-negative bacteria in periodontal disease. I. Topographic distribution in the human dentition. J Periodontal Res 1991;26:301–307.

44. Tonetti MS, Mombelli A, Lehmann B, Lang NP. Impact of oral ecology on the recolonization of locally treated periodontal pockets. J Dent Res 1995;74(special issue):481.

45. Mombelli A, Lehmann B, Tonetti MS, Lang NP. Clinical response to local delivery of tetracycline in relation to overall and local periodontal conditions. J Clin Periodontol 1997;24:470–477.

46. Magnusson I, Lindhe J, Yoneyama T, Liljenberg B. Recolonization of a subgingival microbiota following scaling in deep pockets. J Clin Periodontol 1984;11:193–207.

47. Rosling B, Nyman S, Lindhe J, Jern B. The healing potential of the periodontal tissues following different techniques of periodontal surgery in plaque-free dentitions. A 2-year clinical study. J Clin Periodontol 1976;3:233–250.

48. Nyman S, Lindhe J, Rosling B. Periodontal surgery in plaque-infected dentitions. J Clin Periodontol 1977;4:240–249.

49. Kornman KS, Newman MG, Moore DJ, Singer RE. The influence of supragingival plaque control on clinical and microbial outcomes following the use of antibiotics for the treatment of periodontitis. J Periodontol 1994;65:848–854.

50. Holborow D, Niederman R, Tonetti MS, Cugini M, Goodson JM. Synergistic effects between chlorhexidine mouthwash and tetracycline fibers. J Dent Res 1990;69:277.

51. Niederman R, Holborow D, Tonetti MS, et al. Reinfection of periodontal sites following tetracycline fiber therapy. J Dent Res 1990;69:277.

52. Mombelli A, Tonetti MS, Lehmann B, Lang NP. Topographic distribution of black-pigmenting anaerobes before and after periodontal treatment by local delivery of tetracycline. J Clin Periodontol 1996;23:906–913.

53. Minabe M, Takeuchi K, Nishimura T, et al. Therapeutic effects of combined treatment using tetracycline-immobilized collagen film and root planing in periodontal furcation pockets. J Clin Periodontol 1991;18:287–290.

54. Tonetti MS, Cortellini P, Carnevale G, et al. A controlled multicenter study of adjunctive use of tetracycline periodontal fibers in mandibular Class II furcations with persistent bleeding. J Clin Periodontol 1998;25:728–736.

55. Goodson JM, Haffajee A, Socransky SS. Periodontal therapy by local delivery of tetracyline. J Clin Periodontol 1979;6:83–92.

56. Coventry J, Newman H. Experimental use of a slow release device employing chlorhexidine gluconate in areas of acute periodontal inflammation. J Clin Periodontol 1982;9:129–133.

57. Addy M, Rawle L, Handley R, et al. The development and in vitro evaluation of acrylic strips and dialysis tubing for local drug delivery. J Periodontol 1982; 53:693–699.

58. Friedman M, Golomb G. New sustained release dosage form of chlorhexidine for dental use. J Periodontal Res 1982;17:323–328.

59. Golomb G, Friedman M, Soskolne A, et al. Sustained release device containing metronidazole for periodontal use. J Dent Res 1984;63:1149–1152.

60. Noguchi T, Izumizawa K, Fukuda M, et al. New method for local drug delivery using bioresorbable base material in periodontal therapy. Bull Tokyo Med Dent Univ 1984;31:145–153.

61. Satomi A, Uraguchi R, Noguchi T, et al. Minocycline HCl concentration in periodontal pockets after administration of LS-007. J Japan Periodontal Assoc 1987;29:937–943.

62. Minabe M, Uematsu A, Nishijima K, et al. Application of a local delivery system to periodontal therapy. I. Development of the collagen preparations immobilized tetracycline. J Periodontol 1989;60:113–117.

63. Deasy PB, Collins AE, MacCarthy DJ, Russell RJ. Use of strips containing tetracycline hydrochloride or metronidazole for the treatment of advanced periodontal disease. J Pharm Pharmacol 1989;41:694–699.

64. Passler R, Nossek H. Untersuchungen zur Konzentration und Wirkungsdauer von Metronidazol in der Zahnfleischtasche nach lokaler Applikation. Zahn-, Mund-, und Kieferheilkunde mit Zentralblatt 1989;77:12–16.

65. Eckles TA, Reinhardt RA, Dyer JK, et al. Intracrevicular application of tetracycline in white petrolatum for the treatment of periodontal disease. J Clin Periodontol 1990;17:454–462.

66. Steinberg D, Friedman M, Soskolne A, Sela MN. A new degradable controlled release device for treatment of periodontal disease: In vitro release study. J Periodontol 1990;61:393–398.

67. Higashi K, Morisaki K, Hayashi S, et al. Local ofloxacin delivery using a controlled-release insert (PT-01) in the human periodontal pocket. J Periodont Res 1990;25:1–5.

68. Higashi K, Matsushita M, Morisaki K, et al. Local drug delivery systems for the treatment of periodontal disease. J Pharmacobiodynamics 1991;14:72–81.

69. Norling T, Lading P, Engström S, et al. Formulation of a drug delivery system based on a mixture of monoglycerides and triglycerides for use in the treatment of periodontal disease. J Clin Periodontol 1992;19:687–692.

70. Sauvêtre E, Glupczynsky Y, Labbe M, et al. The effect of clindamycin gel insert in periodontal pockets, as observed on smears and cultures. Infection 1993;21:245–247.

71. Jones AA, Kornman KS, Newbold DA, Manwell MA. Clinical and microbiological effects of controlled-release locally delivered minocycline in periodontitis. J Periodontol 1994;65:1058–1066.

72. Jeong S-N, Han S-B, Lee S-W, Magnusson I. Effects of tetracycline containing gel and a mixture of tetracycline and citric acid containing gel on non-surgical periodontal therapy. J Periodontol 1994;65:840–847.

73. Gates K, Grad H, Birek P, Lee P. A new bioerodible polymer insert for the controlled release of metronidazole. Pharmacol Res 1994;11:1605–1609.

74. Roskos K, Fritzinger B, Rao S, et al. Development of a drug delivery system for the treatment of periodontal disease based on bioerodible poly(ortho esters). Biomaterials 1995;16:313–317.

75. Polson AM, Garrett S, Stoller NH, et al. Multi-center comparative evaluation of subgingivally delivered sanguinarine and doxycycline in the treatment of periodontitis. I. Study design, procedures, and management. J Periodontol 1997;68:110–118.

76. Stoltze K. Concentration of metronidazole in periodontal pockets after application of a metronidazole 25% dental gel. J Clin Periodontol 1992;19:698–701.

Jacob Fleischmann, MD

5

TOPICAL AND SYSTEMIC ANTIFUNGAL AND ANTIVIRAL AGENTS

The onset of the HIV epidemic has spurred intense interest in the development of antiviral drugs. Moreover, the search for newer antifungal drugs has also increased since researchers discovered that fungi are a major cause of opportunistic infections in AIDS patients. As a result, the last decade has seen an increase in the number of agents available for the treatment of fungi and viruses, and many more are currently under development. This chapter covers only drugs already or soon to be released by the FDA as of the writing of this chapter. Drugs are referred to by their generic names.

Antifungal Therapy

IMPORTANT PRINCIPLE

The key to the successful development of an antimicrobial agent is to find a biochemical function that is unique to a pathogen and not present in the host. A chemical interfering with such a process has a good chance of being effective without causing serious side effects. Because fungi are eukaryotes, they are biochemically more similar to mammals than bacteria are; thus the search for such chemicals has not been as productive as has the development of antibacterial drugs. Still, a number of effective agents with fewer side effects have become available, giving clinicians more options for therapy. Additionally, progress is being made in standardizing antifungal testing for these drugs to assist in guiding therapy.

Polyenes

This group includes two drugs, amphotericin B and nystatin (Table 5-1). They exert their effect by binding to ergosterol, the primary sterol in the cell membrane of fungi. Aggregates of this drug in the cell membrane make the cells leaky to cytoplasmic constituents, which leads to their death. They also bind to cholesterol in human cell membranes, probably underlying some of their pharmacology and toxic effects.

Amphotericin B *Indications* Amphotericin B remains the most reliable agent against a wide variety of fungi that cause serious systemic illness.

Distribution The longest and most widely used formulation is amphotericin B deoxycholate (Abd), which has some unusual pharmacological properties. When infused intravenously, peak levels rapidly diminish from circulation and the drug reappears slowly, probably leaking from cell membranes, to plateau at about 0.2–0.5 mg/mL. Higher doses and renal and hepatic failure do not influence this level significantly, and patients on hemodialysis can receive the regular dose.

Adverse effects As effective as amphotericin B is, its usefulness is limited by its toxicity, which includes immediate reactions and long-term effects. During infusion, patients will frequently experience fever and chills and sometimes hypotension, tachypnea, nausea, vomiting, and headaches. Traditionally patients are pretreated with acetaminophen and hydrocortisone to decrease these effects. Meperidine is useful to control the chills when they occur. The most significant long-term and cumulative effect is nephrotoxicity. Volume expansion with normal saline may be protective for the kidneys. Other side effects, with various frequencies, include anemia, hypokalemia, hypomagnesemia, renal tubular acidosis, thrombocytopenia, leukopenia, and weight loss.

Spectrum This includes yeasts such as *Candida* and *Cryptococci* and molds like *Aspergillus*. Some notable exceptions are *Candida lusitaniae* and *Pseudallescheria boydii*, fungi that have inherent amphotericin resistance and are capable of causing serious infection in neutropenic patients.

Drug variations Newer lipid formulations (Table 5-1) have been developed in an attempt to minimize this drug's toxicity. Comparative studies with the deoxycholate form have shown that these formulations do result in a decrease in renal toxicity but do not appear to have an edge in efficacy. They are clearly far more expensive.

An oral suspension of amphotericin B is available. Because it is not absorbed through the gastrointestinal tract, it can not be used for systemic therapy and is usually reserved for oral candidiasis that does not respond to other oral antifungal agents. The usual dose (Table 5-1) is placed directly on the tongue, swished around the mouth, then swal-

Table 5-1 Antifungal drugs

Drugs	Routes*	Usual IV or oral dosages
Polyenes		
Amphotericin B deoxycholate	IV, oral (suspension), topical	IV: 0.5–1.0 mg/kg/day; oral: 100 mg, 4–6 times/day
Amphotericin B lipid complex	IV	5 mg/kg/day
Amphotericin B cholesteryl sulfate	IV	3–4 mg/kg/day
Liposomal amphotericin B	IV	3–5 mg/kg/day
Nystatin	Oral (suspension, troches), topical	200,000–500,000 U, 4–5 times/day
Azoles		
Ketoconazole	Oral, topical	200–400 mg/day
Fluconazole	IV, oral (tablet, suspension)	IV and oral: 200–800 mg/day
Itraconazole	Oral (capsules, suspension)	200–400 mg/day
Miconazole nitrate	IV, topical	200–1000 mg every 8 hours
Clotrimazole	Oral (troches), topical	10 mg, 5 times/day
Econazole nitrate	Topical	
Sulconazole nitrate	Topical	
Oxiconazole	Topical	
Butoconazole nitrate	Topical	
Tioconazole	Topical	
Terconazole	Topical	
Allylamines and benzylamines		
Terbinafine hydrochloride	Oral (tablet), topical	250 mg/day
Naftifine hydrochloride	Topical	
Butenafine	Topical	
Miscellaneous		
Flucytosine	Oral	50–150 mg/kg/day in 4 divided doses
Griseofulvin	Oral	250–500 mg, 2 times/day
Potassium iodide	Oral	1–5 mL, 3 times/day
Ciclopirox olamine	Topical	
Haloprogin	Topical	
Tolnaftate	Topical	
Selenium sulfide	Topical	
Undecylenate	Topical	

*IV—Intravenous.

lowed. Length of therapy is generally guided by clinical response, but 2 weeks usually are required.

Nystatin Nystatin, originally developed in New York state (from which its name is derived), is very active in vitro against a range of *Candida* species and some other yeastlike fungi. It is too toxic to be used as a systemic agent and cannot be used parenterally.

Indications Its use is limited to topical treatments of oral, mucocutaneous, and vaginal candidiasis.

Adverse effects Oral therapy is usually free of significant side effects with only occasional nausea associated with larger doses. Because some of the suspensions contain sucrose, they should be used carefully in diabetics.

Drug form and use A liposomal formulation is in the clinical trial stage of development and may become useful for systemic therapy for a broader range of fungi. Troches that are currently available for oral therapy have improved flavoring and are better tolerated by patients. They should be dissolved slowly and not chewed or swallowed. Oral suspension should be swished around and swallowed to treat possible esophageal involvement. Treatment should continue for 48 hours after symptoms have resolved.

Azoles

This group includes both imidazoles and triazoles, which have similar antifungal actions. They exert their effect by inhibiting ergosterol synthesis by interacting with 14-α demethylase, a cytochrome P-450 enzyme that is necessary for the conversion of lanosterol to ergosterol, although other mechanisms have been postulated. This process increases the permeability of the cell membrane, which leads to the loss of important cellular contents. Also, because of their interaction with the cytochrome system, they can influence the metabolism of a number of drugs, an issue that needs to be considered when prescribing one of the systemically absorbed forms. However, they are active against a broad range of fungi with some variability.

Ketoconazole *Indications* Although it is effective in a number of systemic fungal diseases, including mucocutaneous candidiasis, blastomycosis, histoplasmosis, and coccidioidomycosis, ketoconazole has become relegated to a second-line status because other more effective azoles have better pharmacokinetic profiles and fewer side effects. It has been used successfully in the treatment of advanced prostate cancer.

Distribution It is distributed widely to tissues, with the exception of those associated with the central nervous system.

Adverse effects Side effects include transient nausea and vomiting. Liver enzymes may be elevated and deaths from hepatotoxicity have occurred. It can inhibit sterol synthesis, and this can affect, among other functions, the production of testosterone, possibly resulting in gynecomastia and impotence.

Spectrum Topically it is effective against most common dermatophytes and is available as a cream or shampoo.

Drug form and use Gastric acidity is required for proper absorption of the oral form, and patients with achlorhydria need to dissolve it in acid and drink it with a straw to avoid contact with teeth.

Fluconazole *Indications* Fluconazole, the most commonly prescribed systemic azole, is active against a broad range of fungi. It is used frequently in oropharyngeal and esophageal candidiasis, especially in AIDS patients and others afflicted with resistant yeast strains.

Distribution It is well distributed to all tissues, including the central nervous system, and it has become the drug of choice for coccidioidal meningitis.

Adverse effects Gastrointestinal symptoms such as diarrhea, nausea, vomiting, and mild liver function elevations occur. Headaches are reported in about 10% of patients and dizziness in about 2%. Occasional hypokalemia requires potassium supplementation and, although rare, exfoliative skin reactions can occur. Among the systemic azoles it has the fewest interactions with other drugs.

Spectrum It has become one of the first-line agents for treating systemic candidiasis, coccidioidomycosis, and cryptococcosis and is used as an alternative therapy for blastomycosis, histoplasmosis, and sporotrichosis.

Drug form and use It is available both in oral and intravenous forms, and the two forms have very similar pharmacokinetics. Unlike ketoconazole, it does not require low gastric pH, and food does not impair absorption.

Itraconazole *Indications* A potent azole, itraconazole has become a first-line agent for treating blastomycosis, histoplasmosis, paracoccidioidomycosis, pseudallescheriasis, and sporotrichosis and an alternative treatment for aspergillosis, candidiasis, coccidioidomycosis, and cryptococcosis. It is also effective in treating onychomycosis.

Distribution The drug distributes well to lipophilic tissues but does not cross the blood-brain barrier in significant amounts.

Adverse effects Its side effects are similar to those of other systemic azoles; the most frequent side effects are gastrointestinal symptoms such as nausea. Dermatological problems include rash, alopecia, and pruritus. It is a potent inhibitor of hepatic cytochrome enzymes and will increase the serum level of many drugs when taken concurrently. For example, fatal arrhythmias have occurred among people taking itraconazole with terfenadine, astemizole, or cisapride.

Drug form and use Two oral forms—capsules and suspension—are available; however, because their absorption is different, they are not interchangeable. Food increases the absorption of the capsule form but decreases the absorption of the suspension. Only the suspension should be used for oropharyngeal and esophageal candidiasis. Like ketoconazole, it requires an acidic environment for absorption; therefore, drugs that decrease acidity also decrease the absorption of both forms.

Miconazole nitrate Miconazole nitrate was initially touted as an azole that would replace amphotericin B, but it turned out to be less efficacious and had some serious side effects. Though the intravenous form is still available, it is only rarely used. Miconazole nitrate has been relegated to the topical treatment of skin and vaginal infections and is effective against both the dermatophytes and the *Candida* species.

Clotrimazole *Indications* Clotrimazole is commonly used in oropharyngeal and mild esophageal candidiasis. It is also effective topically against dermatophytes.

Distribution After slow dissolution of an oral troche, clotrimazole is present in saliva for several hours. The azole most likely binds initially with oral mucosa, then is slowly released.

Adverse effects Emergence of resistance in *Candida* has been less frequent to clotrimazole than to fluconazole. Side effects include occasional skin and vaginal irritation.

Spectrum Activity against fungi is similar to that of other azoles. Additionally, it has a number of interesting effects observed in vitro or in animals. These include antibacterial, antiprotozoal, and antitumor effects and a capacity to control even noninfectious diarrhea.

Drug form and use It is available for oral, vaginal, and topical use. A small amount is absorbed via the oral and vaginal routes.

Topical azoles A number of topical azoles with similar effectiveness against dermatophytes and *Candida* are available (Table 5-1). None are useful in treating onychomycosis.

Allylamines and benzylamines

These agents exert their antifungal effect by inhibiting the epoxidation of squalene and thus blocking the formation of ergosterol. They are fungicidal against the dermatophytes, but are less active against *Candida* species; therefore their clinical indication is limited to the former. Terbinafine hydrochloride is the only one of the group available both orally and topically. When taken orally, it is absorbed well and distributes to various tissues, including the skin and nails. In fact, the drug can be detected in these tissues for up to 3 months after cessation of therapy. It is currently the most effective drug in the treatment of onychomycosis and has the lowest relapse rate.

ADVERSE EFFECTS

The most common adverse effects associated with the oral form are gastrointestinal, including abdominal pain, diarrhea, and dyspepsia, as well as rare cases of idiosyncratic hepatobiliary dysfunction. Both topical and oral forms occasionally cause hives and pruritus. Naftifine hydrochloride and butenafine are available as topical agents against dermatophytes.

Miscellaneous antifungal drugs

INFORMATION ABOUT SPECIFIC DRUG

Flucytosine Flucytosine is a fluorinated pyrimidine that is converted to fluorouracil by susceptible fungi cells but not by mammalian cells. It acts as an antimetabolite, disrupting RNA and ultimately protein synthesis. Its use as a single agent has been limited by the fact that resistance to it develops rapidly. It is used in combination with other antifungals, most commonly amphotericin B, to combat *Candida* and *Cryptococci*. One of its major side effects is bone marrow suppression, resulting in anemia, leukopenia, and thrombocytopenia.

INFORMATION ABOUT SPECIFIC DRUG

Griseofulvin Griseofulvin interferes with cell division by disrupting the mitiotic spindle and is effective against dermatophytes. It is available in several different oral formulations, but the ultramicrosize form is the most reliably absorbed. It concentrates in skin, hair, and nails and is useful in onychomycosis. It is not useful topically because it does not penetrate skin well. Transient headaches are common, and a number of potentially serious side effects, such as granulocytopenia, require the careful monitoring of patients who are taking it on a long-term basis.

INFORMATION ABOUT SPECIFIC DRUG

Potassium iodide Potassium iodide is an antithyroid drug that is effective in cutaneous sporotrichosis in nonimmunocompromised hosts. Because of its many side effects, it is considered a second-line drug behind itraconazole for this infection.

Topical agents A number of these are listed at the bottom of Table 5-1. They come in a variety of forms, including powder, cream, lotion, and shampoo, and most are available over the counter. Their effectiveness varies in that they may treat only a few dermatophytes or many, and some are even effective against *Candida* species.

Antiviral (Nonretroviral) Therapy

Viruses are nucleoproteins without the capacity of independent metabolism. Instead, they are capable of capturing a functional host cell and directing its activity toward their own replication. This makes them especially difficult targets when it comes to therapy. As our understanding of viral-cellular interaction at the molecular level increases, so does our capacity to design drugs capable of interfering with this process without significant deleterious effects on the host cell. It is important to remember that while there are a number of drugs capable of modifying viral illnesses, none capable of "curing" any viral illness exist at this point. This section covers nonretroviral agents (Table 5-2) only; retroviral agents are discussed later in the chapter.

Nucleoside and nucleotide analogues

Acyclovir Acyclovir is an analogue of 2'-deoxyguanosine that requires phosphorylation to be active. This is accomplished by means of a virus-induced thymidine kinase (herpes simplex or varicella) or phosphotransferase (cytomegalovirus) since uninfected mammalian cells show only minimal phosphorylation of this compound. The addition of two more phosphates is carried out by cellular enzymes, resulting in acyclovir triphosphate that competes with 2'-deoxyguanosine triphosphate as a substrate for viral DNA polymerase. In addition, acyclovir triphosphate has a far greater affinity than cellular DNA polymerase for viral DNA polymerase. Once inserted into the replicating virus, synthesis stops. All these characteristics make it an effective drug with minimum cellular toxicity.

Indications Acyclovir is most effective in treating primary herpes simplex virus (HSV) infections both 1 and 2. It is less effective for recurrences, but long-term suppressive therapy will decrease their frequency. Varicella zoster (VZV) requires significantly higher doses (Table 5-2). Its role against cytomegalovirus (CMV) is limited to prophylaxis in transplant patients; it is not very effective against the active disease. At higher doses it has been found to be effective in treating hairy leukoplakia, but symptoms recur when therapy is stopped.

Adverse effects Potential adverse effects are abdominal pain, nausea, vomiting, and anorexia. When administered in the intravenous form, the drug can crystallize in urine, leading to tubular obstruction. Adequate hydration minimizes this occurrence. In rare instances, central nervous system effects such as hallucinations, seizures, and coma may occur.

Table 5-2 Antiviral (nonretroviral) drugs

Drugs	Indication for use*	Usual oral doses+ or routes
Nucleoside/nucleotide analogues		
Acyclovir	HSV, VZV, CMV, possibly EBV	HSV: 400 mg tid; VZV: 800 mg 5 times/day
Valacyclovir	HSV, VZV, CMV	HSV: 1 g bid; VZV:1 g tid
Penciclovir	HSV	Topical
Famciclovir	HSV, VZV, possibly HBV	HSV: 250 mg tid; VZV: 500 mg tid
Ganciclovir	CMV, possibly HSV, VZV, EBV, HHV-8	IV, oral form for chronic suppression
Cidofovir	CMV	IV
Vidarabine	HSV	Ophthalmic
Trifluridine	HSV	Ophthalmic
Idoxuridine	HSV	Ophthalmic
Ribavirin	HCV, Lassa fever, and Hantavirus; possibly RSV, parainfluenza, influenza A and B, and measles	Inhaled for RSV; oral for HCV combined with interferon; IV for Lassa fever and Hantavirus
Pyrophosphate analogue		
Foscarnet sodium	CMV, HSV, VZV	IV
Carbon ring amines		
Amantadine	Influenza A	100 mg bid
Rimantadine	Influenza A	200 mg/day
Neuraminidase inhibitors		
Zanamivir	Influenza A and B	Inhaled
Oseltamivir	Influenza A and B	75 mg bid
Recombinant protein		
Interferon-α	HBV, HCV, HHV-8, HPV, possibly HDV	Subcutaneous or intramuscular injection
Antisense oligonucleotide		
Fomivirsen	CMV	Vitreous injection
Monoclonal antibody		
Palivizumab	RSV	Intramuscular injection

*HSV—herpes simplex virus; VZV—varicella zoster virus; CMV—cytomegalovirus; HBV—hepatitis B virus; HCV—hepatitis C virus; HDV—hepatitis D virus; EBV—Epstein-Barr virus; RSV—respiratory syncytial virus; HHV-8—human herpesvirus 8, HPV—human papillomavirus.
+Oral doses listed are for initial episodes in normal hosts. Doses may vary for recurrences and for immunocompromised patients.

Resistance to acyclovir by HSV and VZV is reported, especially in immunocompromised patients.

Drug form and use It is available in topical, oral, and intravenous forms. The topical form is not significantly absorbed and is the least effective. The bioavailability of the oral form is about 20%. It is widely distributed in tissues, including the central nervous system, which reaches 50% of peak serum levels. Immunocompetent patients can be treated with the oral form. Neonates, immunocompromised hosts, and those with encephalitis should be treated with the IV form to achieve reliable therapeutic levels.

Valacyclovir hydrochloride Valacyclovir hydrochloride is the L-valyl ester of acyclovir and is available in oral form only. It is converted in the gastrointestinal tract and liver to acyclovir with a bioavailability at least three times that of oral acyclovir. Its therapeutic range is similar to acyclovir as is its side effects profile. In severely immunocompromised patients, thrombotic thrombocytopenic purpura and hemolytic uremic syndrome have been reported.

Ganciclovir Ganciclovir's mechanism of action is similar to that of acyclovir, but it is a better substrate for CMV-induced phosphotransferase, making it an improved drug for CMV. It is active against other herpesviruses as well, but because of its many and potentially serious side effects, its use is limited to serious CMV infections. It is available for intravenous and oral use and as an intravitreal implant. Serious infection is treated via the intravenous route. Oral therapy is usually limited to maintenance therapy for stable retinitis in AIDS patients and as prophylaxis against CMV infection in solid organ transplants. The intravitreal form is effective in the CMV retinitis seen in advanced AIDS patients and should be replaced every 6 months.

The most common serious side effect is bone marrow suppression, which leads to neutropenia, thrombocytopenia, and anemia. Gastrointestinal problems include nausea, vomiting, diarrhea, and flatulence. Nervous system effects include paresthesia, neuropathy, dizziness, and seizures. It is moderately nephrotoxic and is carcinogenic in animals.

Penciclovir Penciclovir is structurally similar to ganciclovir, but its mechanism of action is similar to that of acyclovir. It is currently available only in topical form for treatment of orolabial herpes infection in immunocompetent patients. No significant side effects have been reported. An intravenous form is under development.

Famciclovir Famciclovir is an oral pro-drug with excellent absorption that is rapidly converted to penciclovir through deacetylation in the gastrointestinal tract and liver. Its spectrum of activity is similar to that of acyclovir, but its intracellular half-life is significantly longer, allowing for less frequent dosing. It is relatively free of side effects; nausea, diarrhea, and headaches are reported at about the same rate as placebo.

Cidofovir Cidofovir is a nucleotide analogue with in vitro activity against a number of DNA viruses, but because of serious side effects, use of the intravenous form is limited to treatment of serious CMV infections. Because it has a phosphate attached to the base-sugar moiety, it remains intracellularly for an extended period, which allows for once-weekly dosing. It has a high affinity for herpesvirus DNA polymerases. Renal toxicity is a major problem; saline loading and probenecid are given to decrease the risk. A topical gel form, which is being tested for mucocutaneous HSV infection, would be effective even against acyclovir-resistant strains.

Vidarabine, trifluridine, and idoxuridine These drugs are currently available as ophthalmic agents for HSV. Their mechanism of action is not fully understood, and evidence for their efficacy is variable. Their main side effect is local irritation.

Ribavirin Ribavirin is a guanosine analogue with in vitro activity against a wide variety of DNA and RNA viruses. Its mechanism of action is not fully understood. Like acyclovir, it gets phosphorylated intracellularly and it interferes with early events of viral transcription. It also interferes with cellular enzymes such as inosine monophosphate dehydrogenase, resulting in a decrease of guanosine, which may underlie some of its toxic effects. While it has been mostly used in the United States as an aerosol for respiratory syncytial virus bronchiolitis, its efficacy for this disease remains controversial. In intravenous form it has been shown to have clinical efficacy against hemorrhagic fever and Hantaviruses, and the oral form shows promise against hepatitis C, especially when combined with an interferon. The systemic form commonly leads to dose-related anemia. The inhaled form can induce bronchospasms. Because it is teratogenic and embryotoxic in animals, pregnant women should avoid caring for children who are receiving the aerosolized form.

Pyrophosphate analogue

Foscarnet sodium Foscarnet sodium is an organic analogue of inorganic pyrophosphate that is capable of forming complexes with viral DNA polymerases. This process prevents them from cleaving pyrophosphate from nucleotide triphosphates, thus blocking DNA chain elongation. It does not appear to have the same effect on cellular polymerases. Because oral absorption is very poor, it is available only in an intravenous form. It is used primarily in serious CMV infections such as retinitis and is also effective in acyclovir-resistant HSV and VZV infections. Among its many side effects, renal insufficiency and electrolyte imbalance are the most common. Hypocalcemia can be life threatening. Other adverse effects include nausea, vomiting, anemia, penile ulcers, seizures, and electrocardiogram changes. Although it is known to leave deposits in bone, the long-term consequences of this have yet to be seen. It can also induce chromosomal changes.

Carbon ring amines

Amantadine and rimantadine Amantadine and rimantadine are two similar drugs in this class that contain the same unique 10-carbon ring. Their antiviral mechanism is not fully understood, but they appear to block the viral M2 protein ion channel, thereby blocking viral uncoating. They are effective only against influenza A virus, both in preventing and treating early infections. The drugs cause similar side effects, namely central nervous system dysfunction, nausea, and anorexia, but they are less frequent with rimantadine.

Neuraminidase inhibitors

Zanamivir and oseltamivir Zanamivir and oseltamivir, the first two drugs developed in this class, were released only this year. Neuraminidase is an enzyme on the surface of influenza viruses that plays an essential role in the release of viruses from infected cells. Crystallographic studies of its structure allowed the development of these two agents by rational drug design. They bind to a conserved active site on the enzyme and block its activity. Zanamivir is available only in an inhalational form and oseltamivir is available only in an oral form. They appear to be effective both in preventing and treating early influenza A and B viral infections. Oseltamivir causes some nausea and vomiting, but side effects appear to be minimal (although our experience with these agents is still limited).

Recombinant protein

Interferon-α Interferon-α represents at least three very similar proteins produced by cells of the immune system in response to viral infections. The recombinant forms available for therapy differ only in that they are not glycosylated. Their mode of action is complex and not well understood. They appear to induce cellular enzymes that interfere with viral protein synthesis, but some of their antiviral properties are likely to result from immune modulation. They need to be injected either intramuscularly or subcutaneously, as oral ingestion would result in proteolytic digestion of these proteins. In vitro, a large number of viruses appear to be susceptible, but clinical responses have been achieved only in a small number of them. About one third of patients with chronic hepatitis B will respond, but relapses are not uncommon once therapy is stopped. A somewhat higher percentage with chronic hepatitis C will respond, and an even higher rate of sustained response can be achieved when interferon-α is combined with ribavirin. Venereal warts caused by papillomaviruses will respond to intralesional injection. Kaposi sarcoma caused by human herpesvirus 8 will also show some response to systemic therapy. Adverse effects are many and troublesome. They include marked flulike symptoms, bone marrow suppression, psychiatric problems such as severe depression, and autoimmune phenomena.

Antisense oligonucleotide

Fomivirsen Fomivirsen is the first approved antiviral agent in this class of drugs, which is designed to combine with specific mRNAs to inhibit gene expression. In the case of fomivirsen, it is approved only for CMV retinitis and is designed to interfere with immediate-early gene transcription. It is injected into the vitreous, and side effects include increased intraocular pressures and inflammation.

Monoclonal antibody

Palivizumab Palivizumab is a humanized murine monoclonal antibody designed to react with the F-protein on the surface of the respiratory syncytial virus. About 95% of the molecule is coded by a human IgG gene while the epitope reactive component remains from original mouse sequences. It is effective in preventing RSV infection in high-risk infants, and side effects so far have been minimal.

Antiviral (Retroviral) Therapy

Treatment of HIV-infected patients is one of the most rapidly evolving areas of medicine, and the pharmacology of their therapy has become very complex. The scope of this chapter allows us to consider only some general principles. Detailed questions are best referred to physicians and pharmacists involved full-time in the care of these patients.

There are currently 16 drugs to choose from. Of those listed (Table 5-3), 15 are already approved and 1 (adefovir) is available on a compassionate basis. They all belong to one of three categories: *(1)* nucleoside/nucleotide reverse transcriptase inhibitors (NRTI), *(2)* nonnucleoside reverse transcriptase inhibitors (NNRTI), and *(3)* protease inhibitors (PI). In addition to the CD4 counts, the capacity to measure virus in blood quantitatively has improved our decision-making process in using these drugs. The general goal of therapy is to reduce the viral load to the lowest achievable level for the longest period of time.

While many questions remain, a number of principles have emerged over the last few years. Because the reverse transcriptase (RT) of HIV is highly error prone (approximately five mistakes per genome) and the replication rate is very high (1 billion to 10 billion copies per day), emergence of resistance is frequent. Therefore, HIV should not be treated with a single agent. The one exception is that HIV-positive pregnant women with high CD4 and low viral load counts should be treated with zidovudine alone to prevent maternal transmission. For the same reason, when resistance necessitates a therapeutic change, at least two drugs should be changed, preferably to types the patient has not received before. Recent developments of genotypic and phenotypic assays for resistance will aid in this choice.

CLINICAL INSIGHT

Clinical data point toward combination drug usage that employs at least three drugs as the best chance for long-term suppression of the virus. These include two NRTIs and one PI or two NRTIs and the NNRTI efavirenz. It is important for the patient to take the appropriate dosages at the appropriate time intervals. Furthermore, the absorption of some of these drugs will be affected by food, and therefore timing of meals becomes important. Finally, these drugs have potential interactions with other drugs, sometimes with serious consequences. Therefore, when one plans to treat a patient already on antiretroviral therapy, drug interactions need to be checked each time. Table 5-3 lists the antiretroviral drugs, their doses, and their most common side effects.

Nucleoside and nucleotide RT inhibitors

In general, these agents need to be phosphorylated intracellularly to be active. Once in their triphosphorylated form they become incorporated into the nascent DNA chain being copied by reverse transcriptase from viral RNA. This terminates the conversion to proviral DNA, leaving the uncoated virus at the mercy of intracellular degradative enzymes. The extent to which NRTIs interact with cellular DNA polymerases is variable and is likely to underlie some of their toxicity. There are NRTI combinations that should be avoided. Zidovudine and stavudine are antagonistic in vivo and have poor clinical outcome. Didanosine and zalcitabine both cause peripheral neuropathy, and their combination increases this risk. Some will have effects against other viruses; for example, lamivudine is effective against HBV. Adefovir is a nucleotide RT inhibitor currently available for compassionate use, but many of its serious side effects, including renal failure, may keep it from approval.

Nonnucleoside RT inhibitors

These drugs do not need any intracellular phosphorylation to be active, and they do not compete with other nucleoside triphosphates. They bind directly to reverse transcriptase, disrupting its catalytic site. Use as single agents results in rapid development of resistance against them, but they can be synergistic with NRTIs.

Protease inhibitors

During the HIV growth cycle, large polyproteins are produced that need to be cleaved by a viral-encoded protease for final assembly of the mature

Table 5-3 Antiretroviral drugs

Drugs*	Main side effects	Usual oral doses
Nucleoside/nucleotide RT inhibitors		
Zidovudine (AZT)	Anemia, neutropenia, headache, nausea, myositis, asthenia	300 mg bid
Didanosine (DDI)	Diarrhea, neuropathy, pancreatitis	200 mg bid
Stavudine (d4T)	Neuropathy, hepatitis, anemia, pancreatitis	40 mg bid
Zalcitabine (ddC)	Neuropathy, rash, aphthous stomatitis, pancreatitis	0.75 mg tid
Lamivudine (3TC)	Only occasional headache, anemia, neutropenia	150 mg bid
Abacavir	Acute drug reaction, do not rechallenge	300 mg bid
Adefovir	Renal failure, nausea, myopathy, hepatitis, encephalopathy	120 mg qd
Nonnucleoside RT inhibitors		
Nevirapine	Rash (can be life threatening), hepatitis	200 mg qd, bid after 2 weeks
Delavirdine	Rash, headaches, hepatitis	400 mg tid
Efavirenz	Dizziness, headache, insomnia, rash	600 mg qd
Protease inhibitors	All cause lipodystrophy, elevated lipids, elevated glucose	
Indinavir sulfate	Nephrolithiasis, hyperbilirubinemia, headache, dizziness	800 mg tid
Nelfinavir mesylate	Diarrhea	750 mg tid
Saquinavir mesylate	Diarrhea, nausea, headache, hepatitis	1200 mg tid
Ritonavir	Nausea, diarrhea, altered taste, renal failure, hepatitis	600 mg bid
Amprenavir	Nausea, diarrhea, rash, oral paresthesia	1200 mg bid
Lopinavir/Ritonavir	Diarrhea, headache, hepatitis	400 mg/100 mg bid
Other		
Hydroxyurea	Cytopenia	500 mg bid

*RT—Reverse transcriptase.

virion and reactivation of the reverse transcriptase for a new round of replication. Protease inhibitors interfere with this process and, in combination with NRTIs, have dramatically improved the care of HIV patients. They can also be used in combination. For example, a combination of ritonavir and saquinavir mesylate at low doses is safe and results in serum levels of saquinavir mesylate far higher than a higher dose of saquinavir mesylate alone. Formulations are also important because soft-gel capsules of saquinavir mesylate have a much better bioavailability than the hard capsules.

Protease inhibitors have varied and complex interactions with the cytochrome P-450 enzyme system, resulting in many confusing adverse drug interactions. Many of their metabolic effects are not understood and can be a source of distress to the patient. Most troublesome is lipodystrophy, which results in peripheral fat wasting and central adiposity. While initially achieving nondetectable viral levels with the "cocktail" of PIs and NRTIs was routine, recent studies show a significant increase in the percentage of patients whose viral load is becoming detectable, again indicating that this is not yet a cure. Finally, when successful viral suppression results in reconstitution of immune function, some patients will develop fever and adenopathy as their immune system deals with latent pathogens. This is important to recognize so that antiretroviral therapy will not be discontinued.

Hydroxyurea Hydroxyurea is a ribonucleotide reductase inhibitor that results in decreased deoxynucleotide triphosphates available for DNA synthesis. It does not have a direct antiviral effect but appears to enhance the effectiveness of NRTIs such as didanosine and stavudine. It appears promising in the primary treatment of HIV in combination with NRTIs and possibly with PIs.

Treatment of Common Oral Fungal and Viral Infections

Fungal infections

A number of fungal infections can involve the oral mucosa as part of the disseminated form of the disease. Examples include histoplasmosis, cryptococcosis, and blastomycosis. Treatment in these cases is achieved through systemic therapy; no specific drugs need to be used for the oral aspect (Fig 5-1). The most common fungal infection that is frequently localized to the oral cavity is candidiasis. *Candida albicans* remains the most commonly isolated species, but others are found with increasing frequency, including *Candida glabrata*.

A number of predisposing factors are recognized as risks for oral candidiasis. These include recent antibiotic therapy, inhaled or systemic steroids, immunosuppressive therapy, malignancies, and AIDS. Normal hosts such as neonates and denture wearers can also be infected. Oral candidiasis can manifest itself as a pseudomembranous form with raised white plaques on the tongue and other oral mucosa. Usually painful, it can also be atrophic with an erythematous shiny appearance of the mucosa. *Candida* species can also be associated with angular cheilitis and denture stomatitis. Therapies, which are similar for all forms, are listed in Table 5-4. The sequence of listing does not imply the superiority of a drug, but in general a topical agent should be tried first. This is true even

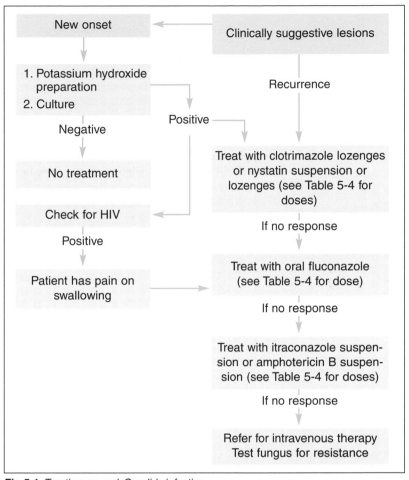

Fig 5-1 Treating an oral *Candida* infection.

Table 5-4 Treatment of oral *Candida* infections

Drugs	Forms and doses	Comments
Clotrimazole	Lozenges, 10 mg 5 times/day up to 14 days*	Dissolve slowly and completely in mouth.
Nystatin	Suspension, 5 mL (500,000 U) 4 times/day up to 14 days* Lozenges, 200,000 U 5 times/day up to 14 days*	Swish and retain in mouth as long as possible, then swallow. Dissolve slowly and completely in mouth.
Amphotericin B	Suspension, 1 mL (100 mg) 4 times/day up to 14 days*	Deposit directly on tongue, swish and swallow.
Fluconazole	Tablets, 100 mg/day up to 14 days*	*C glabrata* and *C krusei* are usually resistant.
Ketoconazole	Tablets, 200 mg/day up to 14 days*	Needs acidic environment for absorption—take with orange juice on empty stomach.
Itraconazole	Suspension, 20 mL (200 mg)/day up to 14 days	Swish solution and swallow 10 mL at a time.

*Immunocompromised patients may require longer therapy. Continue for 48 hours after clinical resolution.

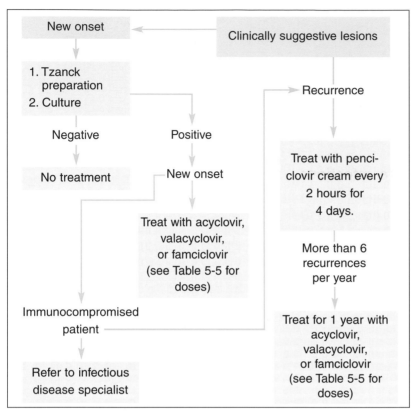

Fig 5-2 Treating an oral herpes infection.

Table 5-5 Treatment of oral herpes simplex infections

Conditions	Drugs (oral or topical) and duration
Normal host	
Primary acute gingivostomatitis	Acyclovir 400 mg, 3 times/day for 10 days
	Valacyclovir hydrochloride 1 g, 2 times/day for 10 days
	Famciclovir 250 mg, 3 times/day for 5–10 days
Recurrences	Penciclovir cream 1% applied every 2 hours for 4 days
Chronic suppression*	Acyclovir 400 mg, 2 times/day up to 1 year
	Valacyclovir hydrochloride 1 g, once/day up to 1 year
	Famciclovir 250 mg, 2 times/day up to 1 year
Immunocompromised host	
Active infection†	Acyclovir 400 mg, 3 times/day for 10 days
	Valacyclovir hydrochloride 1 g, 3 times/day for 7 days
Chronic suppression	Famciclovir 500 mg, 2 times/day for 7 days
	Same as normal host

*More than six recurrences per year.
†For severe infection, use acyclovir intravenously 5 mg/kg every 8 hours for 7 days.

CLINICAL INSIGHT

for AIDS cases, unless the patient also has severe esophagitis, in which case a systemically absorbed agent should be used. There is no role for prophylactic treatment to prevent oral candidiasis in adults with AIDS, but patients with frequent recurrence may benefit from suppressive therapy. Those with angular cheilitis might benefit from application of a topical agent in cream or ointment form directly to the area in addition to the treatment of the oral cavity. Patients with denture stomatitis should have the denture disinfected with an agent such as chlorhexidine in addition to oral therapy.

Viral infections

Similar to fungi, a number of common viral infections, such as varicella zoster, can involve the oral cavity, but no special therapy targeting the mouth is necessary. The one virus that commonly involves the oral cavity and for which useful therapy exists is the herpes simplex virus. Its therapy is outlined in Fig 5-2 and Table 5-5. The majority of cases are caused by HSV type 1, the rest by HSV type 2, but the therapy is the same for both. Therapy will vary depending on the immune status of the patient. Immunocompetent hosts usually acquire their infections during childhood and suffer from recurrences as adults. These can be treated with topical penciclovir. For those who experience more than six episodes per year, chronic suppression with oral agents can be considered for up to 1 year. After a year, therapy should be stopped and the patient should be reassessed. Immunocompromised patients such as those with AIDS, recipients of solid-organ or bone marrow transplants, and those who are receiving chemotherapy should be treated with oral or intravenous agents depending on the severity of the infection. Frequently these patients will benefit from chronic suppressive therapy as well. If a resistant virus is suspected, usually in an immunocompromised host, the intravenous form of foscarnet sodium should be considered.

General References

Abdel-Rahman SM, Nahata MC. Oral terbinafine: A new antifungal agent. Ann Pharmacother 1997;31:445–456.

Abramowicz M (ed). Handbook of Antimicrobial Therapy. New Rochelle, NY: Medical Letter, 1998.

Andriole VT. Current and future therapy of invasive fungal infections. Curr Clin Top Infect Dis 1998;18:19–36.

Christie JM, Chapman RW. Combination therapy for chronic hepatitis C: Interferon and ribavirin. Hosp Med 1999;60:357–361.

Colacino JM, Staschke KA, Laver WG. Approaches and strategies for the treatment of influenza virus infections. Antivir Chem Chemother 1999;10:155–185.

Deeks SG. Practical issues regarding the use of antiretroviral therapy for HIV infection. West J Med 1998;168:133–139.

Fletcher CV. Pharmacologic considerations for therapeutic success with antiretroviral agents. Ann Pharmacother 1999;33:989–995.

Ghannoum MA. Susceptibility testing of fungi and correlation with clinical outcome. J Chemother 1997;9(suppl 1):19–24.

Groll AH, Muller FM, Piscitelli SC, Walsh TJ. Lipid formulations of amphotericin B: Clinical perspectives for the management of invasive fungal infections in children with cancer. Klin Padiatr 1998;210:264–273.

Havlir DV, Lange JM. New antiretrovirals and new combinations. AIDS 1998; 12(suppl A):S165–S174.

Jones PS. Strategies for antiviral drug discovery. Antivir Chem Chemother 1998; 9:283–302.

Keating MR. Antiviral agents for non-human immunodeficiency virus infections. Mayo Clin Proc 1999;74:1266–1283.

Ren S, Lien EJ. Development of HIV protease inhibitors: A survey. Prog Drug Res 1998;51:1–31.

Sheehan DJ, Hitchcock CA, Sibley CM. Current and emerging azole antifungal agents. Clin Microbiol Rev 1999;12:40–79.

Shuter J. Antifungal and antiviral agents: A review. Cancer Invest 1999;17:145–152.

Speed B. A review of antifungal agents. Aust Fam Physician 1996;25:717–719,721.

Weiss B, Davidkova G, Zhou LW. Antisense RNA gene therapy for studying and modulating biological processes. Cell Mol Life Sci 1999;55:334–358.

Section 3

Adverse Reactions

Larry J. Peterson, DDS, MS

6

ALLERGIC AND OTHER SENSITIVITY REACTIONS

Allergy vs Immunity

Clemens Freiherr von Pirquet coined the term "allergy" in the early twentieth century. He used it to describe any altered reaction of the immune system, whether helpful or harmful. In the context of immunology today, *immunity* is thought of as protective and implies enhanced resistance, whereas *allergy* is thought of as harmful and suggests increased susceptibility to a specific substance.

Types of Immunologic Responses

Sensitive vs allergic

We often call unwanted drug reactions or other sensitivity or hypersensitivity reactions "allergic." Allergic reactions are just one type of immunologic reaction (Table 6-1)—the type 1 class.

KEY FACTS

Immunologic reactions are broadly classified into four types:

- Type 1 reactions are often *immediate immunologic* reactions, usually allergic reactions, and usually are mediated by IgE or homocytotropic IgG.
- Type 2 reactions, or *cytotoxic* reactions, occur when an IgG or IgM antibody reacts with cell membranes or antigens associated with cell membranes.

Table 6-1 Types of hypersensitivity

Class	Name	Indicator
Type 1	Immediate	IgE, rarely IgG4
Type 2	Cytotoxic	IgG, IgM, rarely IgA
Type 3	Immune complex	IgG (usually)
Type 4	Delayed	Cellular

- Type 3 reactions are *immune-complex* reactions, in which an antigen and antibody combine to form an immune complex that deposits in the walls of blood vessels, the kidneys, or other selected areas.
- Type 4 reactions, which are *delayed hypersensitivity* or *cell-mediated reactions,* occur when cells interact directly with antigens.

Allergic reactions are only those type 1 reactions mediated by IgE or IgG. When caring for patients, we deal with many reactions of types 2 through 4. Rather than calling these reactions "allergic," as is most often done, we should call them "immunologic."

Type 1: Immediate hypersensitivity

Symptoms Type 1 reactions to drugs predominantly affect the skin and respiratory system. Severe reactions can provoke rash, urticaria, angioedema, respiratory distress and wheezing, and even anaphylaxis and shock. Anaphylaxis is an extreme allergic reaction that can lead to respiratory and cardiovascular collapse.

Agents Penicillin sensitivity can cause classic examples of a type 1 reaction. Other drugs and substances, including allergens used for immunotherapy, xenogeneic sera, insulin, the haptenic metabolites of simple chemical drugs, and certain proteins of biologic products, also can be involved in immediate hypersensitivity type 1 reactions.

Type 2: Cytotoxic reactions

Reaction Cytotoxic reactions are complement dependent and usually involve IgG or IgM antibodies. An antibody-drug-complement complex fixes to a circulating blood cell, causing cell lysis. A blood-type mismatch is an example of a cytotoxic reaction.

Mechanisms There are three mechanisms of cytotoxic blood reactions. In the first, the drug fixes to a cell membrane and an antibody attaches to the drug to form an antibody-antigen complex. Complement is activated and cell lysis occurs. Penicillin-induced immune hemolytic anemia is this type of cytotoxic reaction.

In the second mechanism, the drug, antibody, and complement form a complex before they attach to a cell wall and cell lysis occurs. This is the reaction that results in direct Coombs-positive anti-immune hemolytic anemia, leukopenia, and thrombocytopenia after exposure to certain drugs, including quinidine and sulfonamides.

The third mechanism occurs when the red blood cell membrane is modified by a drug, causing the cell to absorb protein nonspecifically. Cytotoxic cellular destruction results.

Type 3: Immune-complex reactions

Reaction Immunologic sensitivities can be mediated by immune complex reactions. Serum sickness is a reaction of this type and may be caused by heterologous serum or a haptenic drug determinant such as penicillin. The reaction is systemic and can involve multiple organ systems. Complement-dependent vasculitis often results, in which immune complexes are deposited along endothelial surfaces of blood vessels, stimulating inflammation and vascular wall damage.

Symptoms Symptoms of serum sickness, while not as immediately devastating as anaphylactic reactions, are quite serious. They include fever, arthralgia, lymphadenopathy, and rash. Dermatologic manifestations include erythema multiforme; urticaria, which may persist for weeks; and angioedema. A latent period of several days usually passes after the initial administration of a drug before enough antibody to provoke symptoms is produced.

Agents Substances that can invoke immune-complex reactions are foreign sera, penicillin, sulfonamides, thiouracils, diphenylhydantoin, aminosalicylic acid, and streptomycin.

Type 4: Delayed hypersensitivity

Reaction The allergic contact dermatitis that can develop from the use of topical drugs is a cell-mediated, delayed hypersensitivity process. T cells interact directly with antigens.

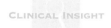

Agents Substances that can cause a delayed hypersensitivity reaction include topical antibiotics, topical antihistamines, topical local anesthetics, and certain additives found in topical medications, including parabens and lanolin. Patch testing can help to establish the agent causing these reactions. However, testing is not always productive and the cause of the reaction may go undetected.

Immunologic Reactions to Drugs

Incidence

Until World War II, serum sickness was the most common allergic drug reaction observed. With the introduction of sulfonamides in the 1930s, more allergic drug reactions were seen. With the increased availability of small-molecular-weight drugs and foreign proteins, the incidence of drug sensitization seems to have increased.

The risk for developing an allergic reaction to most drugs is approximately 2% to 3%. Adverse drug reactions as a whole, including both allergic and nonallergic responses, are experienced by approximately 10% to 15% of *hospitalized* patients. Adults predominate in this group. Less than 7% of the adverse reactions are life threatening.

Examples of common drug reactions

Potential sources of drug reactions and possible allergic problems used in dental patient care are:

- Penicillin and other antibiotics and antimicrobials
- Local anesthetics of the ester type and related drugs
- Adjunctive vasoconstrictors, such as epinephrine
- Other preparations including sedatives, antihistamines, and analgesics.

Clinical vs pharmacological effects

The clinical manifestations of drug allergy differ from the pharmacological effects of the drug. While in most cases pharmacological effects are beneficial, clinical manifestations of drug allergy may be harmful to the body. The clinical response in humans cannot always be predicted from animal tests. Drug allergy involves a small portion of the population and is usually restricted to a limited number of syndromes. Clinically, the patient may develop numerous symptoms (Box 6-1).

Prior exposure

A patient must have been exposed to an agent at least once before to develop an allergic sensitivity to it. It is almost impossible to have an allergic reaction to one's first dose of penicillin. In many cases, the patient may have been exposed to a drug during earlier treatment and had no reaction. After a patient develops sensitivity and the drug is reintroduced into his or her system, the immunologic response may be immediate or may appear after several days. The risk of developing an immunologic response to a drug exists at doses below the therapeutic range. In some cases exposure to a very small amount of drug can trigger an allergic response.

Box 6-1 Clinical manifestations of drug allergy
Urticaria
Angioedema
Rash
Asthma
Systemic anaphylaxis
Fever
Adenopathy
Pulmonary infiltrates

In some cases a patient may have been exposed unknowingly to a drug. For example, a small amount of penicillin naturally occurring in milk can cause sensitivity to develop undetected.

Heredity and genetics

Patients may inherit the tendency to respond favorably as well as to become allergic to drugs. On the other hand, patients experiencing an allergic drug reaction do not necessarily have a history of allergy or atopy. Although it remains speculative, there is evidence for a genetic influence on drug metabolism, and patients who metabolize drugs more slowly are believed to be more likely to develop allergic drug reaction.

Sensitivity Testing

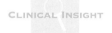
CLINICAL INSIGHT

It is important to consider the basis of the patient's allergic reaction both when deciding whether to continue antibiotic treatment and when managing the reaction itself.

Inconsistent reliability

Immunologic testing to confirm sensitivity or allergy to a drug is not always reliable. Two factors contribute to this:

1. The immunologic bases for many allergic drug reactions have not been clearly defined.
2. The patient may be reacting to a metabolite of a drug or to its dye or capsular material rather than, or in addition to, the drug itself.

Consultation with a specialist

Because of the uncertainties involved in interpreting test results, it is best to consult an allergist or immunologist to clarify the status of a patient with suspected drug sensitivity. The tools for determining the nature of allergic drug reactions are not readily available to all practitioners.

Reliable tests

Tests for low-molecular-weight drugs, such as penicillin, are sufficiently developed so as to yield fairly reliable results. Few drugs responsible for hematologic reactions can be tested reliably.

Positive skin tests are helpful because they verify sensitivity. But only in the case of penicillin are negative skin tests significant. The most conclusive test of sensitivity is to rechallenge the patient, but the risk is usually not justified.

In vivo immunologic tests include immediate skin tests, delayed skin tests, patch testing, and skin window techniques. In vitro tests test for IgE, IgG, and IgM antibodies and for sensitized lymphocytes.

Penicillin Hypersensitivity

KEY FACTS

Penicillin hypersensitivity frequently is a major roadblock in the management of dental infections. The widely used drug can cause almost every known type of sensitivity reaction.

Incidence

Some type of adverse reaction occurs in 3% of penicillin users.

Determinants

Penicilloic acid, a metabolic degradation product, is the major determinant of type 1 reactions and is often primarily responsible for late urticarial reactions and other skin eruptions. Anaphylaxis and immediate urticaria or angioedema can be caused by other antigenic determinants known as minor determinants. These have not yet been fully characterized but seem to be responsible for severe types of immediate allergic reactions such as anaphylaxis. The source of the protein carriers for this haptenic determinant has not been clearly defined. The natures of the antigenic determinants in types 2, 3, and 4 reactions to penicillin are not known.

Manifestations

Skin eruptions The most common manifestation of penicillin allergy is a diffuse erythematous or morbilliform skin eruption. Allergic contact dermatitis may be seen after the topical use of penicillin.

Anaphylaxis Anaphylaxis occurs in about 1 in 10,000 patients using penicillin, accounting for approximately 300 deaths per year in the United States. When urticaria or angioedema appears less than 1 hour after administration, anaphylaxis should be considered. More severe anaphylactic reactions have systemic involvement and compromise breathing. Urticaria that begins days to weeks after penicillin is administered seems to have less serious implications and in some cases may disappear even if penicillin treatment is continued.

Type 3 reactions Immune-complex–mediated reactions, such as serum sickness, will occur occasionally, as will immune hemolytic anemia, which can complicate high-dose intravenous therapy.

Cessation of symptoms

When penicillin is discontinued, the drug reaction subsides. In some cases, urticarial rash may persist for many months and may be triggered occasionally by trace amounts of penicillin in dietary milk. Avoidance of milk products may be helpful in these cases.

Cautions

Concurrent infectious processes can produce an exanthematous eruption that mimics a penicillin sensitivity, possibly causing erroneous diagnosis of penicillin allergy. Awareness of this is especially important when penicillin is given to children with viral or streptococcal respiratory infections. There is some cross-reactivity and cross-allergy between penicillin and the cephalosporins. When cephalosporins are started in a patient with a history of penicillin sensitivity, caution should be exercised. Discussion with the patient's physician is advised.

Diagnosis with skin testing

Detection of determinants Skin testing to detect IgE antibodies to major and minor determinants can be useful in the diagnosis of penicillin allergy. Penicilloyl polylysine (manufactured by several pharmaceutical companies) is marketed to test for the major determinants of this hypersensitivity. A minor determinant mixture is not commercially available, but using penicillin G at 10,000 U/mL serum has correlated well with minor determinants. It is currently the recommended method.

Interpretation of results If the major determinant test is positive, there is a high correlation with skin manifestations such as rash and urticaria. If the minor determinant test is positive, the risk of anaphylaxis is very high. Negative skin test reactions to both major and minor determinants suggest that the patient is *probably* not allergic to penicillin.

Hemagglutination detects serum IgG and IgM antibodies. IgG antibody may function as a "blocking antibody" and may have a protective function. Both IgG and IgM antibodies may produce a type 2 hemolytic anemia if penicillin is given in high dosages intravenously.

When to test Sufficient controversy surrounds this still-developing area so that a clear directive of when to test cannot be given. In the opinion of the author, the best time to perform penicillin skin testing for major and minor determinants is just when the drug becomes needed in treatment. Testing to confirm a previous sensitivity to penicillin at a time when the medication is not required for the treatment of a specific condition is not recommended in most cases because of the possibility that the patient will develop sensitivity in the period between the previous testing and the next exposure.

Emergency Allergic Reactions

Triggers

Most allergic emergencies concerning the dentist are drug-induced anaphylactic reactions. The dentist must also be ready for reactions to anesthetics, vaccines, insect stings, foods, and injected dyes and for transfusion reactions, aspirin sensitivities, hereditary angioedema, and cold- induced urticaria.

Manifestations

Anaphylactic reactions occur when a patient becomes overwhelmed by a sudden release of chemical mediators from mast cells. The onset is usually sudden; can be characterized by bronchospasm, wheezing, laryngeal edema, rash, or hives; and can cause a drop in blood pressure that can lead to life-threatening shock.

Emergency Treatment of Anaphylaxis

While the triggering agent of an acute allergic reaction is variable, the approach to handling the emergency is similar in most cases. The dentist's primary responsibility in an allergic emergency is to stabilize the patient until he or she can be transferred to an emergency facility or until assistance arrives. Whatever the degree of severity, all anaphylactic reactions must be evaluated quickly and carefully. Early treatment usually improves the prognosis and often decreases the severity of the reactions.

Airway and breathing symptoms

The patient's airway must be kept clear. Continual evaluation of the patient's respiratory and cardiovascular status is vital.

Recommended agents Injectable epinephrine 1:1,000 dilution is the first-line drug in patients with bronchospasm and respiratory distress in whom there are no medical contraindications for such therapy.

- Dosage: 0.01 mg/kg body weight, not to exceed 0.3 mL. Dose can be repeated after 10 to 30 minutes if required and if the patient tolerated the previous dose well.
- A bronchodilator such as intravenous aminophylline should also be considered. In addition, oxygen by face mask or nasal prongs should be administered.

Other symptoms

Patients can also have other immediate hypersensitivity reactions such as:

- Hives
- Swelling
- Bronchospasm
- Anaphylactic shock

Patients should be stabilized as quickly as possible and, if indicated, transferred to the nearest emergency facility. A list of emergency telephone numbers and the locations of nearby emergency rooms should be readily available in the dental office. In severe cases, it may be necessary to immediately administer fluids and medications intravenously.

Recommended agents Medications that are most helpful in anaphylactic emergencies include:

- Antihistamines
- Bronchodilators
- Corticosteroids

Antihistamines should be injected intramuscularly at doses appropriate for the patient's body size. Injectable diphenhydramine or hydroxyzine can be used. The drugs are administered intravenously or by subcutaneous or intramuscular injection. Other antihistamines such as chlorpheniramine maleate can be used at the discretion of the clinician.

Corticosteroids can be given either intramuscularly or intravenously. Unlike antihistamines and bronchodilators, which appear to have more immediate effects, corticosteroids usually do not begin to effect a clini-

---

Box 6-2 Emergency treatment of allergic reaction

Immediate allergic reaction

1. Maintain airway, give O$_2$ 6 L/min by mask.
2. Call for medical assistance.
3. Administer 0.2–0.3 mL of 1:1,000 epinephrine subcutaneously.
4. If indicated (condition worsens), administer 50 mg diphenhydramine intramuscularly or intravenously.
5. If indicated (condition worsens), administer 125 mg methylprednisolone intramuscularly or intravenously.
6. If condition continues to deteriorate, repeat epinephrine administration 10 minutes after initial dose.

Delayed reaction

Oral antihistamines may be sufficient treatment.

---

cal change for 8 to 12 hours after their administration. Box 6-2 summarizes emergency treatment of anaphylaxis.

Summary

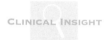

The dentist must stabilize the patient and act quickly and accurately until the patient can be transferred safely to an emergency facility or until assistance arrives. The dental practitioner should remain calm, evaluate the clinical problem quickly and adequately, and then initiate therapy.

Nonimmunologic Drug Reactions

Not all drug sensitivities have allergic or immunologic bases. Many drug reactions are not interactions between antigen and antibody. All persons are at risk to develop nonimmunologic drug reactions. Nonallergic drug reactions are no more likely in atopic than in nonatopic persons.

Some patients develop toxic side effects and unwanted reactions even when taking a drug as directed and within the therapeutic range. Examples of toxic side effects include drowsiness due to antihistamines, muscle tremor from terbutaline sulfate, stomach upset from aspirin or erythromycin, and hyperplasia of the gingiva from phenytoin.

Causes of toxic side effects

Overdose Patients who take a medication in dosages above the therapeutic range may develop symptoms of toxic overdose, such as hemorrhage from the use of an anticoagulant.

Immunosuppressor drugs Any patient is liable to develop an increased susceptibility to candidiasis, *Pneumocystis carinii* pneumonia, or histoplasmosis when taking immunosuppressor drugs.

Drug interactions When two drugs used concurrently have identical binding sites on the same cell, they will compete, one will displace the other, and toxicity will result. Phenylbutazone displaces warfarin and results in bleeding. Phenylbutazone and salicylates displace tolbutamide and result in hypoglycemia. Dentists must be aware of drug interactions. Consult the pharmacist when there is a question.

Altered metabolism In patients with hepatic or renal insufficiencies, toxicity might result from impaired metabolism or excretion of drugs that are metabolized in the liver and in the kidneys. Morphine is detoxified poorly by the cirrhotic patient. Streptomycin, digitalis, and potassium all accumulate during renal failure. When a patient is using digitalis and a diuretic is added, potassium loss may occur. As a result, the patient may develop an increased susceptibility to digitalis and become toxic. Toxicity can occur when asthmatic patients with cirrhosis of the liver take theophylline because clearance of the drug markedly decreases with the liver disorder.

Genetic defects Sometimes genetic defects, such as inherited enzyme deficiency, surface as apparent drug sensitivities. Glucose-6-phosphate dehydrogenase (G6PD) deficiency can result in hemolytic anemia and hyperbilirubinemia after exposure to certain drugs such as antimalarials, sulfonamides, aspirin, and phenacetin.

Symptoms mimicking allergy

"Drug reaction" frequently creates the image of an atopic, wheezing, hives- and shock-prone person. This is not usually the case, although drug reactions sometimes mimic allergic reactions.

Rash A maculopapular rash may develop from viral exanthem when ampicillin is used to treat infectious mononucleosis, certain viral infections, and other diseases. The virus can make the patient temporarily hypersensitive to enteric bacterial products or to the drug itself. Interaction between ampicillin and allopurinol can cause a rash due to hyperuricemia.

Histamine release Morphine, codeine, atropine, pentamidine, polymyxin, meperidine, stilbamidine, and D-tubocurarine, which release histamine directly from cells without antigen-antibody reactions, can cause transient flushing, bronchospasm, urticaria, headache, and hypotension. Although it has not been clearly defined, a possible mechanism for some radiocontrast media reactions is the direct release of histamine from cells.

Aspirin intolerance is an idiosyncratic reaction, sometimes associated with asthma and nasal polyps or sensitivity to indomethacin and other nonsteroidal anti-inflammatory drugs, naproxen, yellow dyes, or tartrazine. Symptoms in these patients, who are usually middle-aged nonallergic women, are similar to those of other idiosyncratic reactions and include wheezing and bronchospasm, transient flushing, and urticaria.

Drug withdrawal

Symptoms Adverse withdrawal reactions and psychological drug reactions can arise when chronic drug treatment is stopped too abruptly. Symptoms associated with opiate withdrawal include nausea, anxiety, abdominal cramps, and hypertension. Withdrawal of diazepam and barbiturates may result in irritability, delirium, seizures, and even death. Amphetamine withdrawal results in a "crash" and often a pattern of lassitude and sleep disturbance. "Rebound rhinitis" and obstruction may result when use of sympathomimetic nose drops is abruptly halted.

Oral steroids Oral steroid medication cutoff risks adrenal insufficiency. An oral surgery patient who has recently stopped taking oral steroids should be covered to prevent acute adrenal insufficiency. Use of steroids for 2 weeks within the previous 2 years usually requires supplemental steroid administration.

Further Reading

de Weck AL. Drug reactions. In: Samter M (ed). Immunological Diseases, ed 3. Boston: Little, Brown, 1978:413–439.

Green GR, Rosenblum AH, Sweet LC. Evaluation of penicillin hypersensitivity: Value of clinical history and skin testing with penicilloyl-polylysine and penicillin G. A cooperative prospective study of the penicillin study group of the American Academy of Allergy. J Allergy Clin Immunol 1977;60:339–345.

Ter AL. In: Fudenberg HH (ed). Basic and Clinical Immunology, ed 2. Los Altos: Lange, 1978:514.

Van Arsdal PP. In: Middleton E Jr (ed). Allergy. St. Louis: Mosby, 1978:1133.

Mariano Sanz, MD, DDS
David Herrera, DDS, Dr Odont

7

Adverse Microbiological Effects

Antibiotics affect not only target bacteria but also the human body microflora. This can lead to overgrowth of opportunistic pathogens, development of resistant strains of bacteria, and an alteration in the body's physiologic mechanisms of resistance to pathogenic bacterial colonization.[1]

Bacterial Resistance

IMPORTANT PRINCIPLE

The use of antibiotics increases the resistance of bacterial microflora by means of one of three processes: pressure selection, acquisition, and random mutation. *Pressure selection* allows only resistant bacteria to survive in a particular niche exposed to the antimicrobial agent. Appropriate mechanisms of resistance are acquired through genetic elements that encode for bacterial resistance *(horizontal acquisition)*. *Random mutation* in the bacterial genome can also serve as a mechanism for resistance.

Bacterial resistance can be either *intrinsic* or *acquired* (Table 7-1). As its name suggests, intrinsic resistance occurs naturally and is inherent to some bacterial species, whereas a particular bacterial strain can acquire resistance to an antimicrobial drug through different mechanisms (Table 7-2).

The organization of bacterial cells in biofilms significantly influences the antimicrobial susceptibility of bacterial cells in these structures. Several factors can explain the lower level of susceptibility of bacteria inside microbial biofilms (Table 7-3).

Table 7-1 Acquisition of antimicrobial resistance[23-25]

Type of resistance	Description	Mechanism
Intrinsic	Naturally occurring	Inherent to many bacterial species
Acquired		
Horizontal acquisition	Most common	Encoded in genetic elements
Transformation		DNA segments are acquired from the surrounding environment
Transduction[22]		DNA is transferred from one bacterium to another through insertion in a bacterial phage
Conjugation		DNA is transferred though cell-to-cell contact from a donor bacterium to a recipient bacterium
Mutation	Random	Chromosomal mutations moderately increase resistance

Table 7-2 Mechanisms of antimicrobial resistance[11,23,25,26]

Mechanism	Example
Alteration of the target site	Enzymes, known as rRNA methylases, modify an adenine residue of the ribosome, preventing macrolides, lincosamynes, and type B streptogramins from binding to the 50 S ribosomal subunit.
Prevention of access to the target site	The blockage of the outer pores of porins avoid the entrance of penicillins in gram-negative bacteria.
Inactivation of the antimicrobial agent	β-lactamase enzymes inactivate β-lactam drugs.
Efflux of the drug	Resistant bacteria pump tetracycline out of the cell.

Table 7-3 Mechanisms of antimicrobial resistance in biofilms[27]

Mechanism	Description
Diffusion limitation of the agent into the biofilm	Deeper areas are more difficult for drug molecules to reach.
Plethora of phenotypes due to spatial gradients	Slow-growing microorganisms inside the biofilm are less susceptible to some antimicrobial drugs.
Selection pressure that favors the less susceptible cells	As susceptible bacteria are destroyed, less susceptible bacteria occupy the niches.
Resistance training with subeffective levels	Due to factors 1 and 2, bacterial cells can be repeatedly exposed to subeffective levels of the drug, which increases the level of resistance.
Biofilm-specific genotype, different from that of planktonic cells	Bacterial cells in biofilms expressed additional genes, probably due to their attachment to a solid surface, which showed a different genotype than planktonic cells, and were characterized by higher levels of resistance to antimicrobial drugs.

There is ample evidence to suggest that resistant bacterial strains emerge following the administration of local or systemic antibiotics.[2–4] This increased resistance appears to be transient,[5] although well-controlled longitudinal studies are needed to clarify this issue. Tetracyclines, for example, have caused clear short-term increases in bacterial resistance,[5,6] but some authors have considered this increment as a selection of naturally resistant species,[5] and the long-term impact remains unclear. Bacterial resistance may start with an increased number of resistant bacteria that compete with the endogenous microflora, which may eliminate or dilute the resistant populations prior to the transfer of resistance. However, some resistant strains may survive and even increase through successful competition with the endogenous bacteria or through the transfer of resistance factors.[7]

Resistant bacteria are not distributed equally throughout the world. Over the past few years, several divergent groups of organisms have caused significant infection morbidity and mortality, mostly because they developed resistance to multiple antimicrobial agents.[8] Several anaerobic bacteria,[9] in particular, have increased in antimicrobial resistance, including multiple drug resistance.[10] The total amount of systemic antibiotics used and compliance to therapy are the two factors that determine the level of bacterial resistance in a population.[11,12]

Changes in the Normal Flora

The resident microflora hamper the colonization of new bacterial species. Through the production of lactic and acetic acids, hydrogen peroxide, and other antimicrobial substances, resident microorganisms possibly contribute to the maintenance of the colonization resistance. They can also improve intestinal immunity by adhering to intestinal mucosa and stimulating local immune responses. Resident intestinal bacteria also play an important role in the development of the immune system.

Changes in the endogenous microflora can also alter the normal homeostasis because endogenous bacteria play a role in multiple physiologic processes of certain metabolic pathways. The normal intestinal microflora play a role in metabolizing nutrients, drugs, endogenous hormones, and carcinogens and influence the metabolism of bilirubin, intestinal mucin, pancreatic enzymes, fatty acids, bile acids, cholesterol, and steroid hormones. The normal microflora of the large intestine synthesize a number of water-soluble vitamins, including riboflavin.

Table 7-4 Antibiotics and superinfections

	Pseudomembranous colitis	Superinfections	Gastrointestinal problems
Cephalosporins	X	Pseudomonads, *Enterobacter*	
Tetracycline	X	*Candida albicans* (gastrointestinal and vaginal tract and oral cavity)	X
Erythromycin		*Enterobacter,* clostridia, yeast (intestines, throat)	X
Clindamycin	X	*Clostridium difficile*	X
Penicillins		*Staphylococcus aureus* (periodontal abscesses)	

Table 7-5 Symptoms of adverse microbiological effects

Microbiological effect	Symptoms
Superinfection	Oral pain
	Xerostomia
	Candidiasis
	Cheilosis
	Black hairy tongue
	Diarrhea
	Enteritis
	Colitis
	Vaginitis
	Pruritus ani
Bacterial resistance	Failure of clinical response
	Deterioration of patient
	Possible resistance of future infections

Superinfections

When prompted by the intake of systemic antimicrobials, changes in the endogenous microflora can lead to superinfections in two ways:

(1) Through overgrowth of potentially pathogenic strains; and
(2) By decreasing the colonization resistance.

Any antibiotic taken orally alters the natural bacterial microflora of the oral cavity and the gastrointestinal/urogenital tracts, but broad-spectrum antibiotics are especially known to result in superinfection by colonization of resistant opportunistic pathogens such as fungi[13] and *Clostridium difficile.*

Several antimicrobials that are widely used in dentistry have been related to superinfections (Table 7-4) and are known to cause a number of different symptoms (Table 7-5).

The use of systemic antibiotics such as doxycycline may give rise to overgrowth of superinfecting microorganisms in the subgingival micro-

KEY FACTS

flora, either by increasing the numbers of preexisting subgingival organisms or by allowing the establishment of these species from other colonized oral sites such as the tongue dorsum and anterior palate.[14]

Periodontal abscesses Periodontal abscesses have been reported after systemic application of penicillins and tetracyclines for nonoral reasons without appropriate subgingival debridement.[4,15,16] Penicillin-resistant *Staphylococcus aureus* has been isolated from periodontal abscesses after penicillin therapy.[15]

Candidiasis *Etiology Candida albicans* is responsible for most common oral fungal infections.[17] A commensal organism in 40% to 65% of the human population, its two main reservoirs are the dorsal surface of the tongue and the palatal mucosa. Candida infections of the oral cavity frequently occur in locally or systemically immunocompromised patients and in patients who have used systemic broad-spectrum antibiotics.[18] The clinical manifestation of oral candidiasis is very heterogeneous and may present in pseudomembranous, atrophic, hyperplastic, and ulcerative forms.[18,19]

Oropharyngeal candidiasis can be treated with nystatin, a classic polyene that is well tolerated and shows low rates of resistance.[20] Systemic azoles are not recommended because of the development of increasing levels of resistance (see chapter 5).

Antibiotic-associated colitis and diarrhea *Etiology Clostridium difficile* is a spore-forming anaerobe that can occur naturally in the human intestine. Changes in the natural composition of the intestinal microflora during or after antibiotic therapy allow this microorganism to multiply in the colon, causing pseudomembranous colitis. *C difficile* may produce enterotoxin-A and/or cytotoxin-B and may result in mild diarrhea or in pseudomembranous colitis, a potentially life-threatening disease. *C difficile*–associated pseudomembranous colitis occurs especially after ampicillin and clindamycin therapy. *C difficile* is resistant to penicillins, cephalosporins, tetracyclines, aminoglycosides, and erythromycin. An incidence of 0.01% to 10% has been reported after clindamycin therapy, and it is associated more with the parenteral phosphate form than with the oral hydrochloride form.

Clinical diagnosis Antibiotic-associated colitis and diarrhea are characterized by mild, inflammatory, and sometimes bloody diarrhea with profuse and watery discharges accompanied by cramps and abdominal pain and are usually complicated by dehydration, hypotension, and hypoalbuminemia. They can be diagnosed by colonoscopic detection of epithelial necrosis, ulceration, and, in the advanced state, by the presence of pseudomembranes.

Treatment Consult a physician. The first step is to discontinue any previous antibiotic therapy. Treatment with metronidazole or vancomycin (500 mg every 6 hours) should then be initiated. A greater number of relapses have been found after vancomycin therapy, and vancomycin resistance among *C difficile* strains has been reported.[21] Additional treatment includes restoration of fluid and electrolyte balance.

Other adverse effects

CLINICAL INSIGHT

Contraceptive failure Certain antibiotics have been blamed for reducing blood concentrations of oral contraceptives, thereby reducing their effectiveness. However, this is controversial since most theories that explain the interference are based on anecdotal reports.

Oral contraceptives combine two components, a semisynthetic estrogen and a semisynthetic progesteron. The first component blocks ovulation by inhibiting the release of follicle-stimulating and luteinizing hormones, whereas progesteron hampers egg implantation by enhancing the viscosity of the cervical fluid and instigating changes in the endometrial lining. The failure rate of oral contraceptives, when used correctly, is less than 1%, but because of human error the common rate is 3%, increasing to 8% in teenagers.[22]

Only the interference of rifampin has been properly documented. It involves the induction of hepatic microsomal activity, which increases the metabolism of different drugs, leading to reduced serum levels of both components in oral contraceptives. Case reports of oral contraceptive failures have also been presented for ampicillin, tetracycline, penicillin, cotrimoxazole, metronidazole, and erythromycin, among others, but evidence of the interference is weak.

Various theories have been proposed to explain the interaction between antibiotics and oral contraceptives. One explanation is related to the estrogen component of the contraceptive drug. Estrogen enters an enterohepatic recirculation, providing additional blood levels. This recirculation can be inhibited by antibiotics that kill colonic bacteria involved in this process. However, different studies that have evaluated oral contraceptive blood concentrations report no significant decreases in plasma level for estrogen or progesteron in women treated with ampicillin, tetracycline, doxycycline, metronidazole, erythromycin, clarithromycin, temafloxacin, or fluconazole.[22]

Adverse drug interactions[22] Erythromycin and tetracyclines interfere with digoxin by reducing the normal gut microflora, which inactivate a significant amount of digoxin in about 10% of patients.

KEY FACTS

Tetracyclines, amoxicillin, and ampicillin affect the normal gut microflora involved in vitamin K production, thereby increasing the anticoagulant activity of warfarin, dicumarol, or anisindione.

References

1. Hooker KD, DiPiro JT. Effect of antimicrobial therapy on bowel flora. Clin Pharm 1988;7:878–888.

2. Olsvik B, Hansen BF, Tenover FC, Olsen I. Tetracycline-resistant micro-organisms recovered from patients with refractory periodontal disease. J Clin Periodontol 1995;22:391–396.

3. Williams BL, Osterberg SK, Jorgensen J. Subgingival microflora of periodontal patients on tetracycline therapy. J Clin Periodontol 1979;6:210–221.

4. Topoll HH, Lange DE, Müller RF. Multiple periodontal abscesses after systemic antibiotic therapy. J Clin Periodontol 1990;17:268–272.

5. Fiehn N-E, Westergaard J. Doxycycline-resistant bacteria in periodontally diseased individuals after systemic doxycycline therapy and in healthy individuals. Oral Microbiol Immunol 1990;5:219–222.

6. Abu Fanas SH, Drucker DB, Hull PS. Amoxycillin with clavulanic acid and tetracycline in periodontal therapy. J Dent 1991;19:97–99.

7. Greenstein G. Clinical significance of bacterial resistance to tetracyclines in the treatment of periodontal diseases. J Periodontol 1995;66:925–932.

8. Doern GV. Antimicrobial resistance among lower respiratory tract isolates of *Haemophilus influenzae*: Results of a 1992–93 Western Europe and USA collaborative surveillance study. The Alexander Project Collaborative Group. J Antimicrob Chemother 1996;38(suppl A):59–69.

9. Rosenblatt JE, Brook I. Clinical relevance of susceptibility testing of anaerobic bacteria. Clin Infect Dis 1993;16(suppl 4):S446–S448.

10. Rasmussen BA, Bush K, Tally FP. Antimicrobial resistance in *Bacteroides*. Clin Infect Dis 1993;16(suppl 4):S390–S400.

11. van Winkelhoff AJ, Herrera Gonzales D, Winkel EG, Dellemijn-Kippuw N, Vandenbroucke-Grauls CMJE, Sanz M. Antimicrobial resistance in the subgingival microflora in patients with adult periodontitis. A comparison between the Netherlands and Spain. J Clin Periodontol 2000;27:79–86.

12. Herrera D, van Winkelhoff AJ, Dellemijn-Kippuw N, Winkel EG, Sanz M. ß-lactamase producing bacteria in the subgingival microflora of adult patients with periodontitis. A comparison between Spain and the Netherlands. J Clin Periodontol 2000;27:520–525.

13. Walker CB. Selected antimicrobial agents: Mechanisms of action, side effects and drug interactions. Periodontol 2000 1996 Feb;10:12–28.

14. Rams TE, Babalola OO, Slots J. Subgingival occurrence of enteric rods, yeasts and staphylococci after systemic doxycycline therapy. Oral Microbiol Immunol 1990;5:166–168.

15. Helovuo H, Hakkarainen K, Paunio K. Changes in the prevalence of subgingival enteric rods, staphylococci and yeasts after treatment with penicillin and erythromycin. Oral Microbiol Immunol 1993;8:75–79.

16. Helovuo H, Paunio K. Effects of penicillin and erythromycin on the clinical parameters of the periodontium. J Periodontol 1989;60:467–472.

17. Zegarelli DJ. Fungal infections of the oral cavity. Otolaryngol Clin North Am 1993;26:1069–1089.

18. Fotos PG, Vincent SD, Hellstein JW. Oral candidosis. Clinical, historical, and therapeutic features of 100 cases. Oral Surg Oral Med Oral Pathol 1992;74:41–49.

19. Epstein JB. Antifungal therapy in oropharyngeal mycotic infections. Oral Surg Oral Med Oral Pathol 1990;69:32–41.

20. Alvarez Alvarez ME, Sanchez-Sousa A, Baquero F. A reevaluation of nystatin in prophylaxis and treatment of oropharyngeal candidiasis. Rev Esp Quimioter 1998;11:295–315.

21. Groschel DH. *Clostridium difficile* infection. Crit Rev Clin Lab Sci 1996;33:203–245.

22. Hersh EV. Adverse drug interactions in dental practice: Interactions involving antibiotics. Part II of a series. J Am Dent Assoc 1999;130:236–251.

23. Roberts MC. Antibiotic resistance in oral/respiratory bacteria. Crit Rev Oral Biol Med 1998;9:522–540.

24. Walker CB. The acquisition of antibiotic resistance in the periodontal microflora. Periodontol 2000 1996;10:79–88.

25. Danziger LH, Pendland SL. Bacterial resistance to ß-lactam antibiotics. Am J Health Syst Pharm 1995;52(6, suppl 2):S3–S8.

26. Nord CE. Mechanisms of ß-lactam resistance in anaerobic bacteria. Rev Infect Dis 1986;8(suppl 5):S543–S548.

27. Gilbert P, Allison DG. Biofilms and their resistance towards antimicrobial agents. In: Newman HN, Wilson M (eds). Dental Plaque Revisited. Oral Biofilms in Health and Disease. Cardiff: BioLine, 1999:125–144.

Section 4

Clinical Application

Sebastian G. Ciancio, DDS
Arie J. van Winkelhoff, PhD

8

ANTIBIOTICS IN PERIODONTAL THERAPY

Periodontal Disease

The most common forms of periodontal disease—gingivitis and periodontitis—are caused by bacteria adjacent to or associated with periodontal structures. These bacteria, along with calculus and other local factors, are the principal components that perpetuate the disease process (see chapter 2). Therapy is focused on identifying, removing, and controlling these factors by a variety of mechanical and chemotherapeutic methods.

In many patients, systemic and local host factors influence the nature and severity of disease. Severe and/or acute periodontal infection may affect the general health status of the patient. Recent studies have suggested that periodontal disease may be a risk factor for preterm, low-birth-weight babies; heart attack; and stroke.[1,2] Periodontal infections can even be life threatening in immunocompromised individuals.

All periodontal diseases are not the same. Gingivitis, defined as inflammation of the gingiva, can be subclassified according to cause, pathogenesis, and host factors. Periodontitis likewise comprises "related but distinct diseases that differ in etiology, natural history, progression and response to therapy"[3] (Table 8-1). The natural course of the disease suggests that destruction of connective tissue attachment to the tooth is associated with alternating periods of active destruction and relative quiescence. Histologically, the periodontal tissues remain chronically inflamed, but clinically the gingiva may or may not exhibit obvious signs of inflammation. Recognition and understanding of the causes and pathogenesis of these diseases are a prerequisite for establishing a rationale for antimicrobial and antibiotic therapy.

Table 8-1 Microbial species associated with various clinical forms of periodontitis[4]

| Species | Forms of periodontitis* | | | |
	Localized juvenile	Early onset	Adult	Refractory
Actinobacillus actinomycetemcomitans	+++	++	++	++
Porphyromonas gingivalis	O	+++	+++	++
Prevotella intermedia/nigrescens	++	+++	+++	+++
Bacteroides forsythus	O	++	+++	++
Fusobacterium species	+	++	+++	++
Peptostreptococcus micros	O	++	+++	++
Eubacterium species	NE	+	++	+
Campylobacter rectus	+	++	++	+
Treponema species	++	+++	+++	++
Enteric rods and pseudomonads	NE	NE	O	+
β-Hemolytic streptococci	?	++	++	++
Candida species	NE	NE	NE	O

* NE—Not elevated in comparison to health; O—occasionally isolated.
+—Less than 10% of the patients positive; ++—less than 50% of the patients positive; +++—greater than 50% of the patients positive.

For common forms of gingivitis and periodontitis, scaling and root planing should always be carried out before antibiotics are administered. In general, antibiotics are seldom necessary for treatment of gingivitis and chronic periodontal diseases. Scaling, root planing, and periodontal surgery (if indicated) are anti-infective measures that may negate the need for antibiotics. A major concern associated with the use of antibiotics is the potential for development of resistant bacterial strains, which is thought to be one of the major therapeutic challenges to face practitioners in the next decade.[5,6] Therefore, antibiotics should not be prescribed unnecessarily. For example, although they are somewhat effective in reducing plaque, antibiotics should never be prescribed for that purpose.

KEY FACTS

Conditions that may call for systemic antimicrobial periodontal therapy are:

- Continuing periodontal attachment loss despite diligent conventional mechanical treatment
- Periodontitis that is refractory to conventional mechanical and surgical periodontal treatment
- Early-onset types of periodontitis
- Medical conditions that predispose patients to periodontitis
- Acute periodontal infections (periodontal abscess, acute necrotizing ulcerative gingivitis/periodontitis)

> **Box 8-1** Antibiotic selection checklist
>
> - Travels readily to the infection site
> - Concentrates in therapeutic levels in the crevicular fluid, gingival tissue, and/or alveolar bone
> - Host and microbial side effects are minimal
> - Benefit-to-risk ratio is positive (ie, more benefit)
> - Clinical effects have been documented for certain types of periodontitis or in certain patient groups

Infecting Microorganisms

The most effective agent against periodontal disease is determined through susceptibility profiles of the dominant microorganisms and the practitioner's clinical diagnosis (Box 8-1). During the initial stages of bacterial colonization, gram-positive bacteria are the ones most commonly associated with gingivitis; however, as the disease becomes more severe, the plaque progressively undergoes ecological changes, and gram-negative bacteria prevail. Anaerobic and motile bacteria also increase as the gingival infection becomes more severe.

In periodontitis, a proliferation of gram-negative capnophilic and anaerobic bacteria (such as *Porphyromonas gingivalis* and *Bacteroides forsythus*) and spirochetes takes place as the pockets deepen.[7] Recent studies strongly suggest that aggressive (juvenile) periodontitis is etiologically related to *Actinobacillus actinomycetemcomitans,* a species found in developing and established pockets associated with the disease[8] (see Table 8-1). Some studies have suggested that in deep pockets bacteria may be found within gingival tissue.[9]

Plaque Formation and Gingivitis

Antibiotic effectiveness

When antibiotics have been used topically or systemically to reduce or prevent plaque formation or gingivitis, the results have been favorable as long as the antibiotic remained in use. In most studies, however, the positive effects ended with cessation of therapy. Long-term use of therapeutic doses of antibiotics is contraindicated because of the increased risk of side effects. The most likely adverse effect is the emergence of resistant bacterial strains.

ADVERSE EFFECTS

Table 8-2 When to use systemic antibiotics

Condition/treatment	When antibiotic use is suggested
Gingivitis	Acute superficial infection associated with bacteremia and septicemia or associated with systemic disease
Acute necrotizing ulcerative gingivitis	When severe and/or systemic signs and symptoms are present
Periodontitis	Early-onset forms nonresponsive to therapy Rapid periodontal destruction Acute, diffuse infection with systemic signs and symptoms
Periodontal surgical therapy	Regenerative periodontal therapies Postsurgical infection
Implant dentistry	During and subsequent to surgical placement (see chapter 14)

Specific conditions

Types of gingivitis that may require antibiotic therapy include acute necrotizing ulcerative gingivitis (ANUG) and streptococcal gingivitis, which is caused by *Streptococcus pyogenes* (Table 8-2). Treatment of severe ANUG may include mechanical debridement, topical use of chlorhexidine, and systemic use of antibiotics, specifically metronidazole. Streptococcal gingivitis, which can be caused by an acute tonsillar infection, may respond well to systemic penicillin therapy.

Systemic and topical antibiotics

Spiramycin, vancomycin hydrochloride, kanamycin, metronidazole, and erythromycin have been tested for effectiveness as both preventive and therapeutic agents against gingivitis and plaque.[10–16] Vancomycin and kanamycin cannot be absorbed through the intestine, which limits their use in general medicine but enhances their potential for topical use in dentistry. Kanamycin and metronidazole have been shown to reduce plaque and gingivitis, but not enough to warrant their general use.[10,11]

Topical antibiotic administration may be less desirable because some antibiotics, notably penicillin, are likely to cause hypersensitivity. Moreover, topical antibiotics can be absorbed through the oral mucosa, which can cause systemic reactions and the development of resistant strains. Vancomycin, erythromycin, kanamycin, tetracycline, and bacitracin have been tested topically with varying degrees of success.[12,14–16] (For a detailed discussion of topical antimicrobials, see chapter 4.)

Periodontitis

Antibiotic use

Antibiotics are used systemically in the treatment of periodontitis as an adjunct to initial periodontal treatment to prevent the need for surgery only after traditional periodontal therapy has failed to achieve an adequate response. Systemic antibiotics are also used as an adjunct to surgical therapy to enhance the success of regenerative procedures. The choice of antibiotic must be made with care, and patients who are taking antibiotics must be closely monitored (Table 8-2). There must be a specific, documentable reason to prescribe antibiotics.

IMPORTANT PRINCIPLE

Microbiological testing

Microbiological analysis of the subgingival plaque may be carried out following initial periodontal treatment or surgical intervention to determine whether a need for antimicrobial therapy exists if the clinical response to the primary therapy is unsatisfactory. In general, culture and susceptibility tests are needed whenever an unusual or recurring infection cannot be diagnosed based on clinical signs and symptoms alone. Microbial testing should include screening for superinfecting microorganisms such as gram-negative enteric rods, pseudomonas, and yeasts.

Sequencing of antibiotic therapy

Rational use of systemic antibiotics in periodontics requires adequate clinical diagnosis of the disease, thorough mechanical debridement, microbiological analysis of the subgingival plaque, and susceptibility testing of target organisms.[4] In other words, antibiotics should be regarded as only one of the tools available in periodontal therapy and as an adjunct to mechanical debridement. Some patients who are at high risk for periodontal breakdown, such as those with aggressive (juvenile) and other early-onset forms of periodontitis, may be treated with antibiotics after the initial mechanical therapy. High posttherapy plaque levels are associated with failure of systemic antibiotic therapy. Box 8-2 presents guidelines for the administration of systemic periodontal antimicrobial therapies.

1. Initial periodontal therapy should include thorough mechanical root debridement combined with surgical access if needed. Supplemental, subgingivally applied, broad-spectrum antiseptic agents may be used. Periodontal abscesses may develop if systemic antibiotics are administered without mechanical debridement.

2. The clinical response is evaluated 1 to 3 months after the completion of mechanical therapy and is deemed unsatisfactory. A microbiological examination of the subgingival microflora may determine the presence and level of remaining putative periodontal pathogens. In vitro susceptibility testing should be carried out to identify feasible systemic antimicrobial therapies.

3. Antibiotics should be prescribed based on the clinical need for further treatment, the microbiological findings, and the medical status and current medications of the patient. Short-term, high-dose antibiotic regimens should be favored.

4. Another microbiological test may be warranted 1 to 3 months after systemic antimicrobial therapy to verify the subgingival elimination of target pathogen(s) and to screen for possible superinfecting organisms. High levels of viridans streptococci, *Actinomyces,* and other bacteria are suggestive of periodontal health or minimal disease.

5. After resolution of the periodontal infection, the patient should be placed on an individually tailored maintenance care program. Good patient home plaque control provides the best clinical and microbiological response to systemic antimicrobial therapy. Recurrence of progressive disease may prompt additional microbiological testing and further therapy targeting the specific periodontal pathogens involved.

Selection of Antibiotic Regimens in Periodontal Therapy

In the complex subgingival microflora, bacteria differ not only in antimicrobial spectra but also in the mechanisms by which they are killed or suppressed. Concentration-dependent drugs—those whose activity depends on the ratio between the peak drug concentration and the minimum inhibitory concentration (MIC) of the pathogen—include aminoglycosides, metronidazole, and the fluoroquinolones. The optimum dosing strategy for a concentration-dependent drug may be a single dose that results in a peak-serum concentration 8 to 10 times above the MIC of a pathogen. Doubling the concentration of a concentration-dependent drug in vitro will kill the same number of organisms in half the time.

Time-dependent, or concentration-independent, drugs kill microorganisms during time periods in which the concentration of the unbound drug remains above the MIC level. β-Lactam antibiotics (penicillins and cephalosporins) are examples of time-dependent antibiotics. Once a threshold drug concentration has been achieved, further increasing the drug concentration does not increase the number of bacteria killed. A time-dependent drug should be continuously administered to maintain a maximum ratio of peak drug concentration to MIC over an appropriate time period.

The post-antibiotic effect of a drug is another important factor in periodontal antibiotic therapy. The post-antibiotic effect represents the period when bacterial growth is inhibited after the drug concentration has fallen below the bacterial MIC. The post-antibiotic effect of a drug differs for gram-positive and gram-negative bacteria, and antimicrobials that inhibit protein synthesis (macrolides and tetracyclines) tend to have a longer post-antibiotic effect than β-lactam drugs. Furthermore, when two antimicrobials are combined, their post-antibiotic effect may be synergistic, indifferent, or antagonistic.[4] Unfortunately, because conclusive studies in this area are lacking, the optimal choice and dosing of antibiotics for various periodontal infections remain to be determined.

Single-drug regimens

Penicillins Systemic administration of penicillin, particularly a broad-spectrum agent such as amoxicillin, is of value as initial therapy (in conjunction with drainage, when possible) in the treatment of a periodontal abscess. It is also useful in the treatment of acute necrotizing ulcerative gingivitis when associated with severe pain, fever, or lymphadenopathy.

Penicillin has a low toxicity and, except for allergic reactions, is one of the safest drugs known. Patients hypersensitive to one penicillin most likely are hypersensitive to all others. Patients with a history of hypersensitivity to cephalosporins, griseofulvin, or penicillamine may show a similar response to penicillins.

Amoxicillin may be useful alone or in combination with clavulanic acid to protect the drug from the bacterial degradation or with metronidazole in the management of patients with refractory or early-onset forms of periodontitis (see "Combination antimicrobial therapy" below). Penicillin G is a narrow-spectrum antibiotic that has no documented clinical effects when used as a single-drug regimen.

Tetracyclines It has been suggested that tetracyclines can concentrate in gingival crevicular fluid at levels five to seven times those in serum.[17,18] Recent data have shown, however, that crevicular fluid levels of tetracyclines do not exceed those of plasma levels in most individuals. Moreover, the gingival crevicular fluid concentration exceeds the antibacterial concentration of 1 μL/mL in only about 50% of the individuals. These observations may account for much of the variability in clinical response to tetracyclines documented in practice.

Tetracyclines may protect collagen and thereby strengthen host resistance by inhibiting the production of collagenase from polymorphonuclear leukocytes.[19,20] Tetracyclines may be effective in the treatment of many young patients with aggressive periodontitis, rapidly advancing cases of periodontitis,[21] and in some cases of periodontitis refractory to conventional therapy,[22–24] but failures after tetracycline therapy have also been documented.[4] Kornman and Robertson[25] evaluated the effects of tetracycline after administration for up to 7 years in 20 patients who were refractory to conventional periodontal treatment. Although many of the patients improved, the organisms associated with periodontal disease returned when treatment was discontinued. High levels of tetracycline-resistant organisms were seen in 4 of the 10 patients. Systemic tetracyclines may not be the optimal choice in early-onset forms of periodontitis, and better guidelines are needed to identify patients who would benefit from long-term tetracycline therapy.

ADVERSE EFFECTS

The major side effects of tetracyclines include gastrointestinal disturbances, photosensitivity, kidney and liver dysfunction, discoloration of mucosa and tooth extraction sockets, discoloration of teeth in children when given during the time of crown formation, and superinfection with *Candida albicans*, particularly in debilitated patients. With the exception of doxycycline, the absorption of tetracyclines is affected by calcium-containing products or metal ions administered within 1 hour of dosing.

INFORMATION ABOUT SPECIFIC DRUG

Minocycline Minocycline is a semisynthetic tetracycline that is effective against a broad spectrum of microorganisms. Unlike other tetracyclines, which generally require administration four times a day, minocycline can be given twice a day and is associated with less renal toxicity and phototoxicity. However, systemic use of minocycline can cause reversible vertigo and may produce a black to gray pigmentation in attached gingiva and adult teeth when used for extended time periods, as in the treatment of acne.[26–29]

ADVERSE EFFECTS

INFORMATION ABOUT SPECIFIC DRUG

Doxycycline Doxycycline has the same spectrum of activity as minocycline and is equally effective against periodontal pathogens. It has the greatest anticollagenase effect of all the tetracyclines, a benefit realized in a low-dosage, subantimicrobial administration of this drug. Because it can be given once daily for a selected time period, doxycycline is associated with high patient compliance.

INFORMATION ABOUT SPECIFIC DRUG

Metronidazole Metronidazole is highly effective against the anaerobic bacteria associated with periodontal disease. Levels of metronidazole in crevicular fluid are slightly higher than those in serum, resulting in concentrations that are lethal to many plaque bacteria.

In some trials, metronidazole has demonstrated a beneficial effect on periodontitis when used in conjunction with good oral hygiene and/or subgingival debridement.[30] A recent study suggests that the clinical benefits of metronidazole combined with scaling and root planing may be maintained for up to 5 years.[31] Research has shown metronidazole to be effective in refractory periodontitis associated with *B forsythus* and *P gingivalis*.[32]

ADVERSE EFFECTS

The major side effects of metronidazole are metallic taste sensations, headache, vertigo, and peripheral neuritis. Alcohol should be avoided altogether by patients taking metronidazole because the interaction often leads to severe gastrointestinal disturbances.

Clindamycin Clindamycin is effective against many of the bacteria associated with periodontal disease. It has shown efficacy in patients with periodontitis who were refractory to tetracycline or metronidazole therapy.[33] Because of its ability to penetrate bone, clindamycin is particularly useful in treating cases of periodontal disease in which bacterial invasion of tissue is suspected.

Levels of clindamycin in crevicular fluid usually are above the MIC for periodontal pathogens.[34] It is almost completely absorbed from the gastrointestinal tract and excreted in urine, feces, and, most importantly, bile. Following oral administration, levels in bone are similar to levels in serum.

The main adverse effects are diarrhea and gastric upset; therefore, it should be taken with food. Ulcerative colitis has occurred during therapy with clindamycin, but less frequently than with ampicillin or cephalosporins. Clindamycin has been shown to be of value in the treatment of cases of periodontitis refractory to conventional therapy.[35-38]

Ciprofloxin Ciprofloxin is a fluoroquinolone that was initially used to treat urinary tract infections. While studies of its value in periodontal therapy are limited, it may be useful in refractory cases.[39] Adverse effects of this drug include gastrointestinal upset, oral candidiasis, headache, restlessness, insomnia, hypersensitivity, hyperpigmentation, and photosensitivity.

Spiramycin The US Food and Drug Administration prohibits use of spiramycin because of the associated high incidence of gastrointestinal problems. Effective mainly against gram-positive organisms, the drug reduces both gingivitis and plaque when administered systemically. Improvement in periodontal parameters has been reported in short-term studies of patients treated with spiramycin even when local therapy was not provided.[40-42]

Combination antimicrobial therapy

Since the subgingival microflora in oral infections may consist of various putative pathogens that differ in antimicrobial susceptibility, the use of a combination of two or more antibiotics may represent a valuable approach in chemotherapeutics (Box 8-3).[4]

It is important to note that a bactericidal antibiotic (β-lactam drugs, metronidazole) should not be used simultaneously with a bacteriostatic agent (tetracyclines) because the bactericidal agent exerts activity during cell division, which is impaired by the bacteriostatic drug.

Amoxicillin and clavulanic acid Clavulanic acid protects amoxicillin from enzymatic degradation by bacterial penicillinase. Although not yet fully identified, the periodontal pathogens affected by protected amoxicillin are known to include both gram-positive and gram-negative bacteria.

> **Box 8-3** Advantages and disadvantages of combination antibiotic therapy
>
> **Advantages**
> - Broadens the antimicrobial range of the therapeutic regimen beyond that attained by any single antibiotic
> - Prevents the emergence of resistant bacteria through overlapping antimicrobial mechanisms
> - Lowers the dose of individual antibiotics by exploiting possible synergy between two drugs against targeted organisms
>
> **Disadvantages**
> - May increase adverse reactions
> - Potential for antagonistic drug interactions with improperly selected antibiotics

This combination has been shown to be of value in the treatment of periodontitis in patients who have been refractory to periodontal therapy.[43–47] However, protected amoxicillin is not effective in adult periodontitis patients with undetermined disease activity.[48] The main side effect of this combination of drugs is gastrointestinal upset.

Doxycycline Because tetracyclines are purported to cause fungal overgrowth in mucous membranes of the gastrointestinal tract and vagina, they are available for prescription in combination with antifungal agents (see chapter 17). However, there is no convincing evidence that such combinations result in decreased fungal infections, although there may be a rational basis for their use in patients who are diabetic, debilitated, or receiving adrenal corticosteroids (see chapter 16).

A more recent study compared the effects of short-term sequential administration of amoxicillin with clavulanic acid and doxycycline to those of short-term systemic administration of doxycycline alone in the treatment of *A actinomycetemcomitans*– and *P gingivalis*–associated periodontitis.[49] The results showed clinical benefits for both regimens.

Metronidazole Studies have suggested that, when combined with amoxicillin or Augmentin, metronidazole may be effective in managing some patients with aggressive (juvenile) and refractory periodontitis.[50,51] Although they are ineffective against *A actinomycetemcomitans*, both metronidazole and its hydroxymetabolite act synergistically with amoxicillin.[52] Metronidazole affects most anaerobes while amoxicillin affects most facultative and aerobic bacteria, making this combination useful for many mixed periodontal infections.[4]

Metronidazole and amoxicillin in vitro exert synergistic activity against *A actinomycetemcomitans* and the combination may suppress markedly or even eliminate *A actinomycetemcomitans* and other subgingival organisms in periodontitis lesions. A metronidazole-amoxicillin combination has also proven to be effective against nonoral infections associated with oral pathogens.[53,54]

Ciprofloxin Ciprofloxin is effective against *A actinomycetemcomitans* when combined with metronidazole, and it also may be used in the treatment of periodontitis associated with enteric rods and/or pseudomonads.[55] Since the combination does not affect most gram-positive facultative bacteria, it may facilitate recolonization of the pocket by facultative streptococci of low periodontopathic potential.

Spiramycin Spiramycin combined with metronidazole can be used as an adjunct to scaling and root planing.[56]

Serial drug regimens

The sequential use of drugs overcomes the potential risk of antagonism between bacteriostatic and bactericidal antibiotics. Serial drug regimens studied to date in periodontics include systemic doxycycline administered initially and then followed by either Augmentin or metronidazole.[49,57,58] Aitken et al[57] indicated that prevention of recurrent periodontitis with metronidazole may be enhanced by previous treatment with doxycycline. Serial use of doxycycline and metronidazole may reduce levels of periodontal pathogens.[58] The value of serial antibiotic therapy in the management of advanced periodontitis merits further studies.

A Final Note: Periodontal Dressings

Some authors have claimed that wound healing improves when antibiotics are applied in periodontal dressings. However, the main advantage appears to be alleviation of the bad taste or odor that patients sometimes experience after periodontal surgery. This limited value does not warrant the use of antibiotics in dressings, especially because applying them to cut surfaces increases the probability of systemic absorption. Moreover, resistant strains may develop from the resultant exposure of body flora to low doses of antibiotics.

References

1. Offenbacher S, Beck J. Periodontitis: A potential risk factor for spontaneous preterm birth. Compend Contin Educ Dent 1998;19:32–39.

2. Genco RJ, Glurich I, Haraszthy V, Zambon JJ, DeNardin E. Overview of risk factors for periodontal disease and implications for diabetes and cardiovascular disease. Compend Contin Educ Dent 1998;19:40–45.

3. American Academy of Periodontology. World Workshop in Clinical Periodontics. Chicago: American Academy of Periodontology, 1996:1–23.

4. van Winkelhoff AJ, Rams TE, Slots J. Systemic antibiotic therapy in periodontics. Periodontol 2000 1996;10:45–78.

5. Murray BE. Problems and dilemmas of antimicrobial resistance. Pharmacotherapy 1992;12(6 pt 2):86S–93S.

6. Tomasz A. Multiple-antibiotic-resistant pathogenic bacteria. A report on the Rockefeller University Workshop. N Engl J Med 1994;330:1247–1251.

7. Lowenguth RA, Chin I, Caton JG, Cobb CM, Drisko CL, Killoy WJ, et al. Evaluation of periodontal treatments using controlled-release tetracycline fibers: Microbiological response. J Periodontol 1995;66:700–707.

8. Mandell RL, Socransky SS. A selective medium for *Actinobacillus actinomycetem-comitans* and the incidence of the organism in juvenile periodontitis. J Periodontol 1981;52:593–598.

9. Saglie R, Newman MG, Carranza FA Jr, Pattison GL. Bacterial invasion of gingiva in advanced periodontitis in humans. J Periodontol 1982;53:217–222.

10. Loesche WJ, Syed SA, Morrison EC, Laughon B, Grossman NS. Treatment of periodontal infections due to anaerobic bacteria with short-term treatment with metronidazole. J Clin Periodontol 1981;8:29–44.

11. Löe H, Theilade E, Jensen SB, Schiott CR. Experimental gingivitis in man. 3. Influence of antibiotics on gingival plaque development. J Periodontal Res 1967;2:282–289.

12. Johnson RH, Rozanis J. A review of chemotherapeutic plaque control. Oral Surg Oral Med Oral Pathol 1979;47:136–141.

13. Ciancio SG, Bourgault PC. Clinical Pharmacology for Dental Professionals, ed 3. Chicago: Year Book Medical, 1989.

14. Hollander L, Hardy SM. The use of aureomycin ointment in dermatology. Am Prac Digest Treat 1950;1:54–57.

15. Jensen SG, Löe H, Schiott CR, Theilade E. Experimental gingivitis in man. 4. Vancomycin induced changes in bacterial plaque composition as related to development of gingival inflammation. J Periodontal Res 1968;3:284–293.

16. Loesche WJ, Nafe D. Reduction of supragingival plaque accumulation in institutionalized Down's syndrome patients by periodic treatment with topical kanamycin. Arch Oral Biol 1973;18:1131–1143.

17. Ciancio SG, Mather ML, McMullen JA. An evaluation of minocycline in patients with periodontal disease. J Periodontol 1980;51:530–534.

18. Gordon JM, Walker CB, Murphy JC, Goodson JM, Socransky SS. Tetracycline: Levels achievable in gingival crevice fluid and in vitro effect on subgingival organisms. Part I. Concentrations in crevicular fluid after repeated doses. J Periodontol 1981;52:609–612.

19. Golub LM, Lee HM, Lehrer G, Nemiroff A, McNamara TF, Kaplan R, Ramamurthy NS. Minocycline reduces gingival collagenolytic activity during diabetes: Preliminary observations and a proposed new mechanism of action. J Periodontal Res 1983;18:516–526.

20. Golub LM, McNamara TF, D'Angelo G, Greenwald RA, Ramamurthy NS, Zambon J, Ciancio S. A non-antibacterial chemically-modified tetracycline inhibits mammalian collagenase activity. J Dent Res 1987;66:1310–1314.

21. Preus HR. Treatment of rapidly destructive periodontitis in Papillon-Lefevre syndrome. Laboratory and clinical observations. J Clin Periodontol 1988;15:639–643.

22. Papli R, Lewis JM. Refractory chronic periodontits: Effect of oral tetracycline hydrochloride and root planing. Aust Dent J 1989;34:60–68.

23. Kornman KS, Karl EH. The effect of long-term low-dose tetracycline therapy on the subgingival microflora in refractory adult periodontitis. J Periodontol 1982;53:604–610.

24. Shapiro A. Healing potential of periodontal osseous defects treated by scaling and root planing. J Dent Que 1990;27:587–592.

25. Kornman KS, Robertson PB. Clinical and microbiological evaluation of therapy for juvenile periodontitis. J Periodontol 1985;56:443–446.

26. Ciancio SG, Mather ML, McMullen JA. An evaluation of minocycline in patients with periodontal disease. J Periodontol 1980;51:530–534.

27. Ciancio SG, Slots J, Reynolds HS, Zambon JJ, McKenna JD. The effect of short-term administration of minocycline HCl on gingival inflammation and subgingival microflora. J Periodontol 1982;53:557–561.

28. Poliak SC, DiGiovanna JJ, Gross EG, Gantt G, Peck GL. Minocycline-associated tooth discoloration in young adults. JAMA 1985;254:2930–2932.

29. Salman RA, Salman DG, Glickman RS, Super S, Salman L. Minocycline induced pigmentation of the oral cavity. J Oral Med 1985;40:154–157.

30. Loesche WJ, Syed SA, Morrison EC, Kerry GA, Higgins T, Stoll J. Metronidazole in periodontitis. I. Clinical and bacteriological results after 15 to 30 weeks. J Periodontol 1984;55:325–335.

31. Söder B, Nedlich U, Jin LJ. Longitudinal effect of non-surgical treatment and systemic metronidazole for 1 week in smokers and non-smokers with refractory periodontitis: A 5-year study. J Periodontol 1999;70:761–771.

32. Winkel EG, van Winkelhoff AJ, Timmerman MF, Vangsted T, van der Velden U. Effects of metronidazole in patients with "refractory" periodontitis associated with *Bacteroides forsythus*. J Clin Periodontol 1997;24:573–579.

33. Tyler K, Walker C, Gordon J, Pappas J, Cohen S. Evaluation of clindamycin in adult refractory periodontitis: antimicrobial susceptibilities. J Dent Res 1985;64(special issue):abstract 1667.

34. Walker CB, Gordon JM, Cornwall HA, Murphy JC, Socransky SS. Gingival crevicular fluid levels of clindamycin compared with its minimal inhibitory concentrations for periodontal bacteria. Antimicrob Agents Chemother 1981;19:867–871.

35. Walker CB, Gordon JM, Magnusson I, Clark WB. A role for antibiotics in the treatment of refractory periodontitis. J Periodontol 1993;64(8 suppl):772–781.

36. Magnusson I, Clark WB, Low SB, Maruniak J, Marks RG, Walker CB. Effect of non-surgical periodontal therapy combined with adjunctive antibiotics in subjects with "refractory" periodontal disease. (I). Clinical results. J Clin Periodontol 1989;16:647–653.

37. Magnusson I, Low SB, McArthur WP, Marks RG, Walker CB, Maruniak J, et al. Treatment of subjects with refractory periodontal disease. J Clin Periodontol 1994;21:638–637.

38. Walker C, Gordon J. The effect of clindamycin on the microbiota associated with refractory periodontitis. J Periodontol 1990;61:692–698.

39. Slots J, Rams TE. Rational use of antibiotics. J Calif Dent Assoc 1990;18(5):21–23.

40. Quee TC, Chan EC, Clark C, Lautar-Lemay C, Bergeron MJ, Bourgouin J, Stamm J. The role of adjunctive Rodogyl therapy in the treatment of advanced periodontal disease. A longitudinal clinical and microbiologic study. J Periodontol 1987;58:594–601.

41. Chin Quee T, Al-Joburi W, Lautar-Lemay C, Chan EC, Iugovaz I, Bourgouin J, Delorme F. Comparison of spiramycin and tetracycline used adjunctively in the treatment of advanced chronic periodontitis. J Antimicrob Chemother 1988;22(suppl B):171–177.

42. Bain CA, Beagrie GS, Bourgoin J, Delorme F, Holthius A, Landry RG, et al. The effects of spiramycin and/or scaling on advanced periodontitis in humans. J Can Dent Assoc 1994;60:209, 212–217.

43. Collins JG, Offenbacher S, Arnold RR. Effects of a combination therapy to eliminate *Porphyromonas gingivalis* in refractory periodontitis. J Periodontol;1993;64:998–1007.

44. Walker CB, Gordon JM, Magnusson I, Clark WB. A role for antibiotics in the treatment of refractory periodontitis. J Periodontol 1993;64(8 suppl):772–781.

45. Magnusson I, Clark WB, Low SB, Maruniak J, Marks RG, Walker CB. Effect of nonsurgical periodontal therapy combined with adjunctive antibiotics in subjects with "refractory" periodontal disease. (I). Clinical results. J Clin Periodontol 1989;16:647–653.

46. Magnusson I, Marks RG, Clark WB, Walker CB, Low SB, McArthur WP. Clinical, microbiological and immunological characteristics of subjects with "refractory" periodontal disease. J Clin Periodontol 1991;18:291–299.

47. Magnusson I, Low SB, McArthur WP, Marks RG, Walker CB, Maruniak J, et al. Treatment of subjects with refractory periodontal disease. J Clin Periodontol 1994; 21:628–637.

48. Winkel EG, van Winkelhoff AJ, Barendregt DS, van der Weijden GA, Timmerman MF, van der Velden U. Clinical and microbiological effects of initial periodontal therapy in conjunction with amoxicillin and clavulanic acid in patients with adult periodontitis. A randomised double-blind, placebo-controlled study. J Clin Peridontol 1999;26:461–468.

49. Matisko MW, Bissada NF. Short-term sequential administration of amoxicillin/clavulanate potassium and doxycycline in the treatment of recurrent/progressive periodontitis. J Periodontol 1993;64:553–558.

50. van Winkelhoff AJ, Rodenburg JP, Goené RJ, Abbas F, Winkel EG, de Graaff J. Metronidazole plus amoxycillin in the treatment of *Actinobacillus actinomycetemcomitans*–associated periodontitis. J Clin Periodontol 1989;16:128–131.

51. van Winkelhoff AJ, Tijhof CJ, de Graaff J. Microbiological and clinical results of metronidazole plus amoxicillin therapy in *Actinobacillus actinomycetemcomitans* associated periodontitis. J Periodontol 1992;63:52–57.

52. Pavicic MJAMP, van Winkelhoff AJ, de Graaff, J. Synergistic effects between amoxicillin, metronidazole and the hydroxymetabolite of metronidazole against *Actinobacillus actinomycetemcomitans*. Antimicrob Agents Chemother 1991;35:961–966.

53. van Winkelhoff AJ, Abbas F, Pavicic MJ, de Graaff J. Chronic conjunctivitis caused by oral anaerobes and effectively treated with systemic metronidazole plus amoxicillin. J Clin Microbiol 1991;29:723–725.

54. van Winkelhoff AJ, Overbeek BP, Pavicic MJ, van den Bergh JP, Ernst JP, de Graaff J. Long-standing bacteremia caused by oral *Actinobacillus actinomycetemcomitans* in a patient with a pacemaker. Clin Infect Dis 1993;16:216–218.

55. Slots J, Feik D, Rams TE. In vitro antimicrobial sensitivity of enteric rods and pseudomonads from advanced adult periodontitis. Oral Microbiol Immunol 1990; 5:298–301.

56. Quee TC, Chan EC, Clark C, Lauter-Lemay C, Bergeron MJ, Bourgouin J, Stamm J. The role of adjunctive Rodogyl therapy in the treatment of advanced periodontal disease. A longitudinal clinical and microbiologic study. J Periodontol 1987;58: 594–601.

57. Aitken S, Birek P, Kulkarni GV, Lee WL, McCulloch CA. Serial doxycycline and metronidazole in prevention of recurrent periodontitis in high-risk patients. J Periodontol 1992;63:87–92.

58. Birek D, Kulkarni GV, Lee WK, et al. Effect of serial doxycycline/metronidazole on recurrent periodontitis pathogens [abstract 864]. J Dent Res 1989;68(special issue): 373.

Sushma Nachnani, MS

ORAL MALODOR

Oral malodor (OM) has been recognized in the literature since ancient times, but only in the last 5 to 6 years has it come to the forefront of public and dental professional awareness.[1] Approximately 40% to 50% of dentists report seeing six or seven self-described OM patients per week.[2] Routine diagnosis and treatment of OM have not been established either in the dental or medical field; however, pioneering researchers and clinicians have established reputable clinics dealing with this condition, evidence that the transfer of knowledge is increasing.

At least 50% of the population[3] suffers from a chronic OM condition, causing personal discomfort and social embarrassment that often lead to emotional distress. Moreover, the consequences of OM may be more than social in that it may be a symptom of serious local or systemic conditions. Recent research has shown that sulfur-producing bacteria could be the primary source of this condition.

This chapter outlines a basic overview of OM and describes most of the antimicrobial agents presently involved or suggested in its treatment.

Oral and Nonoral Causes of Oral Malodor

Oral malodor can be caused by a number of localized and systemic disorders. When the cause is a normal physiological process, the condition is usually transitory. Transient or nonpathologic OM may be the result of hunger, low levels of salivation during sleep, food debris, prescription drugs, or smoking.[4] Chronic or pathological halitosis may have oral or nonoral causes. The mucosa of the mouth and the upper respiratory tract

> **Box 9-1** Seven common sources of oral malodor
>
> 1. Mouth and tongue
> 2. Nasal, nasopharyngeal, sinus, and oropharyngeal
> 3. Xerostomia
> 4. Primary lower respiratory tract and lung
> 5. Systemic disease
> 6. Gastrointestinal diseases and disorders
> 7. Odiferous ingested foods, fluids, and medications

are used to expel volatile compounds from the body, including gases and metabolic end products of the diet (garlic, alcohol, etc). These volatile compounds are produced in extraoral cavities as well as in the oral cavity. In advanced cases this condition is described as oral malodor.

There appear to be several other metabolic conditions involving enzymatic and transport anomalies (such as trimethylaminuria) that lead to systemic production of volatile malodors that manifest themselves as halitosis and/or altered chemoreception.[5] Some of the oral causes are periodontitis, gingivitis, and plaque coating on the dorsum of the tongue. Oral malodor may be aggravated by a reduction in salivary flow. Radiation therapy, Sjögren syndrome, lung cancer, peritonsillar abscess, cancer of the pharynx, and cryptic tonsils can also contribute to OM.[5] Nasal problems, such as postnasal drip at the posterior dorsum of the tongue, may exacerbate an OM condition. Odor generated in this manner can easily be distinguished from mouth odor by comparing the two odors.[6]

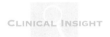

The nonoral causes of OM include diabetic ketosis, uremia, gastrointestinal conditions, irregular bowel movement, hepatic and renal failure, and certain types of carcinomas such as leukemia. The accurate clinical labeling and interpretation of different OMs contribute to the diagnosis and treatment of underlying disease[8] (Box 9-1). Taste and smell can be altered due to facial injuries, cosmetic surgery, radiation, and an olfactory epithelium located on the dorsal aspect of the nose.[8] A relationship between gastrointestinal diseases, such as gastritis, and OM has not been established. However, OM has been reported in patients with a history of gastritis or duodenal or gastric ulcers.[10]

Oral malodor has a basis in bacterial putrefaction (Fig 9-1), the degradation of proteins, and the resulting amino acids produced by microorganisms.[11] While many patients with a chief complaint of OM have a level of gingival and/or periodontal pathology sufficient to be the etiology, periodontol pathology clearly is not a prerequisite for production of OM.[12] Medications such as antimicrobial, antirheumatic, and antihypertensive agents; antidepressants; and analgesics may cause altered taste and xerostomia.

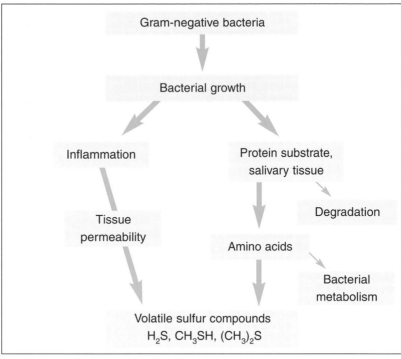

Fig 9-1 Production of volatile sulfur compounds.

Oral malodor in healthy patients arises from the oral cavity and generally originates on the dorsum of the tongue.[6,13–16] The volatile sulfur compounds (VSCs) producing anaerobic bacteria appear to be the primary source of these odors.[16] The bacteria hydrolyze the proteins to amino acids, three of which contain sulfur groups and are the precursors to VSCs. These gaseous substances consist primarily of hydrogen sulfide (H_2S), dimethyl sulfide ($[CH_3]_2S$), methylmercaptan (CH_3SH) and sulfur dioxide (SO_2).[11,13,15,16] Cadaverine levels have been reported to be associated with oral malodor, and this association may be independent of VSC.[17] Subjects without a history of oral malodor who rinsed with cysteine produced high oral concentrations of VSC, suggesting that cysteine is a major substrate for VSC production. The other sulfur-containing amino acids had much less effect on VSC production. It was found that the tongue was the major site for VSC production.[18]

The tongue plaque coating

Research suggests that the tongue is the primary site in the production of OM (Fig 9-2). The dorsoposterior surface of the tongue has been identified as the principal location of the intraoral generation of VSCs.[20] The tongue is an excellent site for the growth of microorganisms since

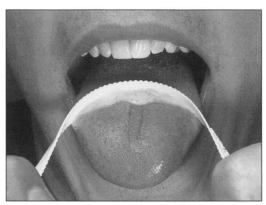

Fig 9-2 Plaque coating on the surface of the tongue.

the papillary nature of the tongue dorsum creates a unique ecological site that provides an extremely large surface area, favoring the accumulation of oral bacteria. The proteolytic, anaerobic bacteria that reside on the tongue play an essential part in the development of OM. The presence of tongue coating has been shown to have a correlation with the density or total number of bacteria in the tongue-plaque coating.[21] The weight of the tongue coating in periodontal patients was elevated to 90 mg, while the VSC was increased by a factor of 4 and the CH_3SH/H_2S ratio was increased thirtyfold when compared with individuals with healthy periodontium.[20] This high ratio of amino acids can be due to free amino acids in the crevicular fluid when compared with those of L-cysteine.[20] The benzoyl–DL-arginine-2 napthylamide (BANA) test has been used to detect *Treponema denticola*, *Porphyromonas gingivalis*, and *Bacteroides forsythus*. The three organisms that may contribute to OM can easily be detected by their capacity to hydrolyze BANA, a trypsinlike substrate. BANA scores are associated with a component of OM, which is independent of volatile sulfide measurements, and suggest its use as an adjunct test to volatile sulfide measurement.[22] Higher mouth odor organoleptic scores are associated with heavy tongue coating and correlate with the bacterial density on the tongue and with the BANA-hydrolyzing bacteria *T denticola*, *P gingivalis*, and *B forsythus*.[23]

KEY FACTS

Microflora associated with oral malodor

The bacterial species that cause OM have yet to be isolated from among the more than 300 bacterial species in the mouth. Putrefaction is thought to occur under anaerobic conditions, involving a range of bacteria such as *Fusobacterium*, *Veillonella*, *T denticola*, *P gingivalis*, *Bacteroides*, and *Peptostreptococcus*.[23,24] Studies have shown that essentially all odor production is a result of gram-negative bacterial metabolism and that the gram-positive bacteria contribute very little odor (see Fig 9-1).[24]

IMPORTANT PRINCIPLE

Fusobacterium nucleatum, one of the predominant organisms associated with gingivitis and periodontitis, produces high levels of VSCs. The nutrients for the bacteria are provided by oral fluids, tissue, and food debris. Methionine is reduced to methylmercaptan and cysteine and the latter is reduced to cystine, which, in the presence of sulfhydrase-positive microbes, is further reduced to hydrogen sulfide. This activity is favored at a pH of 7.2 and inhibited at a pH of 6.5.[11,13,15,16] Isolates of *Klebsiella* and *Enterobacter* emitted foul odors in vitro that resembled bad breath with concomitant production of volatile sulfides and cadaverine, both compounds related to bad breath in denture wearers.[26] The amount of VSCs and the methylmercaptan/hydrogen sulfide ratio in mouth air from patients with periodontal infection was reported to be eight times greater than that of control subjects.[16]

Oral Malodor Assessment Parameters

Organoleptic measurements

One major research obstacle is the lack of an established "gold standard" for rapidly measuring an OM condition. The best objective assessment of OM is still the human sense of smell (direct-sniffing organoleptic method), but more quantifiable measures are being developed. At present, confidante feedback and expert odor (organoleptic) judges are the most commonly used approaches. Both assessments use a 0 to 5 scale to quantify the odor (0 = no odor present, 1 = barely noticeable odor, 2 = slight but clearly noticeable odor, 3 = moderate odor, 4 = strong offensive odor, 5 = extremely foul odor). Individuals are instructed to refrain from using any dental products, eating, or using deodorants or fragrances 4 hours prior to the visit to the clinic. They are also advised to bring their confidante or friend to assess their oral malodor (Box 9-2).

KEY FACTS

KEY FACTS

To create a reproducible assessment, a subject is instructed to close his or her mouth for 2 minutes and to refrain from swallowing during that period. After 2 minutes the subject breathes out gently at a distance of 10 cm from the nose of their counterpart, and the organoleptic odors are assessed.[27] To reduce interexaminer variations, a panel consisting of several experienced judges is often employed. A study on the interexaminer reproducibility indicates that there is some correlation, albeit poor.[28] Gender and age influence the performance of an organoleptic judge. The olfactory sense is generally better in females, and it decreases with age. Dentists and periodontists may not be ideal judges if they do not use masks on a daily basis.[29]

Oral malodor can be analyzed using gas chromatography (GC) coupled with flame photometric detection,[30] which allows separation and quantitative measurements of the individual gases. However, because the equipment necessary is cumbersome and expensive, only skilled personnel may operate it, and analysis of the results is time-consuming. As a result, GC cannot be used in the dental office and is not always used in OM clinical trials.

Portable sulfide meter

The portable sulfide meter (Halimeter, Interscan, Chatsworth, CA) has been widely used over the last few years in OM testing (Fig 9-3). The portable sulfide meter is an electrochemical, voltmetric sensor that generates a signal when exposed to sulfide and mercaptan gases and measures the concentration of hydrogen sulfide gas in parts per billion. The Halimeter is portable and does not require skilled personnel for operation. The main disadvantages of using this instrument are the necessity of periodic recalibration and its sensitivity to perfume, hairspray, deodorant, and other odor-causing products.[28] This limitation does not allow the assessment of mouthwash efficacy until after these components have dissipated.

Electronic nose

The electronic nose is a handheld device being developed to rapidly classify the chemicals in unidentified vapor. This device is based on sensor technology that can "smell" and produce unique profiles for distinct odors. Preliminary data indicate that this device has a potential to be used as a diagnostic tool to detect odors. It is hoped that this technology will be inexpensive, miniaturizable, and adaptable to practically any odor-detecting task.[31] If the electronic nose can learn to "smell" in a quantifiable and reproducible manner, this tool could be a revolutionary assessment technique in the field of OM.

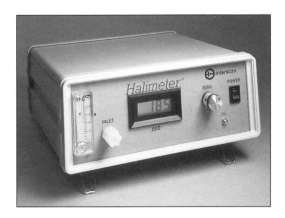

Fig 9-3 Halimeter used for measurement of hydrogen sulfide.

Spoon test

Scrapings from the posterior dorsum of the tongue are obtained using a small disposable spoon, and the odor of these scrapings is assessed after 5 seconds. Nasal odor is distinguished from oral odor by asking the subject to close his or her mouth and exhale through the nose. Odors are assessed according to the following scale: 0 = no odor present; 1 = barely noticeable odor; 2 = slight but clearly noticeable odor; 3 = moderate odor; 4 = strong, offensive odor; and 5 = extremely foul odor.

Management of Oral Malodor

Large numbers of "breath clinics" are offering diagnostic and treatment services for patients complaining of OM. However, because standards of care for these services are lacking, the clinical protocols vary widely. A thorough medical, dental, and halitosis history is necessary to determine whether a patient's complaint of bad breath is due to oral or other causes (Fig 9-4).[32] It is important to determine the source of oral malodor. Complaints about bad taste should be noted because these patients may not have bad breath but rather some other disorder.[32] It has been reported that in approximately 8% of individuals the odor was caused by tonsilitis, sinusitis, or a foreign body in the nose.[35] Approximately 80% to 90% of the oral malodor originates from the dorsum of the tongue. Therefore, treatments targeted toward reduction of the oral malodor will require antimicrobial agents directed against the tongue microflora.

Treatment of OM is important not only because it improves patients' self-confidence but also because evidence indicates that VSCs can be toxic to periodontal tissues even at extremely low concentrations.[35] The

CLINICAL INSIGHT

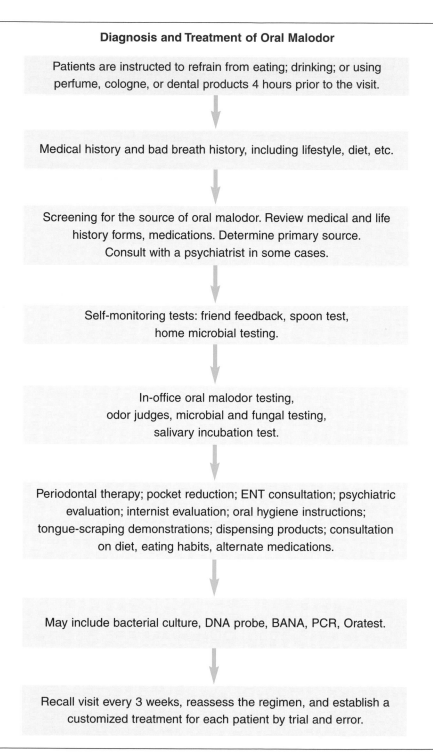

Diagnosis and Treatment of Oral Malodor

Patients are instructed to refrain from eating; drinking; or using perfume, cologne, or dental products 4 hours prior to the visit.

Medical history and bad breath history, including lifestyle, diet, etc.

Screening for the source of oral malodor. Review medical and life history forms, medications. Determine primary source. Consult with a psychiatrist in some cases.

Self-monitoring tests: friend feedback, spoon test, home microbial testing.

In-office oral malodor testing, odor judges, microbial and fungal testing, salivary incubation test.

Periodontal therapy; pocket reduction; ENT consultation; psychiatric evaluation; internist evaluation; oral hygiene instructions; tongue-scraping demonstrations; dispensing products; consultation on diet, eating habits, alternate medications.

May include bacterial culture, DNA probe, BANA, PCR, Oratest.

Recall visit every 3 weeks, reassess the regimen, and establish a customized treatment for each patient by trial and error.

Fig 9-4 Diagnosis and treatment of oral malodor.

Box 9-3 Management of oral and nonoral malodor

1. Local chemical/antibacterial methods
2. Systemic antibacterial methods
3. Mechanical debridement
4. Salivary stimulation and/or substitutes
5. Nasal mucus-control methods
6. Avoidance of foods, fluids, and medications
7. Correction of anatomical abnormalities
8. Medical management of systemic diseases

---

best way to treat OM is to ensure that patients practice good oral hygiene and that their dentition is properly maintained (Box 9-3).[36] Traditional procedures, such as scaling and root planing, can be effective for patients with OM caused by periodontitis.[37] All patients should be instructed in proper tooth brushing, flossing, and tongue cleaning. Mouthrinses should be recommended based on scientifically proven efficacy; caution should be exercised and professional advice sought as to administration and type of mouthrinse to be used. Proper tongue scraping should be demonstrated to and by patients. A combination of flexible tongue scrapers and tongue scrapers with handles is recommended since the tongue has a tendency to curl up during scraping.

Saliva functions as an antibacterial, antiviral, antifungal, buffering, and cleaning agent,[38] so any treatment that increases saliva flow and tongue action, including the chewing of fibrous vegetables and sugarless gum, will help to decrease OM.[39] Finally, oral rinses can be used to supplement oral hygiene practices (see below).

Antimicrobial agents

Mouthwashes have been used as a chemical approach to combatting OM. Mouth rinsing is a common oral hygiene measure dating back to ancient times.[39] Antibacterial components such as cetylpyridinium chloride, chlorhexidine, triclosan, essential oils, quaternary ammonium compounds, benzalkonium chloride, hydrogen peroxide, sodium bicarbonate,[41] zinc salts, and combinations of these compounds have been considered along with mechanical approaches to reducing OM (Box 9-4). Any successful mouthrinse formulation must balance the elimination of the responsible microbes with maintenance of the normal flora and prevention of an overgrowth of opportunistic pathogens. Most commercially available mouthrinses merely mask odors and provide little antiseptic function. Even when they do contain antiseptic substances, the effects of these mouthrinses are usually not long-lasting.[42,43] Thick layers of plaque and mucus protect the microbes from antiseptic attacks.[13]

Box 9-4 Antimicrobial agents used in the treatment of oral malodor

1. Cetylpyridinium chloride
2. Triclosan
3. Essential oils
4. Hydrogen peroxide
5. Sodium bicarbonate
6. Chlorine dioxide
7. Benzalkonium chloride/sodium chloride
8. Zinc salts

Many commercially available rinses contain alcohol as an antiseptic and flavor enhancer. The most prevalent problem with ethanol is that it can dry the oral tissues, which is in itself a risk factor for OM. In addition, there is some debate as to whether the use of alcohol rinses is associated with oral cancer.[44,45] The FDA has found no evidence to support the removal of alcohol from over-the-counter products, but alcohol-free mouthrinses are becoming increasingly popular.

Zinc rinses

Clinical trials conclude that zinc mouthrinses are effective in reducing OM in patients with good oral health.[39] Available in chloride, citrate, or acetate form, zinc rinses have been found to reduce oral VSC concentrations for more than 3 hours. The zinc ion may counteract the toxicity of the VSCs, and it inhibits odor by preventing disulfide group reduction to thiols and by reaction with the thiols groups in VSCs. One study reported that a zinc-based rinse was more effective than a chlorine dioxide–based rinse when both rinses were used twice a day for 60 seconds over a 6-week period.[46] Zinc chewing gum has been shown to reduce OM.[47]

Chlorhexidine rinses

Chlorhexidine digluconate is one of two active ingredients in mouthrinses that have been shown to reduce gingivitis in long-term clinical trials and appears to be the most effective antiplaque and antigingivitis agent known today.[13,48]

The efficacy of chlorhexidine as a mouthrinse to control OM has not been extensively studied. The primary side effect of chlorhexidine is discoloration of the teeth and tongue. In addition, an important consideration for long-term use is its potential to disrupt the oral microbial balance, causing some resistant strains, such as *Streptococcus viridans*, to flourish.[49]

The effect in periodontitis patients of one-stage full-mouth disinfection—that is, scaling and root planing of all pockets within 24 hours combined with chlorhexidine application to all intraoral niches followed by chlorhexidine rinsing for 2 months—resulted in a significant improvement in OM when compared to a conventional periodontal therapy.[50] While these open-design clinical studies suggest that chlorhexidine is clinically effective, it is an agent that should not be used routinely or for long periods of time in the control of OM because of its side effects. A mouthrinse containing chlorhexidine, cetylpyridium chloride, and zinc lactate was evaluated in a clinical study for 2 weeks. The eight subjects who participated in this pilot study showed improvement in organoleptic scores and a trend to reduce tongue and saliva microflora.[51]

Antimalodor properties of chlorhexidine spray 0.2%, chlorhexidine mouthrinse 0.2%, and sanguinaria-zinc mouthrinse were evaluated on morning breath. Oral malodor parameters were assessed before breakfast and 4 hours later following lunch. Results indicated that a sanguinaria-zinc solution had a short effect compared to that of chlorhexidine.[52]

Chlorine dioxide rinses

Chlorine dioxide (ClO_2) is a strong oxidizing agent that has a high redox capacity with compounds containing sulfur. Used in water disinfection and in the sanitation of food-processing equipment, it functions best at a neutral pH. Sodium chlorite is the solution used in commercially available rinses because chlorine dioxide readily loses its activity.[39] Further independent clinical investigations are needed to substantiate the effectiveness of sodium chlorite rinses for the control of OM. In fact, although sodium chlorite is the agent most widely touted on the Internet, no clinical studies have been published to substantiate claims that it is effective in reducing OM. Benzalkonium chloride in conjunction with sodium chlorate has been shown to be effective in reducing OM in a pilot study. Subjects with mild to severe periodontitis were instructed to use the mouthwash twice a day for 6 weeks, and periodontal and oral malodor parameters were then assessed.[53] Results indicated a trend toward reduction in pocket depths and bleeding on probing.

Triclosan rinses

Triclosan (2, 4, 4'-trichloro-2'-hydroxydiphenylether) is a broad-spectrum, nonionic antimicrobial agent. This lipid-soluble substance has been found to be effective against most types of oral bacteria.[54] A combined zinc and triclosan mouthrinse system has been shown to have a cumulative effect; that is, the reduction of malodor increases with the duration of the product use.[39]

The FDA has approved a triclosan toothpaste (Total) manufactured by Colgate. In two studies conducted by Colgate, Total (in combination with fluoride) was shown to reduce plaque by 11.9% in the first trial and by 19.3% in the second trial. The same studies showed a reduction in gum disease by 19.3% and 29%, respectively. Total also contains another ingredient (Gantrez) that allows triclosan to remain active between brushings. However, it is not fully understood how triclosan works in the mouth.

The American Dental Association (ADA) has given Total its seal of acceptance for fighting cavities (and bad breath), reducing plaque, controlling tartar, and helping to prevent periodontal disease. While other toothpastes carry the ADA's seal of approval, Total is the only one approved to help prevent periodontal disease. There are some mouthrinses that can make such a claim, but no toothpastes.

Two-phase rinses

Two-phase oil-water mouthrinses have been tested for their ability to control OM. A clinical trial reported significant long-term reductions in OM from the whole mouth and the tongue dorsum posterior.[55] The rinse is thought to reduce odor-producing microbes on the tongue because of the polar attraction between the oil droplets and the bacterial cells. The two-phase rinse has been shown to significantly decrease the level of VSCs 8 to 10 hours after use, although not as effectively as a 0.2% chlorhexidine rinse.[56] Positive controls that had previously shown an effect in reducing organoleptic scores, such as chlorhexidine and Listerine (Warner Lambert), were used in these clinical studies.

Hydrogen peroxide

The potential of hydrogen peroxide to reduce levels of salivary thiol precursors of oral malodor has been investigated. Using analytical procedures, reduction in salivary thiol levels posttreatment was found to be 59%.[57]

Topical antimicrobial agents

Azulene ointment with a small dose of clindamycin was used topically in eight patients with maxillary cancer to inhibit OM originating from a gauze tamponade applied to the postoperative maxillary bone defect. The malodor was markedly decreased or eliminated in all patients. Anaerobic bacteria involved in the generation of malodor, such as *Porphyromonas* and *Peptostreptococcus,* also became undetectable.[58]

Other products

Breathnol, a proprietary mixture of edible flavors, was evaluated in a clinical study and found to reduce OM for at least 3 hours.[59] Lozenges, chewing gums, mints, and oxidizing lozenges containing Breathnol have all been reported to reduce tongue dorsum malodor.[60]

Alternative remedies

Some of the natural controls for OM include gum containing tea extract. Also recommended are natural deodorants such as copper chlorophyll and sodium chlorophyllin. Alternative dental health services also suggest the use of chlorophyll oral rinses in addition to spirulina and algae products that contain antimicrobial properties.

Conclusions

Many of the mouthrinses available today are being used for the prevention and/or treatment of OM. Much more research is required to develop an efficacious mouthrinse for the alleviation of this condition. The treatment of OM is a relatively new field in dentistry, and many of the treatments have involved a trial-and-error approach, but the knowledge and experience gained so far should facilitate clinical investigations in this field and eventually lead to improved diagnostic techniques and treatment products.

References

1. Nachnani S. Oral malodor: A brief review. CDHA J 1999;14:13–15.
2. Survey conducted at ADA reveals interesting trends. Dent Econ 1995;Dec:6.
3. Gerlach RW, Hyde JD, Poore CL, et al. Breath effects of three marketed dentifrices: A comparative study evaluating single use and cumulative use. J Clin Dent 1998;9: 83–88.
4. Scully C, Porter R, Greenman J. What to do about halitosis? Brit Med J 1994;308:217–218.
5. Preti G, Clark L, Cowart BJ, et al. Nonoral etiologies of oral malodor and altered chemosensation. J Periodontol 1992;63:790–796.
6. Young K, Oxtoby A, Field EA. Halitosis: A review. Dent Update 1993;20:57–61.
7. Rosenberg M. Clinical assessment of bad breath: Current concepts. JADA 1996; 127(4): 475–482.
8. Touyz LZ. Oral malodor–A review. J Can Dent Assoc 1993;Jul(7):607–610.
9. Ship JA. Gastatory and olfactory considerations. Examination and treatment in general practice. JADA 1993;31:53–73.
10. Tiomny E, Arber N, Moshkowitz M, et al. Halitosis and *Helicobacter pylori*. J Clin Gastroenterol 1993;15:236–237.
11. Klienberg I, Westbay G. Salivary metabolic factors involved in oral malodor formation. J Periodontol 1992;63:768–775.
12. Newman MG. The role of periodontitis in oral malodor. In: van Steenberghe D, Rosenberg M (eds). Clinical Perspectives on Bad Breath: A Multidisciplinary Approach. Leuven: Leuven University Press, 1996.
13. Rosenberg M, ed. Bad Breath: Research Perspectives. Tel Aviv: Ramot, 1995.
14. Tessier JF, Kulkarni GV. Bad breath: Etiology and treatment. Periodontics Oral Health 1991;Oct:19–24.
15. Tonzetich J. Production and origin of oral malodor: A review of mechanisms and methods of analysis. J Periodontol 1977; 48:13–20.

16. Yaegaki K, Sanada K. Biochemical and clinical factors influencing oral malodor in periodontal patients. J Periodontol 1992;63:783–789.

17. Clark G, Nachnani S, Messadi D. Detecting and treating oral and nonoral malodors [review]. CDA J 1997; 25:133–144.

18. Goldberg S, Kozlovsky A, Gordon D, et al. Cadaverine as a putative component of oral malodor. J Dent Res 1994;73:1168–1172.

19. Waler S. On the transformation of sulfur–containing amino acids and peptides to volatile sulfur compounds (VSC) in the human mouth. Eur J Oral Sci 1997;105(5 pt 2):534–537.

20. Yaegaki K, Sanada K. Volatile sulfur compounds in mouth air from clinically healthy subjects and patients with periodontal disease. J Periodontal Res 1992; 27:223–238.

21. De Boever EH, Loesche WJ. The tongue microflora and tongue surface characteristics contribute to oral malodor. In: van Steenberghe D, Rosenberg M (eds). Clinical Perspectives on Bad Breath: A Multidisciplinary Approach. Leuven: Leuven University Press, 1996: 111–121.

22. Kozlovsky A, Gordon D, Gelernter I, et al. Correlation between BANA test and oral malodor parameters. J Dent Res 1994;73:1036–1042.

23. De Boever EH, Loesche WJ. Assessing the contribution of anaerobic microflora of the tongue to oral malodor. JADA 1995;126:1384–1393.

24. Klienberg L, Codipilly M. The biological basis of oral malodor formation. In: Rosenberg M (ed). Bad Breath: Research Perspectives. Tel Aviv: Ramot, 1995:13–39.

25. McNamara TF, Alexander JF, Lee M. The role of microorganisms in the production of oral malodor. Oral Surg 1972;34:41.

26. Rosenberg M, Septon I, Eli I, et al. Halitosis measurement by an industrial sulfide monitor. J Periodontol 1991;62:487–489.

27. Rosenberg M, Kulkarni GV, Bosy A, McCulloch CAG. Reproducibility and sensitivity of oral malodor measurements with a portable sulfide monitor. J Dent Res 1991;11:1436–1440.

28. Doty RL, Green PA, Ram C, Yankel SL. Communication of gender from human breath odors: Relationship to perceived intensity and pleasantness. Norm Behav 1982:16:13–22.

29. Tonzetich J, Richter VJ. Evaluation of volatile odiferous components of saliva. Arch Oral Biol 1964;9:39–45.

30. Gibson.TD, Prosser O, Hulbert JN, et al. Detection and simultaneous identification of microorganisms from headspace samples using an electronic nose. Sensors Actuators 1970:B44:413–422.

31. Neiders M, Brigette R. Operation of bad breath clinics. Proceedings of the Third International Conference on Breath Odor. Quintessence Int 1999;30:295–301.

32. Deems DA, Doty RL, Settle RG, et al. Smell and taste disorders: A study of 750 patients from University of Pennsylvania Smell and Taste Centre. Arch Otolaryngol Head Neck Surg 1991;117:519–528.

33. Delanghe G, Ghyselen J, Feenstra L, van Steenberghe D. Experiences in a Belgium multidisciplinary breath odour clinic. In: van Steenberghe D, Rosenberg M (eds). Clinical Perspectives on Bad Breath: A Multidisciplinary Approach. Leuven: Leuven University Press, 1996:199–208.

34. Johnson PW, Yaegaki K, Tonzetich J. Effect of volatile thiol compounds on protein metabolism by human gingival fibroblast. J Periodontal Res 1992;27:533–561.

35. Rosenberg M. Bad breath: Diagnosis and treatment. Univ Tor Dent J 1990;3:7–11.

36. Ratcliff PA, Johnson JW. The relationship between oral malodor, gingivitis, and periodontitis. A review. J Periodontal Res 1999;70:485–489.

37. Spielman A, Bivona P, Rifkin BR. Halitosis: A common oral problem. NY State Dent J 1996 Dec; 63(10):36–42.

38. Nachnani S. The effects of oral rinses on halitosis. CDA J 1997;25:2.

39. Mandel ID. Chemotherapeutic agents for controlling plaque and gingivitis. J. Clin Periodontol 1988;15:488–498.

40. Grigor J, Roberts AJ. Reduction in the levels of oral malodor precursors by hydrogen peroxide in vitro and in vivo assessments. J Clin Dent 1992;3:111–115.

41. Moneib NA, El-Said MA, Shibi AM. Correlation between the in vivo and in vitro antimicrobial properties of commercially available mouthwash preparations. J Chemother 1992;4(50):276–280.

42. Pitts G, Brogdon C, Hu L, et al. Mechanism of action of an antiseptic, anti-odor mouthwash. J Dent Res 1983;62:738–742.

43. Gagari E, Kabani S. Adverse effects of a mouthwash use. Oral Surg Oral Med Oral Pathol Oral Radiol Endod 1995;80:432–439.

44. Elmore JG, Horwitz RJ. Oral cancer and mouthwash use: Evaluation of the epidemiological evidence. Otolaryngol Head Neck Surg 113;30:253–261.

45. Nachnani S, Anson D. Effect of Orasan on periodontitis and oral malodor [abstract]. J Dent Res 1998;77(6).

46. Nachnani S.Reduction of oral malodor with zinc-containing chewing gum [abstract]. J Dent Res 1999;78.

47. Beiswanger BB, Mallet ME, Jackson RD, et al. Clinical effects of a 0.12% chlorhexidine rinse as an adjunct to scaling and root planing. J Clin Dent 1992;3:33–38.

48. Lauri H, Vaahtoniemi LH, Karlqvist K, et al. Mouth rinsing with chlorhexidine causes a delayed temporary increase in the levels of oral viridans streptococci. Acta Odontol Scand 1995;53:226–229.

49. Quirynen M, Mongardini C, van Steenberghe D. The effect of 1-stage full mouth disinfection on oral malodor and microbial colonization of the tongue in periodontitis. A pilot study. J Periodontol 1998;69:374–382.

50. Roldan S, Herrera D, Sanz M. Clinical and microbiological effects of an antimicrobial mouthrinse in oral mouthrinse [abstract]. Fourth International Conference on Breath Odor, UCLA, 1999.

51. van Steenberghe D, Avontroodt B, Vandekerkhove A. A comparative evaluation of a chlorhexidine spray, a chlorhexidine mouthrinse and a sanguinarine-zinc mouthrinse on morning breath odour [abstract]. Fourth International Conference on Breath Odor, UCLA, 1999.

52. Gaffar A, Sheri D, Afflito J, Coleman EJ. The effect of triclosan on mediators of gingival inflammation. J Clin Periodontol 1995;22:480–48.

53. Kozlovsky A, Goldberg S, Natour I, et al. Efficacy of a two phase oil water mouthrinse in controlling oral malodor, gingivitis and plaque. J Periodontol 1996;67:577–578.

54. Rosenberg M, Gelentre I, Barki M, et al. Daylong reduction of oral malodor by two-phase oil water mouthrinse as compared to chlorhexidine and placebo rinses. J Periodontol 1992;63:39–43.

55. Ogura T, Urade M, Matsuya T. Prevention of malodor from intraoral gauze with the topical use of clindamycin. Oral Surg Oral Med Oral Pathol 1992;74:58–62.

56. Rosenberg M, Barkim, Goldberg-Levitan S, et al. Oral reduction by Breathanol [abstract]. Fourth International Conference on Breath Research. UCLA, Los Angeles, 1999.

57. Greenstein RB, Goldberg S, Marku-Cohen S, et al. Reduction of oral malodor by oxidizing lozenges. J Periodontal 1997;68:1176–1181.

J. Craig Baumgartner, DDS, MS, PhD

10

ANTIBIOTICS IN ENDODONTIC THERAPY

Endodontic Infections

Microorganisms have been implicated in endodontic infections since 1890, when Miller[1] first observed microorganisms associated with inflamed pulpal tissue. The relationship was confirmed in 1965 when Kakehashi et al[2] demonstrated that pulpal necrosis and the development of periapical inflammatory lesions occur only in conventional rats—not in germ-free rats—after exposure of the dental pulp to the oral cavity. Once the pulpal tissue becomes necrotic and loses its blood supply, the root canal system becomes a reservoir for microorganisms and their byproducts. Because the necrotic pulp lacks circulation, the root canal is insulated from the normal host defense mechanism of the body.

Pathways of endodontic infection

KEY FACTS

Dentinal tubules Dental caries is the most common route by which microorganisms reach the dental pulp. Multiplying as the caries progresses, microbes may reach the dental pulp via dentinal tubules exposed by enamel lamellae or dental procedures or from pressure on dentinal tubules produced by impression or restorative materials.

Pulpal exposure Microorganisms may also reach the pulp via a pulpal exposure caused by either a traumatic injury or an operative procedure.

Lateral or furcation canals Lateral or furcation canals exposed by either disease or dental treatment also may serve as portals by which microorganisms enter the root canal system of a tooth. Deep periodontal infections may expose these canals to large numbers of bacteria. Teeth adjacent to periodontal lesions may have periodontal bacteria deep within the dentinal tubules.

Other There may be direct extension of an infection from an adjacent tooth or an anachoretic transport of microorganisms through the blood to an area of pulpal inflammation.[3]

Microflora in infections of endodontic origin

Ecosystem The microbial ecosystem in a root canal is very complex and not fully understood. Determining which bacteria are present in an infected root canal depends on several factors, including the method used to sample the root canal, the timing of the culture, the type of media (ie, transport, selective, or nonselective), the incubation conditions (ie, aerobic or anaerobic), the use of microscopy (ie, phase or darkfield), and the use of bacterial smears (ie, Gram stain). Because culturing techniques through the 1960s were inadequate for the growth of strict anaerobes, the most common bacteria cultured from infected root canals were aerobic and facultative anaerobes such as α-hemolytic streptococci. Then, in the early 1970s, a significant breakthrough in culturing occurred with the development of obligate anaerobic incubation of microorganisms. The advent of anaerobic techniques demonstrated that the predominant flora of infected root canal systems were strict anaerobes. The incidence of anaerobes varies with sample site and the disease state of the subject being cultured. Anaerobic infections occur where there is necrotic tissue or a compromised blood supply and in tissue with reduced oxidation-reduction potential following infections by aerobes and facultative microorganisms.

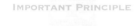

Polymicrobial infections It has been well documented that infected root canals are polymicrobial in nature with several predominant anaerobic microorganisms. As detailed in Box 10-1, black-pigmented bacteria received a lot of attention because of their association with symptomatic endodontic infections. While microorganisms inhabiting an infected root canal are mostly anaerobic, large numbers of facultative microorganisms also may occur.

Black-pigmented bacteria In 1976 the first study establishing a correlation between the presence of a specific microorganism isolated from a root canal and clinical signs or symptoms was conducted when Sundqvist[8] isolated anaerobic black-pigmented bacteria from seven patients with acute pain. Several more recent studies have demonstrated the presence of black-pigmented bacteria in endodontic infections as well, although none of these has established an absolute correlation to specific clinical signs and symptoms.[9–14] For example, in a recent study by Baumgartner et al,[14] 17 of 40 infected root canals contained purulent

> **Box 10-1** Genera of microorganisms commonly isolated from endodontic infections
>
> **Anaerobic genera:** Prevotella, Porphyromonas, Peptostreptococcus, Eubacterium, Fusobacterium, Actinomyces, Veillonella, Propionibacterium, Lactobacillus (anaerobic)[4–7]
>
> **Facultative anaerobic genera:** Streptococcus (Enterococcus), Lactobacillus (aerobic), Staphylococcus

material, and 9 (62%) of the purulent samples were positive for the growth of black-pigmented bacteria. In the same study, 16 of 22 (73%) canals positive for the growth of black-pigmented bacteria were associated with either purulence in the root canal or drainage from a sinus tract (suppurative apical periodontitis). Coincidentally, Sundqvist et al[12] also found that 16 of 22 root canals containing black-pigmented bacteria were associated with abscesses and purulent drainage.

The oral black-pigmented bacteria, formerly of the genus *Bacteroides,* have been reclassified within the *Porphyromonas* or *Prevotella* genus. *Porphyromonas* includes species previously identified as asaccharolytic black-pigmented *Bacteroides,* such as *P asaccharolytica, P gingivalis,* and *P endodontalis.*[15] Saccharolytic black-pigmented bacteria in the *Prevotella* genus include *P nigrescens, P intermedia, P melaninogenica, P denticola, P loescheii, P corporis,* and *P tannerae.*[16,17] Gharbia et al and Bae et al have shown that the most commonly isolated black-pigmented bacteria from infected root canals are *P nigrescens.*[17,18]

Although the above microorganisms have been associated with infections of endodontic origin, no single microbe or group of microbes has been proven to be more pathogenic than others. From a clinical viewpoint, it is still best to consider all infections of endodontic origin as polymicrobial and treat them accordingly.

Periapical pathoses Once the dental pulp becomes necrotic, microbial infection of the root canal system may contribute to a localized periapical inflammatory lesion, an abscess, or a diffuse cellulitis. The growth of microorganisms within the root canal system and subsequent irritation of the periapical tissue by their by-products will continue indefinitely or until the source of the irritation is removed. On occasion, bacteria overcome the host defenses and invade the periapical tissues. When this occurs, the inhabitants of infected root canal systems can be cultured from the aspirates of abscesses of endodontic origin.[13,19–21] Even without direct invasion, bacteria produce by-products that diffuse into the periapical tissues via apical and lateral canals, provoking both specific and nonspecific inflammatory reactions. The inflammatory response may give rise to both protective and immunopathogenic effects. The developing periapical inflammatory reaction to the irritants may be destructive to surrounding tissue and contribute to adverse signs and symptoms. Serious infections may develop, depending on the pathogenicity of the microorganisms involved and the resistance of the host.

Treatment of Endodontic Infections

Debridement and drainage

IMPORTANT PRINCIPLE

The key to successful management of infections of endodontic origin is chemomechanical debridement of the infected root canal system and drainage from both soft and hard tissues (Table 10-1).

- The root canal system of the infected tooth should be allowed to drain and be debrided to the working length of the root canal. Because debridement of the root canal must be accomplished aseptically, a rubber dam and sterile instruments should be used to prevent further microbial contamination. The maintenance of a patent apical foramen with a small endodontic instrument (eg, no. 15) will act as a vent for drainage from the periapical tissues through the root canal.
- The objectives for treatment of infections of endodontic origin are removal of the pathogenic microorganisms, their by-products, and pulpal debris from the infected root canal system that caused the periapical pathosis and establishment of conditions favorable for the lesion to resolve. Because the microorganisms are found in tubules and in parts of the canal system that cannot be reached by endodontic instruments, an irrigating solution with antimicrobial and tissue dissolution properties, such as sodium hypochlorite, should be used.
- After drainage and debridement, the root canal system should be filled with calcium hydroxide and sealed with a temporary restoration that will prevent coronal leakage of bacteria. If drainage from the root canal continues for more than 30 minutes or if time is short, the canal may be left open until the next day. In general, it is best not to leave the canal open for drainage for more than 24 hours because further contamination by the oral microflora will result.

Soft tissue incision for drainage Localized soft tissue swelling of endodontic origin should be incised and drained concurrently with chemomechanical debridement of the root canal system. In most cases a latex drain placed in the incision for 24 hours will allow for adequate drainage. Drainage reduces the accumulated irritants and inflammatory mediators to a level that allows otherwise healthy patients to heal on their own. A regimen of antibiotics is not indicated in an otherwise healthy patient unless there is cellulitis or systemic signs and symptoms of infection (Table 10-2).

KEY FACTS

Table 10-1 Treatment of infections of endodontic origin

Clinical findings	Treatment approach
Uncomplicated endodontic lesion • No compromised host resistance • Pain resolves with drainage through canal • No swelling	• Debridement of root canal system • Antibiotics not indicated
Soft tissue swelling of endodontic origin • Well-localized swelling • No systemic signs such as fever, malaise, or cellulitis	• Debridement of root canal system • Soft tissue incision for drainage • Antibiotics not indicated
Endodontic lesion confined to bone • No soft tissue swelling • Exquisite pain • No drainage through root canal	• Trephination of bone to relieve pressure and speed healing • Antibiotics not indicated
Endodontic lesion / soft tissue swelling • Compromised host response or evidence of systemic involvement or spread of infection such as fever, malaise, cellulitis, trismus, lymphadenopathy	• Debridement of root canal system and incision for drainage • Systemic antibiotics indicated (see Table 10-3)

Table 10-2 Indications for adjunctive antibiotics (antimicrobial therapy)

Indications	Signs and symptoms
Systemic involvement	• Fever greater than 100°F • Malaise • Lymphadenopathy • Trismus
Progressive infection	• Increased swelling • Cellulitis • Osteomyelitis

Trephination In some cases a patient will present with exquisite pain with no evidence of soft tissue swelling. Treatment may have been delayed if the lesion is not evident radiographically, and, as a result, the restraint of fluids may have caused such extreme pressure that drainage through the root canal would be inadequate. If left untreated, the inflammatory mediators and purulent drainage will follow the pathway of least resistance and eventually perforate the cortical plate and elevate the periosteum. In such cases, consideration should be given to the use of trephination, that is, direct surgical penetration through the bone to the periapical lesion. This usually provides the patient with immediate relief.

Antibiotic treatment of endodontic infections

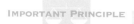

Patients requiring antibiotics to treat endodontic infections Antibiotics (antimicrobials) are considered adjunct chemotherapy to aid the host defenses in the elimination of microorganisms that have overwhelmed the host. Bactericidal rather than bacteriostatic agents are recommended for immunocompromised patients and patients with life-threatening infections. Whenever possible, narrow-spectrum antimicrobials should be pre-

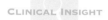

scribed because extended-spectrum or broad-spectrum antibiotics produce more alterations in normal gut microflora, resulting in more side effects. In addition, an extended- or broad-spectrum antibiotic selects for resistant organisms. Narrow-spectrum antibiotics useful in endodontic infections include penicillin VK, metronidazole, clindamycin, and erythromycin analogues (clarithromycin, azithromycin). Selection of the appropriate antimicrobial without susceptibility tests is based on knowledge of the organisms usually involved in endodontic infections.

Antibiotic therapy is indicated when there is systemic involvement or evidence of the spread of infection to adjacent facial spaces. Signs and symptoms suggesting systemic involvement or a progressive infection include fever above 100°F, malaise, cellulitis, unexplained trismus, and swelling beyond simple mucosal enlargement that affects the soft palate, the floor of the mouth, or another anatomic space (see Table 10-2).

Patients should receive a dose of antibiotic that exceeds the minimum inhibitory concentration (MIC) by a factor of 2 to 8 to compensate for barriers limiting the diffusion of antibiotic. Such barriers also can be offset by accompanying antimicrobial therapy with an incision for drainage. Antibiotics move via a diffusion gradient through the edematous fluid and the purulent exudate that accumulates in an anatomic space. An incision for drainage removes purulent material containing bacteria, bacterial by-products, disintegrated inflammatory cells, enzymes (spreading factors), and other inflammatory mediators, thus improving circulation to the area and increasing the likelihood of an MIC of the antibiotic reaching the area.

Because infections of endodontic origin are polymicrobial, no single antibiotic is likely to be effective against all strains of microorganisms in an infection. However, if the antibiotic is effective against some of the strains, it will disrupt the microbial ecosystem.

Systemic administration of the appropriate dosage is usually given for about 5 to 7 days. Clinical signs and symptoms of the infection should diminish significantly within 2 to 4 days of diagnosis and initiation of treatment. Patients should continue to take the antibiotic for an additional 2 to 3 days after the clinical signs and symptoms of the infection have diminished. Patients should be carefully monitored until the infection is controlled. If there is any question about the patient's health (ie, they are medically compromised) or if the patient's condition deteriorates, consultation is advised and referral to a specialist should be considered. Clinicians must be very familiar with the antibiotics they prescribe.

Contraindications or adjustments in dosage for medically compromised patients or interactions of the agents with other medications must be ascertained (see chapters 6 and 7).

Patients not requiring antibiotics Evaluating the patient and accurately diagnosing the source of the infection are of utmost importance. It also is important to evaluate the host defenses, noting any disease states or medications that might adversely affect treatment. The following types of patients do not require antibiotics:

- Healthy patients who present with a localized, fluctuant, intraoral swelling of endodontic origin without systemic signs or symptoms.
- Healthy patients with a symptomatic pulpitis, symptomatic apical periodontitis, or a draining sinus tract. In such cases, debridement of the root canal system, which is the reservoir of the infection, combined with drainage of both soft and hard tissues (as discussed above) is the treatment of choice.

Antibiotics should not be substituted for root canal debridement and drainage of soft and hard tissues.

Empiric selection of an antibiotic (Table 10-3) *Penicillin VK* In general, the antibiotic with the narrowest effective spectrum of activity for the bacteria most often associated with endodontic infections should be used. Penicillin remains the drug of choice because most of the bacteria encountered are susceptible to penicillin and it is well tolerated. However, a complete medical history must be obtained because penicillin is the most common cause of drug allergies. Penicillin VK is effective against numerous facultative and anaerobic microorganisms associated with endodontic infections. The anaerobic spectrum of penicillin includes *Fusobacterium, Peptostreptococcus, Actinomyces,* and some black-pigmented bacteria. Depending on the species of bacteria producing the infection, steady-state blood levels are important with β-lactam antibiotics. Penicillin VK should be administered every 4 to 6 hours to achieve a steady state.[22]

Because the MIC levels usually are not known, dosing should be on the high side and the dosing intervals should be short.[22] However, increasing the dose of penicillin greater than 4 to 5 times the MIC does not necessarily result in the destruction of more bacteria.[22] Penicillin VK remains the antibiotic of choice because of its effectiveness, low toxicity, and low cost. A loading dose of 1,000 mg of penicillin VK should be administered orally followed by 500 mg every 4 to 6 hours for 5 to 7 days. With concurrent debridement of the root canal system and drainage of purulence, significant improvement of the infection should be seen within 48 to 72 hours.

Table 10-3 Systemic antibiotics for adjunctive treatment of endodontic infections

Agent	Special instructions	Dosage
Penicillin VK	Agent of first choice Confirm no allergies to penicillin	Loading dose: 1000 mg followed by 500 mg every 4–6 h for 5–7 days
Amoxicillin	Alternative to penicillin VK for medically compromised patients and when rapid sustained serum level is desired	Loading dose: 1000 mg followed by 500 mg every 8 h for 5–7 days
Metronidazole	Add to penicillin for increased efficacy Only effective against anaerobes	Loading dose: 1000 mg followed by 500 mg every 6 h for 5–7 days
Clindamycin	Use for patients with a serious infection who are allergic to penicillin	Loading dose: 600 mg followed by 300 mg every 6 h for 5–7 days
Clarithromycin	Alternative antibiotic for patient allergic to penicillin	Loading dose: 500 mg followed by 500 mg every 12 h for 5–7 days

INFORMATION ABOUT
SPECIFIC DRUG

KEY FACTS

Amoxicillin Amoxicillin is absorbed more rapidly and has a longer half-life than penicillin, which is reflected in higher and more sustained serum levels. Amoxicillin may be preferred for more serious infections, especially if the patient is immunocompromised. However, against enteric bacteria not usually associated with endodontic infections, amoxicillin has an extended spectrum that selects for additional resistant strains of bacteria. Amoxicillin with clavulanate potassium (Augmentin, SK Beecham, Philadelphia, PA) is not recommended for endodontic infections because it has been shown to be no more effective than amoxicillin alone in susceptibility tests.[23]

INFORMATION ABOUT
SPECIFIC DRUG

Cephalosporins Cephalosporins are usually not indicated for the treatment of endodontic infections. The second-generation cephalosporin cefuroxime (Ceftin, GlaxoWellcome, Research Triangle Park, NC) is the only cephalosporin that includes an effective spectrum of activity against the anaerobes usually involved in endodontic infections. However, because of its high cost and its potential for cross-allergenicity with penicillins, it is not recommended.

INFORMATION ABOUT
SPECIFIC DRUG

CLINICAL INSIGHT

Metronidazole in combination with penicillin If the patient's clinical signs and symptoms have not significantly improved 48 to 72 hours after treatment with penicillin, the addition of metronidazole to the continued dose of penicillin should be considered. It is of utmost importance to review the diagnosis and treatment to confirm that the management of the infection has been appropriate. Metronidazole is a synthetic antimicrobial agent that is bactericidal and has exceptional activity against many anaerobes, including *Porphyromonas, Prevotella, Fusobacterium, Eubacterium, Peptostreptococcus,* and *Veillonella*.[24] However, unlike penicillin, metronidazole lacks activity against aerobes and facultative anaerobes, so it is important that the patient continue to take penicillin. Metronidazole is rapidly absorbed, although food may delay peak serum levels. Mild side effects include gastrointestinal disturbances, a metallic taste, and an innocuous darkening of the urine. Patients must be warned that an "antabuse" reaction (nausea, vomiting, abdominal cramps) may occur if alcohol is ingested.

The usual oral dosage for metronidazole is a 1,000 mg loading dose followed by 500 mg every 6 hours for 5 to 7 days. When patients fail to respond to treatment, consultation with an endodontist or oral surgeon is recommended.

Clindamycin Clindamycin is primarily effective against gram-positive facultative microorganisms, but it is also effective against anaerobes, including black-pigmented bacteria, *Fusobacterium* species, *Peptostreptococcus* species, *Actinomyces* species, and other species associated with endodontic infections. Penicillin and clindamycin also have been shown to produce similarly positive results in treating odontogenic infections.[25] Clindamycin is well distributed throughout most body tissues and reaches a concentration in bone approximating that of plasma. The oral adult dosage for serious endodontic infections is a 600 mg loading dose followed by 300 mg every 6 hours for 5 to 7 days. Food may be taken with the antibiotic to avoid stomach upset. Clindamycin therapy has been associated with pseudomembranous colitis; however, antibiotic-associated colitis/pseudomembranous colitis is more commonly associated with patients treated with ampicillin and cephalosporins and only rarely associated with dental therapy.[26] When patients fail to respond to treatment, consultation with an endodontist or oral surgeon is recommended.

Macrolides Erythromycin is a macrolide that has traditionally remained the antibiotic of choice for patients allergic to penicillin. Erythromycin has a spectrum of activity similar to that of penicillin for gram-positive microorganisms, but it is not effective against the anaerobes usually involved in dental infections. Because of this poor spectrum of activity and its side effects, including significant gastrointestinal upset, erythromycin is no longer recommended for treatment of endodontic infections.

The newer macrolides include clarithromycin and azithromycin, which are effective against some of the anaerobes involved in endodontic infection and offer improved pharmacokinetics. Food slows down but does not reduce the bioavailability of clarithromycin; however, food and heavy metals may inhibit the absorption of azithromycin. These antibiotics have not had much clinical use and should be reserved for patients who have a penicillin allergy and relatively mild infections.

Prophylactic antibiotics for medically compromised patients When treating medically compromised patients, follow the American Heart Association recommendations for prophylactic antimicrobial therapy[27] (see chapter 15). Although the incidence of bacteremia is low, studies using aerobic and anaerobic culturing report that a transient bacteremia can result when microorganisms extrude beyond the apex of a root as a result of instrumentation of a root canal.[28],[29] Patients requiring prophylactic treatment include those with prosthetic cardiac valves, previous bacterial endocarditis, complex cyanotic congenital heart disease, surgically constructed shunts, congenital cardiac malformations, acquired valval dysfunction, and mitral valve prolapse with valval regurgitation.[29] The standard regimen for antibiotic prophylaxis is 2 g amoxicillin administered 1 hour before the dental procedure.[30]

The American Dental Association and the American Academy of Orthopaedic Surgeons have also issued an advisory statement on the use of antibiotic prophylaxis for dental patients with total joint replacement.[30] Patients at potential increased risk of hematogenous total joint infection include immunocompromised or immunosuppressed patients with inflammatory arthropathies, such as rheumatoid arthritis and systemic lupus erythematosus, or disease-, drug-, or radiation-induced immunosuppression. Other patients that require prophylactic antibiotics include those with insulin-dependent (Type I) diabetes; previous prosthetic joint infections; malnourishment; and hemophilia; and those who had a joint replacement within the last 2 years.

When and How to Culture

Indications for microbial sampling

Medically compromised patients For patients at high risk for infections, especially those who are not immunocompetent, a culture of the infecting organisms with susceptibility testing may be indicated. Identification of anaerobes and results of susceptibility tests may take several days to 2 weeks, depending on the microorganisms involved in an infection. A microbial sample should be taken when an otherwise healthy patient has persistent symptoms following surgical or nonsurgical root canal therapy. Persistent symptoms may include tenderness to touch (percussion) and palpation, swelling, and drainage from the root canal or a sinus tract.

Processing a microbial sampling

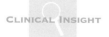

Communication with the laboratory Good communication with a laboratory will ensure that the sample is properly collected, transported, cultured, and identified. Request a Gram stain of the sample to determine what types of microorganisms are predominant. Emphasize to the laboratory personnel that the culture results should report specifically each of the predominant isolated microorganisms (opportunistic pathogens)—they should not be grouped merely as "normal oral flora."

Sampling exudate from a root canal The tooth to be sampled must be effectively isolated with a rubber dam and the field disinfected with sodium hypochlorite or another disinfectant. Antimicrobial solutions should not be used after access to the root canal system has been made. Sterile burs and instruments should be used to gain access to the pulp cavity. If exudate is present in the tooth, it may be sampled with a sterile paper point and immediately placed in a prereduced transport medium provided by a laboratory. If there is copious drainage, it may be aspirated into a sterile syringe with an 18- or 20-gauge needle. Air should be vented from the syringe and the aspirate injected into the prereduced transport medium. Some laboratories will accept the sample in the syringe if it can be transported to the laboratory within a few minutes.

Sampling microbes from a dry root canal Use a sterile syringe to place some prereduced transport medium in the canal. A sterile endodontic instrument can be used to scrape the walls of the canal to get microorganisms into the medium. The medium in the canal can either be sampled with a sterile paper point or aspirated into a sterile syringe and then deposited in the transport medium tube.

Sampling exudate from a submucosal swelling Before an incision is made, an 18- or 20-gauge needle and syringe should be used to aspirate the exudate. After air is vented from the syringe, the needle is inserted through the sealed cap of the sample tube and the exudate is injected into prereduced transport medium. If a sample cannot be aspirated, it can be collected on a swab after the incision for drainage is made. Care must be taken not to contaminate the swab with saliva. The swab used should be from an anaerobic swab tube. After the sample has been collected, the swab should be quickly placed into another prereduced tube for transport to the laboratory.

Identification and antibiotic susceptibility Once growth of the microorganisms is observed, colonies are subcultured both aerobically and anaerobically to determine if the isolate is facultative. The microorganisms then can be identified and antibiotic susceptibility testing undertaken to establish the MIC of the antibiotics available. Antibiotics usually can be chosen to treat anaerobic infections based on the identification of the isolates and without susceptibility testing. Because most infections of endodontic origin are polymicrobial, it is difficult to perform anaerobic susceptibility tests for all the isolated species within a short time period. Moreover, many laboratories do not have the capability to do susceptibility testing for strict anaerobes. It is therefore recommended that antibiotics be chosen based on the microbial pattern and that susceptibility testing be performed only if the laboratory routinely tests for antibiotic susceptibility of anaerobes.

References

1. Miller WD. Microorganisms of the Human Mouth. Philadelphia: S.S. White Dental, 1890.

2. Kakehashi S, Stanley HR, Fitzgerald RJ. The effects of surgical exposures of dental pulps in germfree and conventional laboratory rats. J South Calif Dent Assoc 1966; 34:449–451.

3. Allard U, Nord CE, Sjoberg L, Stromberg T. Experimental infections with *Staphylococcus aureus, Streptococcus sanguis, Pseudomonas aeruginosa,* and *Bacteroides fragilis* in the jaws of dogs. Oral Surg Oral Med Oral Pathol 1979;48: 454–462.

4. Gomes BP, Drucker DB, Lilley JD. Positive and negative associations between bacterial species in dental root canals. Microbios 1994;80:231–243.

5. Yoshida M, Fukushima H, Yamamoto K, Ogawa K, Toda T, Sagawa H. Correlation between clinical symptoms and microorganisms isolated from root canals of teeth with periapical pathosis. J Endod 1987;13:24–28.

6. Heimdahl A, von Konow L, Satoh T, Nord CE. Clinical appearance of orofacial infections of odontogenic origin in relation to microbiological findings. J Clin Microbiol 1985;22:299–302.

7. Drucker DB, Lilley JD, Tucker D, Gibbs AC. The endodontic microflora revisited. Microbios 1992;71:225–234.

8. Sundqvist GK. Bacteriological Studies of Necrotic Dental Pulps [Odontological Dissertation No. 7]. Umea, Sweden: University of Umea, 1976.

9. Haapasalo M, Ranta H, Ranta K, Shah H. Black-pigmented *Bacteroides* spp. in human apical periodontitis. Infect Immun 1986;53:149–153.

10. Haapasalo M. Black-pigmented gram-negative anaerobes in endodontic infections. FEMS Immunol Med Microbiol 1993;6:213–217.

11. Griffee MB, Patterson SS, Miller CH, Kafrawy AH, Newton CW. The relationship of *Bacteroides melaninogenicus* to symptoms associated with pulpal necrosis. Oral Surg Oral Med Oral Pathol 1980;50:457–461.

12. Sundqvist GU, Johansson E, Sjögren U. Prevalence of black-pigmented *Bacteroides* species in root canal infections. J Endod 1989;15:13–19.

13. Van Winkelhoff AJ, Carleé AW, de Graaff J. *Bacteroides endodontalis* and other black-pigmented *Bacteroides* species in odontogenic abscesses. Infect Immun 1985;49: 494–497.

14. Baumgartner JC, Watkins BJ, Bae KS, Xia T. Association of black-pigmented bacteria with endodontic infections. J Endod 1999;25:413–415.

15. Shah HN, Collins MD. Proposal to restrict the genus *Bacteroides* (Castellani and Chalmers) to *Bacteroides fragilis* and closely related species. Int J Syst Bacteriol 1989;39:85–87.

16. Shah HN, Collins DM. Prevotella, a new genus to include *Bacteroides melaninogenicus* and related species formerly classified in the genus *Bacteroides.* Int J Syst Bacteriol 1990;40:205–208.

17. Gharbia SE, Haapasalo M, Shah HN, Kotiranta A, Lounatmaa K, Pearce M, et al. Characterization of *Prevotella intermedia* and *Prevotella nigrescens* isolates from periodontic and endodontic infections. J Periodontol 1994;65:56–61.

18. Bae KS, Baumgartner JC, Shearer TR, David LL. Occurence of *Prevotella nigrescens* and *Prevotella intermedia* in infections of endodontic origin. J Endod 1997;23: 620–623.

19. Chow AW, Roser SM, Brady FA. Orofacial odontogenic infections. Ann Intern Med 1978;88:392–402.

20. Brook I, Grimm S, Kielich RB. Bacteriology of acute periapical abscess in children. J Endod 1981;7:378–380.

21. Williams BL, McCann GF, Schoenknecht FD. Bacteriology of dental abscesses of endodontic origin. J Clin Microbiol 1983;18:770–774.

22. Pallasch TJ. Pharmacokinetic principles of antimicrobial therapy. Periodontol 2000 1996;10:5–11.

23. Le Goff A, Bunetel L, Mouton C, Bonnaure-Mallet M. Evaluation of root canal bacteria and their antimicrobial susceptability in teeth with necrotic pulp. Oral Microbiol Immunol 1997;12:318–322.

24. Sutter VL, Jones MJ, Ghoneim AT. Antimicrobial susceptibilities of bacteria associated with periodontal disease. Antimicrob Agents Chemother 1983;23:483–486.

25. Gilmore WC, Jacobus NV, Gorbach SL, Doku HC, Tally FP. A prospective double-blind evaluation of penicillin versus clindamycin in the treatment of odontogenic infections. J Oral Maxillofac Surg 1988;46:1065–1070.

26. Jaimes EC. Lincocinamides and the incidence of antibiotic-associated colitis. Clin Ther 1991;13:270–280.

27. Dajani AS, Taubert KA, Wilson W, Bolger AF, Bayer A, Ferrieri P, et al. Prevention of bacterial endocarditis: Recommendations by the American Heart Association. JAMA 1997;277:1794–1801.

28. Baumgartner JC, Heggers JP, Harrison JW. Incidence of bacteremias related to endodontic procedures. II. Surgical endodontics. J Endod 1977;3:399–402.

29. Debelian GJ, Olsen I, Tronstad L. Anaerobic bacteremia and fungemia in patients undergoing endodontic therapy: An overview. Ann Periodontol 1998;3:281–287.

30. Antibiotic prophylaxis for dental patients with total joint replacements. American Dental Association; American Academy of Orthopaedic Surgeons [advisory statement]. J Am Dent Assoc 1997;128:1004–1008.

Larry J. Peterson, DDS, MS

11

ANTIBIOTICS FOR ORAL AND MAXILLOFACIAL INFECTIONS

IMPORTANT PRINCIPLE

Infections of the oral and maxillofacial region, although commonly encountered by dentists, can be challenging to manage. Such infections usually arise from necrotic dental pulp caused by dental decay. While most of these infections are minor and can be managed easily through the administration of appropriate antibiotics and minor surgical procedures, on rare occasions these infections become severe and require management by a specialist, sometimes in the hospital setting. This chapter presents guidelines for using a combination of antibiotics and surgery to manage minor orofacial and odontogenic infections in the office setting.

Microbiology of Odontogenic Infections

Over the last decade, microbiological studies have clearly isolated the etiological bacteria in odontogenic infections.[1] Most of these studies have been performed on pus aspirated percutaneously from an odontogenic abscess. Obligate aerobes are rarely found in the oral cavity; therefore, most of the oral bacteria that are grown in air are facultative anaerobic, which means that they are able to grow with or without oxygen. The facultative anaerobic bacteria are primarily streptococci, but a wide variety of other organisms are also found. The anaerobic bacteria are primarily obligate anaerobic gram-positive cocci, mainly *Peptostreptococcus* species, and obligate anaerobic gram-negative bacilli such as *Fusobacterium* and *Prevotella* species.[2]

In approximately 5% of infections only facultative anaerobic bacteria are found, while in 35% only obligate anaerobic bacteria are recovered. Most odontogenic infections (60%) are composed of a combination of facultative anaerobic and obligate anaerobic bacteria.[3]

157

Because obligate anaerobic bacteria tend to produce pus with greater frequency than facultative anaerobic bacteria, the abscess stage of the infection, which tends to be later, is caused primarily by obligate anaerobic bacteria. In the early stage of an odontogenic infection (the phase without pus formation), facultative anaerobic bacteria may dominate. This concept has been fairly well established by researchers studying experimental infections in animals and by clinicians managing odontogenic infections.

Natural Course of Odontogenic Infections

Once an infection is established, its course can be predicted fairly reliably based on the type of bacteria, its inherent invasiveness, and the host's resistance. For example, certain bacteria, like streptococci, tend to spread rapidly without producing pus while other bacteria, such as the obligate anaerobic bacteria, tend to have a slow, insidious onset and produce pus.

Initial stage: Cellulitis

The initial phase, when bacteria first gain access to the underlying tissues through odontogenic sources, is usually cellulitis (Table 11-1). The cellulitis usually is acute, has diffuse borders, and does not produce pus. In its early stages it has a soft, doughy consistency when palpated, the overlying skin is likely to appear erythematous, and the patient usually has significant pain. As the cellulitis progresses, the swelling becomes larger and harder until it becomes indurated. Induration results from the extravasation of fluid from the vascular space into the interstitial tissue, producing tension in the tissue that compresses blood vessels and thereby compromising the vascular supply to the local area. When the cellulitis is in the indurated stage, the patient almost always has significant pain and an elevated temperature. At this point the infection is usually quite serious.

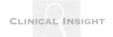

The bacteria that cause the cellulitis stage are usually facultative anaerobic bacteria such as streptococci. Therefore, antibiotic treatment that targets these bacteria should be used at this stage of an infection.

Second stage: Abscess

Abscess usually marks the second stage of the infection. At this point the body is able to mobilize its defenses sufficiently to wall off the infection and limit its spread. The resulting accumulation of polymorphonuclear leukocytes produces part of the pus. More chronic in nature than the cellulitis, the abscess—a localized collection of pus within a tissue space—frequently has well-defined borders and fluctuates to palpation. Although some abscesses are serious, the presence of a well-defined chronic abscess usually indicates that the host defenses have been sufficiently potent to wall off and contain the infectious process.

Table 11-1 Natural course of odontogenic infections

Stage of infection	Characteristics
I. Cellulitis	Phase 1 Erythema Diffuse swelling Pain Doughy consistency
	Phase 2 Increased swelling Hard consistency Induration Significant pain Elevated temperature (in most cases)
II. Abscess	Well-defined borders Pus accumulation in tissues fluctuant to palpation
III. Sinus tract	Abscess ruptures to produce a draining sinus tract

The bacteria responsible for abscess formation are predominately obligate anaerobic bacteria. Although facultative anaerobic bacteria such as streptococci are frequently found in pus specimens from abscesses, their role in the abscess process is relatively minor.

In serious odontogenic infections that appear to be primarily in an advanced stage of cellulitis with induration, it is very common to find small or even sizeable areas of abscess formation—that is, an abscess frequently will exist within a large area of cellulitis. In these situations, both obligate anaerobic and facultative anaerobic bacteria are playing important roles, which should be considered when selecting an antibiotic treatment.

Third stage: Sinus tract

The third stage of the infectious process is the formation of a sinus tract. In these situations the abscess ruptures intraorally or, occasionally, extraorally, establishing a chronic draining sinus tract. As long as this sinus tract continues to drain, no overt signs of infection such as swelling, pain, or temperature will be visible. If the patient is treated with antibiotics the sinus tract usually will cease to drain, but it will open again after withdrawal of the antibiotic. The method of treatment in this situation is to remove the source of the infection, either by endodontic therapy or by tooth extraction.

IMPORTANT PRINCIPLE

Table 11-2 Most common locations for spread of odontogenic infections

Location of spread	Original location of infection
Buccal vestibule	Maxilla Mandibular anterior teeth and premolars
Buccal space	Maxilla (if infection perforates bone superior to attachment of buccinator muscle)
Submandibular space	Mandibular posterior teeth
Fascial spaces (posteriorly and inferiorly into the neck)	If left untreated, infection can spread from any space and produces major risks

Summary

Odontogenic infections begin when mixed bacterial flora invade the underlying tissue. In the early stages the facultative anaerobic bacteria such as streptococci are predominant and cellulitis is established. If the infection is treated at this point, there will not be a progression to an abscess. If the infection is left untreated, the cellulitis will progress from the soft doughy swelling to a harder, indurated swelling. During this process the oxidation-reduction potential in the local tissue becomes such that the hypoxic, acidotic environment favors the overgrowth of obligate anaerobic bacteria while hindering the growth of facultative anaerobic bacteria.[1] This change in the bacterial population, coupled with the increased response in the host, results in abscess formation.

At this point the cellulitis is primarily a facultative anaerobic infection that does not produce pus but tends to be rapidly progressive and has the potential to become quite serious if not treated promptly. The abscess, on the other hand, is primarily an obligate anaerobic infection, which is usually chronic, has more well-defined margins, is fluctuant, and produces pus. These two stages of the infection are treated quite differently, as will be discussed in subsequent sections.

Spread of infection

IMPORTANT PRINCIPLE

Once an infection has been established in the periapical area, it will spread through the bone and involve the adjacent tissues (Table 11-2). The direction of the spread of the infection is determined primarily by the thickness of the overlying bone and the position of the muscle attachment in relation to the infection. For example, in the maxilla, the labial-buccal cortical bone is quite thin; consequently, most maxillary infections spread to the facial aspect and almost always result in a vestibular abscess. However, if the infection erodes through the bone superior to the attachment of the buccinator muscle, as it does occasionally in the molar region, a buccal space infection may result.

In the mandible, the labial-buccal bone is likewise relatively thin around the anterior teeth and premolars. Therefore, the most common location for infection is in the buccal vestibule. However, in the posterior region the lingual cortical plate is thinner, and the attachment of the mylohyoid muscle is relatively high in relationship to the apex of the molars; the result is a submandibular space infection.

Infection from these spaces can continue posteriorly and inferiorly into the neck and possibly even into the thorax. Infections that involve fascial spaces should be treated vigorously, and the patient should be referred to a specialist early for combined antibiotic and surgical treatment.

Depressed Host Defenses

Patients with odontogenic infections who have a decreased ability to mobilize normal host defenses will have increased need for early and more aggressive antibiotic and surgical treatment. A variety of conditions will compromise these host defenses (see chapter 16); these must be identified in the patient's history to ensure proper modification of treatment.

Chemotherapy

One of the most common causes of depressed host defenses is chemotherapy, which is given for treatment of a variety of cancers. Cancer chemotherapeutic agents target all rapidly dividing cells, including not only cancerous cells but also those found in bone marrow. The result is that the patient has fewer polymorphonuclear leukocytes to combat infection.

Metabolic diseases

A second common cause of compromised host defenses is severe uncontrolled metabolic diseases such as diabetes, uremia, and cirrhosis of the liver. These metabolic diseases, when uncompensated and severe in nature, result in depressed leukocyte function and depressed immunoglobulin and complement function.

Organ transplants

Patients who have received organ transplants such as kidney, liver, or heart often receive cyclosporin for immunosuppression to increase the chances of graft survival. This immunosuppressive drug inhibits the immune system, thereby prolonging graft life but also making the patient more likely to develop an infection.

Myeloproliferative diseases

A final cause of depressed host defenses is the group of diseases referred to as the myeloproliferative diseases, such as leukemia and lymphoma. They interfere in the function of leukocytes, causing the patient to be more susceptible to infection.

Treatment

IMPORTANT PRINCIPLE

The patient with depressed host defenses will have impaired antibacterial defenses, an increased risk of infection, and an increased rate of spread when infection occurs. Because there is lack of adequate support from the defenses, these infections are also more difficult to treat. Therefore, these patients should be treated with bactericidal antibiotics.

Dental-Spectrum Antibiotics

Because the bacteria responsible for odontogenic infections have been carefully isolated (facultative anaerobic streptococci, obligate anaerobic gram-positive cocci [ie, *Peptostreptococcus*], and obligate anaerobic gram-negative rods), the proper choice of an antibiotic to treat such infections usually can be made without culture and sensitivity testing. The antibacterial spectrum of a variety of antibiotics will kill or inhibit the growth of the causative organisms (see chapter 3). The following antibiotics are most commonly used in managing odontogenic infections.

Penicillin

INFORMATION ABOUT SPECIFIC DRUG

Orally administered penicillin V is the drug of choice for most mild to moderate odontogenic infections. A bactericidal drug that kills streptococci and most oral anaerobic bacteria, it has low toxicity and is well tolerated by most patients. Although approximately 3% of the patient population is allergic to penicillin, severe allergic reactions are relatively uncommon when this drug is administered orally. Penicillin is also a drug of choice for the prophylaxis of subacute bacterial endocarditis in the nonallergic patient. About 50% of the *Prevotella* species are resistant to penicillin.[4]

Extended-spectrum penicillins

INFORMATION ABOUT SPECIFIC DRUG

Biochemical alteration of the basic structure of the penicillin molecule has resulted in a variety of penicillinlike antibiotics. These antibiotics have extended antibacterial activity and presumably are more useful for infections. Ampicillin and amoxicillin are two commonly recommended antibiotics that have a broader spectrum; however, they have more limited additional activity against streptococci or oral anaerobes than penicillin V.

Because their extended spectrum is almost exclusively in the area of aerobic gram-negative rods such as *Haemophilus influenzae, Escherichia coli, Salmonella, Shigella,* and *Proteus* organisms, they rarely are indicated in the management of odontogenic infections. If culture and sensitivity tests obtained from an infection reveal that the causative organism is *H influenzae,* then amoxicillin might be considered in its management. Amoxicillin is recommended for prophylaxis of bacterial endocarditis due to its excellent absorption, slow excretion, and prolonged high plasma levels.

Cephalosporins

INFORMATION ABOUT SPECIFIC DRUG

An antibiotic family with a molecular structure similar to that of penicillin is the cephalosporin group. Like penicillin, cephalosporins are bactericidal and have a low toxicity, but their antibiotic spectrum is generally broader than that of penicillin, and they tend to be more expensive. There is a large number of cephalosporins available, but only a few can be administered orally. The two that are most popular in dentistry, cephalexin and cefadroxil, are effective against streptococci, staphylococci, oral anaerobes, and some aerobic gram-negative rods such as *E coli, Proteus,* and *Klebsiella* species. Cephalosporins have been shown to

ADVERSE EFFECTS

produce allergic reactions in 5% to 15% of patients who are allergic to penicillin. In general, neither of these agents should be used in patients with a history of anaphylactic allergic reaction to penicillin. Despite these concerns, cephalosporins may be useful in the penicillin-allergic patient who has compromised host defense mechanisms and requires a bactericidal antibiotic. After administration of the first dose, the patient must be monitored carefully in the office by a specialist and/or physician who is comfortable with the management of acute allergic reactions.

Erythromycin

INFORMATION ABOUT SPECIFIC DRUG

Erythromycin is a bacteriostatic antibiotic that is effective against streptococci, staphylococci, and some oral anaerobes. It is also effective against several other organisms that rarely cause odontogenic infections. Erythromycin is useful primarily by the oral route and has a relatively low toxicity when taken at doses below 2 g per day. This low dose requirement limits its usefulness in treating more serious infections and allows for the potential for moderate bacterial resistance. The primary indica-

KEY FACTS

tion of erythromycin is for treatment of mild odontogenic infections in healthy penicillin-allergic patients.

Clarithromycin

INFORMATION ABOUT SPECIFIC DRUG

Clarithromycin is a bacteriostatic antibiotic that is effective against *Streptococcus, Staphylococcus,* obligate anaerobes, and many common sinus and pulmonary pathogens. It usually is given orally and has a relatively low incidence of toxicity and side effects. Like erythromycin, it is a macrolide antibiotic, but it has fewer side effects, most notably a lower incidence of nausea. While clarithromycin is more expensive than erythromycin, it is given on a twice-per-day dosage schedule instead of a four-times-per-day dosage schedule, which may result in increased patient compliance. The primary indication for clarithromycin is for the treatment of mild odontogenic infections in immunocompromised patients who are allergic to penicillin. Clarithromycin is now preferred over erythromycin as a second antibiotic choice for routine odontogenic infections.

KEY FACTS

Clindamycin

INFORMATION ABOUT SPECIFIC DRUG

Clindamycin is effective against streptococci, staphylococci, and essentially all anaerobic bacteria. It is bacteriostatic in most situations and has a relatively high toxicity. It is substantially more expensive than penicillin; therefore, it is usually not considered as a first-line drug for odontogenic infections. However, it has been found to be a useful and effective drug in chronic low-grade infections that have been resistant to previous treatment with penicillin or erythromycin. Diarrhea may occur in 20% to 30% of the patients treated with clindamycin, but it is reversible and subsides rapidly when therapy is discontinued. Clindamycin may cause antibiotic-associated colitis, as do amoxicillin and oral cephalosporins. However, this rarely occurs in nonhospitalized, ambulatory patients.

Tetracycline

INFORMATION ABOUT SPECIFIC DRUG

The family of tetracycline antibiotics has been available since the mid-1950s. Its original spectrum included streptococci, staphylococci, oral anaerobes, and a variety of gram-negative aerobic rods. However, because it is a bacteriostatic drug that has been widely prescribed, there is a high degree of bacterial resistance to it at this time. The drug has relatively mild toxicities and is inexpensive. Its main indication in the maxillofacial area is for treatment of a mild odontogenic infection in a patient who has severe allergy to penicillins and cephalosporins and cannot tolerate erythromycinlike drugs.

Metronidazole

INFORMATION ABOUT SPECIFIC DRUG

Metronidazole is bactericidal against all obligate anaerobic bacteria but has no activity against facultative anaerobic bacteria such as streptococci. Therefore, metronidazole is an effective antibiotic for managing chronic infections that are caused primarily by obligate anaerobic bacteria, but it has little or no indication in the cellulitis stage of an infection. Metronidazole is very effective when combined with penicillin, and the two are often used in mixed infections dominated by obligate anaerobes.

KEY FACTS

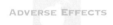
Fluoroquinolones

The fluoroquinolones are a relatively new group of antibiotics that may have occasional application in odontogenic infections. These bactericidal antibiotics have a broad antibacterial spectrum and can be administered either orally or parenterally. The first group of fluoroquinolones that were clinically useful included drugs like ciprofloxacin. However, these drugs had poor activity against streptococcus and anaerobes and therefore had little usefulness in odontogenic infections. The third generation of fluoroquinolones have antistreptococcus and antianaerobic activity and therefore may be useful in odontogenic infections. Fluoroquinolones such as trovafloxacin mesylate are administered on a once-per-day dosage, which may help increase patient compliance.

Trovafloxacin mesylate is well absorbed orally and has mild toxicity. Its primary indication is to treat chronic anaerobic infections. Drugs such as trovafloxacin mesylate also are indicated for immunocompromised patients who have a history of severe allergy to penicillin and are therefore unable to receive β-lactam antibiotics and require a bactericidal antibiotic.

Antibiotic selection summary

The selection of an antibiotic for the initial management of an odontogenic infection can be made with great predictability because the antibacterial pattern has been so well described (Table 11-3). Penicillin remains the drug of choice for odontogenic infections. An oral cephalosporin such as cephalexin is useful in patients who are allergic to penicillin and require a bactericidal drug. (Caution: 5% to 15% of patients who are allergic to penicillin will have cross-reacting allergies to cephalosporins such as cephalexin.) Clarithromycin is effective in the treatment of a mild odontogenic infection in a patient who is allergic to penicillin and does not require a bactericidal antibiotic. Clindamycin is primarily useful in a chronic infection thought to be caused by anaerobic bacteria that has not responded to penicillin. Metronidazole is an effective drug for treating a chronic, well-established abscess and perhaps in combination with penicillin for a serious infection. Tetracycline has a very limited role in the management of odontogenic infections.

Table 11-3 Antibiotic selection summary for odontogenic infections

Drug	Indications	Notes
Penicillin V	Drug of choice for most mild to moderate odontogenic infections	Bactericidal Approximately 3% of the patient population is allergic to penicillin
Clarithromycin	Mild odontogenic infections in immunocompromised patients who are allergic to penicillin	Bacteriostatic
Cephalosporins	Use with caution in case of penicillin allergy; may produce allergic reactions in 5–l5% of patients allergic to penicillin	Bactericidal Broader antibiotic spectrum than penicillin
Tetracycline	Mild odontogenic infection in a patient who has severe allergy to penicillins and cephalosporins and cannot tolerate erythromycinlike drugs	Bacteriostatic
Fluoroquinolones (third generation, ie, trovafloxacin mesylate)	Odontogenic infection in an immuno-compromised patient who has a history of severe allergy to penicillin	Bactericidal
Clindamycin	Chronic low-grade infections that have been resistant to previous treatment with penicillin or erythromycin	Bacteriostatic
Metronidazole	Chronic infections that are caused primarily by obligate anaerobic bacteria. Very effective in combination with penicillin in mixed infections dominated by obligate anaerobes	Bactericidal No activity against facultative anaerobic bacteria such as streptococci

Principles of Therapy

The approach to managing odontogenic infections should be systematic and logical to ensure that important pieces of information are not omitted and the progress of the patient is carefully monitored (Table 11-4).[4]

Determination of severity

IMPORTANT PRINCIPLE

The first step is to determine the severity of the infection. This is accomplished by taking a thorough history of the onset and progress of the infection and by performing a physical examination. The history of the pain and its spread from the local area are important to note. It is also important to note the infection's rate of progression. An infection that progresses rapidly in a matter of hours is considered more serious than an infection that develops and spreads over a period of days or weeks. On physical examination, swelling should be evaluated from both a quantitative and qualitative point of view—that is, how large is the swelling and how does it feel to palpation? A soft, doughy, early cellulitis, for example,

Table 11-4 Principles of managing odontogenic infections

Step	Substeps
1. Determine severity	Assess history of onset and progression Perform physical examination of area: (1) Determine character and size of swelling (2) Establish presence of trismus
2. Evaluate host defenses	Evaluate: (1) Diseases that compromise the host (2) Medications that may compromise the host
3. Perform surgery	Remove the cause of infection Drain pus Relieve pressure
4. Select antibiotic	Determine: (1) Most likely causative organisms based on history (2) Host defense status (3) Allergy history (4) Previous drug history Prescribe drug properly (route, dose and dosage interval, and duration)
5. Follow up	Confirm treatment response Evaluate for side effects and secondary infections

probably can be managed through antibiotic therapy and treatment of the offending tooth. An indurated cellulitis or a fluctuant abscess will require incision and drainage as well as antibiotic therapy. The presence of trismus (limitation of opening) is also important. Trismus usually indicates involvement of the muscles of mastication and is therefore a serious sign.

Evaluation of host defenses

IMPORTANT PRINCIPLE

KEY FACTS

The next step is to evaluate the patient's host defenses. Immunocompromising diseases and medications that were discussed earlier should be identified. If the patient presents with any factors that may decrease host defenses, the infection may spread more rapidly and has an increased chance of becoming severe. In patients with compromised host defenses, bactericidal antibiotics will be necessary and removal of the offending tooth is more likely to be indicated than conservative endodontic therapy. Moreover, in severe cases, early referral to a specialist and early hospitalization may be indicated.

Surgical treatment

IMPORTANT PRINCIPLE

The first treatment modality in managing infections is surgical. The three primary goals of surgical treatment are to remove the cause (ie, the necrotic pulp of the tooth), drain pus that has accumulated in any abscess space, and relieve pressure in the indurated cellulitis situation. Surgical treatment may be as simple as opening a tooth and removing the necrotic pulp or it may be as complex as making an extensive incision and draining the soft tissue involved in the infection.

Antibiotic choice

An antibiotic that will be effective against the likely causative organisms should be chosen. When deciding which antibiotic to prescribe, factors such as host defenses, allergy status, and previous drug history are important. In general, a narrow-spectrum antibiotic is preferred over a broad-spectrum antibiotic so that the alteration of the normal host microflora will be kept to a minimum. Of course, the drug with the lowest toxicity also should be preferred. One should be aware of the cost of the drugs since two drugs with equal effectiveness and toxicity may vary dramatically in their cost to the patient.

Antibiotic administration

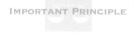

Once an antibiotic is selected, it must be administered properly. This means that the drug should be given by the proper route (usually the oral route in mild to moderate odontogenic infections), in the proper dose, and at the proper dosage interval. These last two factors are well delineated in reference books, package inserts, and the *Physicians' Desk Reference*.[5] The antibiotic should be prescribed for an adequate length of time, usually for at least 2 days after the major clinical symptoms disappear. In most mild odontogenic infections that have appropriate antibiotic and surgical care, a dramatic improvement will be seen within 2 days and major resolution within 4 or 5 days. Therefore, the usual prescription should be written for 7 days.

Follow-up

The patient should be followed carefully after the initial appointment. In most cases, the patient should return for a follow-up visit the following day or at least check in with a follow-up telephone call. The purpose of such follow-ups is to look for an appropriate treatment response. For example, if the patient is treated with antibiotics alone, there might be little improvement at the first follow-up, but the patient should not be worse. By the second or third day, the patient's condition should begin to improve significantly. However, if the patient received both surgical treatment and antibiotic treatment, the first postoperative day should bring marked improvement.

Side effects and secondary infection

The doctor also will need to watch the patient for allergic reactions, toxicity reactions, and side effects typical for the antibiotics being given. Because gastrointestinal distress is a common side effect of erythromycin, for example, patients should be advised to take the antibiotic with small amounts of food, which will tend to make the drug more tolerable. Secondary infections are another common problem that should be watched for during antibiotic therapy. Oral or vaginal candidiasis is the most common secondary infection that occurs as the result of management of odontogenic infection, usually after 10 to 14 days of antibiotic therapy. (See chapters 5 and 17 for further discussion of antifungal therapy.)

Wound Infection Prophylaxis

Some patients, especially those with compromised host defenses, will need antibiotics to prevent infection in the operative wound when surgical procedures are performed in the mouth. The guidelines for antibiotic prophylaxis in this situation have been well defined.[6,7] (See chapters 15 and 16.)

Antibiotic selection

The first guideline is to choose an appropriate antibiotic. For surgery in the mouth, the antibiotic chosen should be the same one used for therapy—that is, penicillin or an alternative drug depending on the patient's allergic status. Moreover, it is best to use a bactericidal drug for prophylaxis.

Plasma level

The plasma level of the antibiotic should be higher than it would be for treatment of infection, which means twice the usual dose. For example, if the normal dose of penicillin is 500 mg, the prophylactic dose should be 1 g.

Correct administration

The antibiotic administration must be timed correctly. The first dose should be given before the surgery begins. If the surgery is long (ie, over 2 hours), an additional dose should be given in the middle of the operation.

Antibiotic exposure

The final guideline for effective use of prophylaxis is to use the shortest antibiotic exposure that is effective. The universal conclusion of animal and human clinical studies is that the final dose of the antibiotic should be given at the end of the surgical procedure. Therefore, for most surgery done in the office setting, a patient should be given 1 g of penicillin 1 hour before the operation and a second 1-g dose of penicillin before the patient leaves the office. If the procedure lasts for 3 hours, an interim dose of 1 g could be given approximately 2 hours after the first dose.

Special Considerations

In the course of dental practice, there will be some therapeutic and prophylactic clinical situations in which the need for antibiotics is not clear.

Sinus perforations

When extracting teeth from a maxillary arch with a large maxillary sinus, the possibility exists that a small piece of bone may be removed with the root, resulting in a perforation of the maxillary sinus. The most common tooth involved in such inadvertent perforations is the maxillary first molar. When this happens, attention should be directed at preventing the formation of a chronic fistulous tract, or communication, between the maxillary sinus and the oral cavity. Almost all perforations are small; in fact, a large number go unrecognized. If the perforation is large—as when the bone encasing all three roots of the maxillary first molar is removed with the tooth—an aggressive surgical approach must be taken to close the perforation. In this situation a referral to an oral and maxillofacial surgeon would be indicated.

In the case of a small perforation, a relatively well-established regimen will prevent the formation of a chronic fistula. Every effort should be made to maintain a proper blood clot, possibly with the use of collagen preparations or sutures over the top of the socket. The patient should be cautioned against sneezing, sucking through a straw, and other maneuvers that would create a differential pressure between the mouth and sinus. Sinus decongestants are frequently prescribed as well. Some clinicians also prefer to prescribe an antibiotic to decrease the chance for an infection, although it is very unlikely that one would occur. Since the bacteria that would cause such an infection would be primarily the normal mouth bacteria, penicillin is the drug of choice (clarithromycin in the case of a penicillin-allergic patient). If the decision is made to use antibiotics, they should be administered as soon as possible after the perforation is noted and continued for approximately 5 days.

Avulsed teeth

Management of avulsed teeth is a complex problem that requires a variety of different decisions. Fundamental to success is placing the avulsed tooth back into the socket as quickly as possible and stabilizing it to adjacent teeth in such a way as to allow a minimal amount of movement. Care should be taken to avoid injury to the root and cementum of the tooth, which could result in resorption and/or ankylosis. The question of whether antibiotics should be used is again one of clinical opinion. While no controlled studies have been performed to define whether antibiotics should be prescribed for such patients, it is common clinical practice to use antibiotics. The drug of choice in these situations is penicillin (erythromycin in the case of a penicillin-allergic patient). The antibiotics should be administered as soon as possible and continued for 5 to 7 days. In situations in which there has been extensive soft tissue and bone injury, the clinician may decide to use antibiotics for a longer period of time.

Osteomyelitis

Osteomyelitis of the jaws is an infrequent occurrence, but it usually has several predisposing parameters. It is seen primarily in patients who are debilitated by systemic disease, most commonly alcoholism. Moreover, it is often precipitated by a traumatic event such as fracture of the mandible followed by extraction of the tooth, which leads to a nonhealing dry socket. The diagnosis and management of osteomyelitis of the jaw is a complex topic. Generally, however, osteomyelitis causes pain, draining sinus tracts (either intraorally or extraorally), and destruction of bone that is obvious on the radiograph. Frequently it is very difficult to eradicate.

Aggressive surgical intervention and precise antibiotic choices are necessary for prompt resolution of this disease. The antibiotic of choice in these situations is a drug that is effective primarily against the anaerobic bacteria of the mouth but also has effectiveness against *Streptococcus*. While *Staphylococcus* has been implicated as a causative bacterium in osteomyelitis of the jaws, recent investigations have established that it is not a major causative organism. Therefore, a drug like clindamycin, which is excellent against anaerobes, would be one of the first-line drugs. Penicillin, alone or in combination with metronidazole, may also be useful for the management of osteomyelitis of the jaws. This infection usually would be managed by a specialist such as an oral and maxillofacial surgeon.

Dry socket

KEY FACTS

The postoperative complication known as "dry socket" or "alveolar osteitis" occurs in approximately 10% of patients who undergo removal of a mandibular third molar. This complication is most likely the result of a bacteria-induced lysis of the blood clot, which results in exposed bone and moderate to severe pain. Dry socket can best be prevented through copious intraoperative irrigation. Moreover, topical antibiotics (placed directly in the socket at the end of a procedure) may reduce the incidence by approximately 50%. There is also evidence that preoperative and postoperative rinsing with chlorhexidine may reduce the incidence of dry socket. Once this complication has occurred, however, antibiotics are essentially ineffective and therefore unnecessary. Irrigation of the socket to remove loose debris and placement of a sedative dressing are all that is required for its management.

Pericoronitis

The partially erupted third molar frequently will have a soft tissue operculum, which may give rise to the special periodontal infection known as *pericoronitis*. In this situation, the deep periodontal pocket caused by the operculum becomes mildly to severely infected. If the patient presents for treatment when the symptoms are very localized (ie, local pain and swelling without trismus, extraoral swelling, or temperature), the most effective method of management is to irrigate the periodontal pocket with hydrogen peroxide, saline, or chlorhexidine. Occasionally, removal of the hypererupted maxillary third molar is of great benefit as well. Antibiotics are not necessary in these mild situations. If the patient presents for treatment after developing trismus, extraoral swelling, and temperature, however, irrigation and removal of the maxillary third molar will need to be supplemented by administration of antibiotics. The drug of choice in this situation continues to be penicillin (clarithromycin or cephalexin for penicillin-allergic patients).

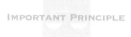

Routine extractions

Questions frequently arise as to whether patients should receive antibiotics for routine extraction of teeth. However, this is almost never necessary in patients with normal host-defense mechanisms. Antibiotics should be used prophylactically only when the patient has a history of diseases or drug usage, such as cancer chemotherapeutic agents, that would depress host defenses.

Impacted third molars

Similar questions have been raised about the removal of impacted third molars. As with other dentoalveolar surgery, if the patient is healthy, prophylactic antibiotics are not necessary for routine third molar extractions. If, on the other hand, the patient has an acute pericoronitis, administration of short-term prophylactic antibiotics may be of some benefit in preventing postoperative infection. However, if the pericoronitis is very mild or if it has been resolved with irrigation and/or antibiotic therapy in the period preceding the extraction, antibiotics are not necessary.

References

1. Aderhold L, Knothe H, Frenkel G. The bacteriology of dentogenous pyogenic infections. Oral Surg Oral Med Oral Pathol 1981;52:583–587.

2. Bartlett JG, O'Keefe P. The bacteriology of perimandibular space infections. J Oral Surg 1979;37:407–409.

3. Labriola JD, Mascaro J, Alpert B. The microbiologic flora of orofacial abscesses. J Oral Maxillofac Surg 1983;41:711–714.

4. Peterson LJ. Principles of management and prevention of odontogenic infections. In Peterson LJ (ed). Contemporary Oral and Maxillofacial Surgery, ed 3. St. Louis: Mosby, 1997:392–417.

5. Physicians' Desk Reference. Oradell, NJ: Medical Economics, 1986.

6. Conover MA, Kaban LB, Mulliken JB. Antibiotic prophylaxis for major maxillocraniofacial surgery. J Oral Maxillofac Surg 1985;43:865–869.

7. Peterson LJ. Antibiotic prophylaxis against wound infections in oral and maxillofacial surgery. J Oral Maxillofac Surg 1990;48:617–620.

Robert Lindemann, DDS, MEd, MS
Douglas Harrington, DDS

12

PEDIATRIC CONSIDERATIONS

Qualities of the Young Patient

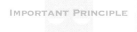

Pediatric antibiotic therapy shares many of the general principles that have been applied to adults in the preceding chapters. However, for treatment purposes, the child cannot be considered a small adult. Although the child patient benefits from the resiliency of youth, it is important to remain aware of the dangers of unchecked orofacial infection. Regardless of the age of the patient, infection can spread quickly with dramatic changes in signs and symptoms.

Pharmacokinetics, which involves the absorption, biotransformation, and elimination of specific drugs, functions differently in children than in adults. Children also differ physiologically and anatomically from adults, primarily in body size and fluid volume.[1] Simple standard formulas, such as Clark's rule or Young's rule, which calculate pediatric dosage based only on weight and age, are not always appropriate for prescribing antibiotics for children.[2] Understanding differences in pharmacokinetics, physiology, anatomy, microflora, and cognitive processes will enable the dentist to treat the child confidently and successfully.

Cognition

During the early stages of their development, children are busy collecting the experiential knowledge that will be incorporated in the creation of their unique personalities. They frequently need understanding and extra patience from the dentist to make dental visits as pleasant as possible. This especially is true if the child presents with an infection or condition that elicits pain or is uncomfortable.

175

Microflora

At their first dental encounters, pediatric patients with primary dentition present with many of the same endogenous bacteria found in the normal microflora of adults. Children undergo a progressive addition of oral bacteria after their first exposure during passage through the maternal birth canal and with the eruption of primary teeth.[3] For example, *Streptococcus mutans*, the organism primarily responsible for dental caries, is thought to appear after the emergence of the primary dentition during a discrete window of infectivity. Moreover, it is believed that the child's *S mutans* levels positively correlate with the mother's levels.[4]

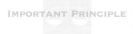

Occasions when antibiotic therapy will benefit the child are discussed in this chapter. However, because of the variety of systemic conditions and the constantly emerging advances in medical treatment of those conditions, it is important to consult with the child's pediatrician before prescribing antibiotic treatment. The goals of this chapter are twofold: *(1)* to reinforce the application of appropriate antibiotic therapy for the child, and *(2)* to alert the reader to the required modifications of therapy.

Pediatric Antibiotic Therapy: Indications and Treatment

The primary source of orofacial infection in children is odontogenic. The causative agents of these infections tend to be a mix of aerobic and anaerobic bacteria. After identifying the source of infection, treatment should be directed toward providing adequate drainage through pulpal therapy, extraction, and/or incision. Antibiotic therapy is advised in addition to local treatment when the infection extends beyond the dentoalveolar structure. Children are susceptible to infections from periodontal diseases or trauma, and they may also be at risk from cardiac disease.

Acute odontogenic infections

Dangers Wide marrow spaces in children can allow permanent-tooth germs and critical growth centers of the jaws to be threatened by intraosseous infection.[5] Children are also susceptible to the life-threatening consequences of rapidly spreading odontogenic infections, including cavernous sinus thrombosis, brain abscess, septicemia, airway obstruction, and mediastinitis.[6] Use of antibiotics therefore is advised when the infection extends beyond the dentoalveolar structures, concomitant with the primary treatment of pulpectomy or extraction to eliminate the source of the infection. Dehydration, which complicates recovery, is also a potential danger since children with orofacial infections may refuse to drink sufficient liquids because of oral pain.

Table 12-1 Average doses* recommended for children under 60 lb (27 kg)

Antibiotic	Usual oral dose
Ampicillin	50–100 mg/kg per day in 4 divided doses up to 250 mg/dose
Cephalexin	25–50 mg/kg per day in 4 divided doses (maximum of 3 g per day)
Clindamycin	10–25 mg/kg per day in 3–4 divided doses (maximum adult dose of 1.8 g per day)
Erythromycin	30–40 mg/kg per day in 4 divided doses (maximum of 2 g per day)
Penicillin V	25–50 mg/kg per day in 4 divided doses (maximum of 3 g per day)

*Actual doses should be based on infection severity, child's age, and renal and hepatic clearances.

INFORMATION ABOUT SPECIFIC DRUG

Penicillin Once the location and source of the infection is determined, penicillin V is the empiric drug of choice because of the effectiveness of oral administration against gram-positive anaerobes typically associated with odontogenic infections (see Table 12-1 for recommended dosages). To achieve and maintain high serum and tissue levels, penicillin V should be prescribed for a minimum of 7 days. The importance of compliance should be stressed to the patient and the responsible adult. The culture techniques used for adults (see chapter 2) also may be performed on children.

INFORMATION ABOUT SPECIFIC DRUG

KEY FACTS

Amoxicillin Amoxicillin is a penicillin-based, broad-spectrum antibiotic that is more effective than penicillin against gram-negative bacteria.[7] The use of amoxicillin for pediatric patients has become increasingly popular because the taste of its elixir is more agreeable than that of penicillin. However, penicillin V is still considered the drug of choice for odontogenic infections. Amoxicillin should be reserved for gram-negative infections such as nonodontogenic maxillary sinusitis[5] and prophylaxis for infective endocarditis.

ADVERSE EFFECTS

Penicillin allergy Children with documented penicillin allergy can be prescribed erythromycin or clindamycin for the treatment of acute odontogenic infections. Recommended erythromycin and clindamycin dosages are listed in Table 12-1. However, because therapy with clindamycin carries a risk of pseudomembranous colitis, consultation with the patient's physician is recommended before prescribing the agent.

Periapical abscess Clinical research has implicated anaerobic micro-organisms in the etiology of acute periapical abscess in children.[8] This discovery was made possible by meticulous sampling techniques that avoided contamination with normal flora. Because these anaerobes have been associated with serious infections that arise from an oral focus, appropriate antimicrobial therapy is indicated. Fortunately, most of the anaerobic pathogens isolated from the abscesses are sensitive to penicillin. However, patients who do not show signs of improvement after instituting penicillin therapy may be infected with β-lactamase–producing organisms, possibly *Bacteroides* species and other organisms.[9] Antimicrobial agents effective against these strains, such as metronidazole, may be required in serious cases.[10] In conjunction with judicious antimicrobial therapy, dental surgical intervention also may be indicated.

IMPORTANT PRINCIPLE

Severe infections Severe infections require more aggressive treatment, including parenteral administration of antibiotics and, in extreme cases, hospitalization. Close cooperation between the dentist and pediatrician is essential. Initial cultures from the odontogenic abscess become critically important in cases that do not respond to therapy because failure may be caused by the development of resistant strains.

Chemoprophylaxis

Bacteremia It has been firmly established that bacteremias do occur in children following dental prophylaxis, local anesthetic injections, and extraction of normal and diseased primary or permanent teeth.[11–13] Antibiotic prophylaxis is indicated in children (and adults) with most congenital heart diseases, rheumatic or acquired valvular heart disease, and prosthetic heart valves or vessels[14,15] (see chapter 15). Antibiotics are not necessary, however, during the spontaneous exfoliation of primary teeth or the simple adjustment of orthodontic appliances.

KEY FACTS

American Heart Association guidelines In 1997, the American Heart Association (AHA) updated its recommendations regarding bacterial endocarditis prophylaxis prior to dental procedures (see chapter 15). Note, however, that adjustments according to the child's weight may need to be made.[14] According to the new guidelines, erythromycin is no longer recommended for penicillin-allergic patients. Alternative antibiotics include cephalexin, azithromycin, and clindamycin. These alternative prophylaxis regimens should also be considered for patients who are currently taking antibiotics, such as amoxicillin, for other medical conditions.

IMPORTANT PRINCIPLE

It is important to remember that AHA guidelines are recommendations only. Close cooperation between dentist and pediatrician is essential for optimal prophylaxis. Keeping current on changes in the AHA's or other regulatory agencies' regimens is the best way to prevent the high morbidity and mortality of bacterial endocarditis.[16]

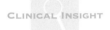

Resistance A careful history of antibiotic therapy should be taken from those patients requiring chemoprophylaxis. Recent history of penicillin or clindamycin therapy alerts the practitioner to the possibility of resistant organisms. Because children receive frequent regimens of antibiotics for childhood illnesses, close monitoring becomes even more critical to prevent untoward sequelae of infection by those resistant strains.[17]

Periodontal disease

Local debridement remains the major treatment for most periodontal diseases in children. However, in the clinical management of aggressive forms such as aggressive periodontitis, tetracycline therapy may enhance success. A combination of antibiotics, amoxicillin and metronidazole, has also been proposed for *Actinobacillus*-associated periodontal disease.[18] In most cases, a combined therapy of surgery and systemic antibiotics is recommended[19] (see chapter 8).

Trauma

Pediatric patients with face lacerations, through-and-through lip lacerations, puncture wounds, dog bites, or electrical burns of the orofacial complex should receive antibiotics in addition to meticulous surgical management. Consultation and/or referral to an oral surgeon or emergency room are indicated in most cases. Tetanus immunization history must be taken into account. Antibiotics may be considered in addition to chlorhexidine rinses and analgesics in cases of trauma involving displacement or complete luxation of permanent teeth.[20] However, some experts question the benefit of antibiotic usage following dental trauma.[21]

Special Considerations

Problems swallowing pills

Children, like some adults, often have difficulty swallowing capsules or tablets. Elixirs of penicillin V are available in dosages of 125 mg/5 mL and 250 mg/5 mL in either 100- or 200-mL bottles. Erythromycin is available in two oral suspensions as well—200 mg/5 mL and 400 mg/5 mL—both in pint bottles. They are flavored for palatability. Clindamycin is available in flavored granules for oral solution in the equivalent of 75 mg/5 mL (100- or 200-mL reconstituted bottles).

Noncompliance

If a child does not respond favorably to antibiotic treatment, noncompliance may be a factor. A child who refuses to accept his or her medications, vomits shortly after ingestion, or is suspected of removing the

CLINICAL INSIGHT

IMPORTANT PRINCIPLE

tablet after it is administered is a candidate for the parenteral route. Fortunately, noncompliance is unusual, particularly if palatable elixir forms are administered.

Childhood systemic diseases

Many childhood diseases have orofacial manifestations (eg, chicken pox, measles, and mumps) and should be considered in a differential diagnosis before an antibiotic regimen is prescribed for a problem of presumed odontogenic or periodontal etiology.

Chronic systemic disease The following special circumstances of systemic disease in pediatric patients require consideration. Attention should be given to reducing the potential for an oral focus of infection in these patients.

- Routine systemic antibiotic prophylaxis of HIV-positive patients is not recommended unless warranted by coexisting cardiac conditions because the use of broad-spectrum antibiotics may enhance the probability of fungal infections in these patients.[22]
- Consultation with the patient's pediatrician is recommended for the immunosuppressed child, who may need antibiotic prophylaxis prior to dental procedures. As an adjunct, 0.12% chlorhexidine gluconate rinse may be effective in reducing dental-plaque bacteria. Nystatin oral suspension, Mycostatin pastilles (Bristol Meyers) or clotrimazole troches (Mycelex; Bayer) may be used to eliminate *Candida* infections, which are frequently reported in the immunocompromised host (see chapters 5 and 16). Mycelex is recommended for children under 3 years of age.
- During the first 3 months following liver transplantation (regardless of whether the transplant was accepted), immunosuppression and graft anastomoses that are not fully epithelialized may put patients at risk for bacterial endarteritis.[23] Consequently, antibiotic prophylaxis is required for these patients. Similarly, the chronic renal failure patient (possibly on dialysis or posttransplant) may also be at risk for infection from dental sources; therefore, consultation is recommended.[24]
- Judicious home care and regular dental examinations help reduce the threat of infection in the diabetic child. However, some pediatricians believe that antibiotics are warranted before surgical procedures.
- Children with Down syndrome have a high incidence of congenital heart defects. Patients with positive cardiac findings after a physical exam should be prescribed antibiotic prophylaxis according to current AHA guidelines. For the child with hydrocephalus, the scientific literature has clearly demonstrated the need for antibiotic prophylaxis if a ventriculovenous shunt has been placed; however, recent literature questions the need for prophylaxis if a ventriculoperitoneal shunt has been placed.[25]

Tetracycline staining

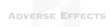

Children are susceptible to staining of their primary and permanent dentition when tetracycline is prescribed during critical developmental periods. The first of these periods is from approximately 4 months in utero to 9 months postpartum for primary incisors and canines. The second sensitive period is from 3 to 5 months postpartum until about the seventh year for permanent incisors and canines.[26] An alternative antibiotic should be given to preclude unsightly staining.

References

1. Anderson JA. Physiologic principles in pediatric dentistry. In: Pinkham JR (ed). Pediatric Dentistry: Infancy Through Adolescence. Philadelphia: WB Saunders, 1994:82–84.

2. Picozzi A, Lewis VA. Prescription writing and drug regulations. In: Yagiela JA, Neidle EA, Dowd FJ (eds). Pharmacology and Therapeutics for Dentistry. St. Louis: Mosby, 1998:701.

3. Minah GE. Dental plaque. In: Forrester DJ (ed). Pediatric Dental Medicine. Philadelphia: Lea & Febiger, 1981.

4. Caufield PW, Cutter GR, Dasanayake AP. Initial acquisition of mutans streptococci by infants: Evidence for a discrete window of infectivity. J Dent Res 1993;72:37–45.

5. Wilson S, Montgomery RD. Local anesthesia and oral surgery. In: Pinkham JR (ed). Pediatric Dentistry: Infancy Through Adolescence. Philadelphia: WB Saunders, 1994:95.

6. Kaban LB. Infections of the maxillofacial region. In: Kaban LB (ed). Pediatric Oral and Maxillofacial Surgery. Philadelphia: WB Saunders, 1990:163–188.

7. Montgomery EH. Principles and mechanisms of antibiotic therapy. In: Yagiela JA, Neidle EA, Dowd FJ (eds). Pharmacology and Therapeutics for Dentistry. St. Louis: Mosby-Year Book, 1998:487.

8. Brook I, Grimm S, Kielich RB. Bacteriology of acute periapical abscess in children. J Endod 1981;7:378–380.

9. Brook I, Calhoun L, Yocum P. Beta-lactamase producing isolates of *Bacteroides* species from children. Antimicrob Agents Chemother 1980;18:164–166.

10. Scully BE. Metronidazole. Med Clin North Am 1988;72:613–621.

11. Roberts GJ, Simmons NB, Longhurst P, Hewitt PB. Bacteraemia following local anaesthestic injections in children. Br Dent J 1998;185:295–298.

12. Roberts GJ, Holzel HS, Sury MR, Simmons NA, Gardner P, Longhurst P. Dental bacteremia in children. Pediatr Cardiol 1997;18:24–27.

13. Coulter WA, Coffey A, Saunders ID, Emmerson AM. Bacteremia in children following dental extraction. J Dent Res 1990;69:1691–1695.

14. Dajani AS, Taubert KA, Wilson W, Bolger AF, Bayer A, Ferrier P, et al. Prevention of bacterial endocarditis. Recommendations by the American Heart Association. JAMA 1997;277:1794–1801.

15. Lindemann RA, Henson JL. The dental management of patients with vascular grafts placed in the treatment of arterial occlusive disease. J Am Dent Assoc 1982;104:625–628.

16. Brooks SL. Survey of compliance with American Heart Association guidelines for prevention of bacterial endocarditis. J Am Dent Assoc 1980;101:41–43.

17. Lampe RM, Cheldelin LV, Brown J. Brain abscess following dental extraction in a child with cyanotic congenital heart disease. Pediatrics 1978;61:659–660.

18. van Winkelhoff AJ, Rodenburg JP, Goené RJ, Abbas F, Winkel EG, de Graaff J. Metronidazole plus amoxycillin in the treatment of *Actinobacillus actinomycetemcomitans*–associated periodontitis. J Clin Periodontol 1989;16:128–131.

19. Newman MG. Localized juvenile periodontitis (periodontosis). Pediatr Dent 1981;3: 121–126.

20. Nowak AJ. Trauma. In: Nowak AJ (ed). Handbook of Pediatric Dentistry, ed 2. Chicago: American Academy of Pediatric Dentistry, 1999:96.

21. Andreason JO, Andreason FM. Avulsions. In: Andreason JO, Andreason FM (eds). Textbook and Color Atlas of Traumatic Injuries to Teeth. St. Louis: Mosby, 1994:400.

22. Dougherty MA, Slots J. Periodontal diseases in young individuals. J Calif Dent Assoc 1993;21:55–69.

23. Douglas LR, Douglass JB, Sieck JO, Smith PJ. Oral management of the patient with end-stage liver disease and the liver transplant patient. Oral Surg Oral Med Oral Pathol Oral Radiol Endod 1998;86:55–64.

24. Svirsky JA, Nunley J, Dent CD, Yeatts D. Dental and medical considerations of patients with renal disease. J Calif Dent Assoc 1998;26:761, 763–770.

25. Helpin ML, Rosenberg HM, Sayany Z, Sanford RA. Antibiotic prophylaxis in dental patients with ventriculo-peritoneal shunts: A pilot study. ASDC J Dent Child 1998; 65:244–247.

26. Moffitt JM, Cooley RO, Olsen NH, Hefferren JJ. Prediction of tetracycline-induced tooth discoloration. J Am Dent Assoc 1974;88:547–552.

Perry R. Klokkevold, DDS, MS

CHEMOTHERAPEUTIC AGENTS IN RESTORATIVE DENTISTRY

KEY FACTS

Recent advances in restorative materials and techniques have had a remarkable impact on our ability to realistically replicate (or improve upon) the appearance of "natural" teeth in dental restorations. As a result of these achievements, patient demand for esthetic restorations has increased. Today, one of the major challenges for dentists who provide esthetic dental restorations is management of the soft tissues, sometimes referred to as the "pink" esthetics of dentistry. Proper management of periodontal soft tissues and control of gingival inflammation are critically important to achieving optimal esthetics.

Chemotherapeutic agents, which traditionally are used to reduce gingival inflammation and prevent periodontal infections, are also useful in the enhancement of the soft tissue aspect of restorative dentistry. The creative incorporation of these agents into prosthodontic procedures facilitates optimal esthetics via improved periodontal soft tissue health. This chapter describes how clinicians can use today's chemotherapeutic agents for improvement and long-term maintenance of the periodontal tissues surrounding dental restorations. In addition, the chapter discusses the diagnosis and management of microbial infections that can develop in conjunction with restorative dental procedures.

Importance of Periodontal Health for Fixed Prosthodontics

As the cornerstone of long-lasting fixed prosthodontic restorations, sound periodontal health influences:

- Diagnosis
- Treatment planning
- Therapeutic procedures
- Installation of final restorations
- Esthetics
- Long-term maintenance

The esthetics and predictability of every case are improved when optimal gingival health is established and maintained.

The performance of prosthetic procedures, most notably the taking of impressions, is more effective and efficient when periodontal tissues are healthy. Unfortunately, however, the placement of "esthetic" crowns has been associated with the occurrence of iatrogenic periodontal disease.[1,2] Traumatic soft tissue management either during or after fixed prosthetic procedures can adversely affect the appearance of final restorations as well as long-term periodontal health.

Gingival bleeding during tooth preparation, gingival retraction, and impression procedures not only creates difficulty in obtaining a good impression, but it can severely compromise the quality of master stone dies and final crown margin integrity. Unhealthy tissues that bleed easily also are more likely than healthy tissues to be traumatized by prosthetic procedures. Since bleeding from inflamed tissues results in failed impressions, repeated attempts at gingival retraction and impressions are needed, which can negatively affect the long-term stability and predictability of the gingival tissue level in relation to esthetic anterior crown margins.

The marginal integrity and emergence profile of fixed restorations must be compatible with gingival health. Unsightly gingival inflammation (erythema and swelling) around provisional and permanent crowns is most often caused by bacterial plaque accumulation. Several factors related to the fit and form of fixed prosthetics contribute to plaque accumulation:

- Crowns that have poor-fitting margins or that are made with a rough surface finish (porous acrylic provisional restorations or exposed unglazeable opaque near the margin of permanent crowns) provide a nidus for plaque growth.[3]
- Oral hygiene is impaired and gingival health is compromised when restorations are overcontoured in the cervical third or when crown margins are placed too close to the periodontal attachment apparatus.

- Crowns with open or rough margins that are placed either in close proximity to the gingiva or below it (subgingival) are difficult for patients to clean effectively. Consequently, plaque accumulation is localized at the tissue level, where it has the greatest potential to elicit a destructive inflammatory response.

Left undisturbed, bacterial plaque matures from a predominantly gram-positive, facultative, "healthy" flora to one that is predominantly gram-negative, anaerobic, and disease-causing in nature. In individuals who are relatively resistant to periodontal disease, the extent of gingival inflammation and periodontal destruction may be rather minimal; conversely, in individuals who are more susceptible, inflammation may cause periodontal pocket formation, bone loss, and gingival recession. The resultant exposed root surfaces and crown margins are unsightly and unacceptable.

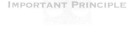

Crowns with excellent marginal adaptation, proper contours, and smooth surfaces should always be used to ensure the maintenance of good oral hygiene and gingival health.[4] Effective antimicrobial mouthrinses, used adjunctively, can further limit plaque accumulation, thus enhancing long-term gingival health.[5–7]

Topical Agents for Restorative Dentistry

IMPORTANT PRINCIPLE

Patients with extensive fixed prostheses who have suffered from periodontal disease with associated gingival recession and exposure of root surfaces are at higher risk for additional periodontal destruction and recurrent caries. Patient education and individualized oral hygiene instructions are imperative for long-term maintenance and predictability.

Fluorides

- Fluoride solutions have been proven effective in reducing cariogenic plaque.[8,9]
- Stannous fluoride (SNF_2) can function as a weak antimicrobial agent against some periodontopathic organisms.[10–12] A 0.4% SNF_2 gel applied in a stent will aid in preventing secondary caries around abutment teeth.
- Most adults with moderate to extensive restorative or postperiodontal treatment are susceptible to recurrent caries and will benefit from long-term, low-dose fluoride rinses. A low-concentration, over-the-counter fluoride rinse (eg, 0.05% NaF_2) should be recommended for long-term use.
- As a preventive measure, long-term topical application of fluorides either directly with a brush or indirectly with custom-formed stents is advocated. With a stone cast, a vacuum-made stent can be fabricated easily and will last for several years.

Table 13-1 Diagnostic and treatment regimen for fixed prosthodontic procedures

Assessment	Diagnostic and treatment regimen
Periodontal pocket depths of 4 mm or greater	Should be treated first or referred to a periodontist
Bleeding on probing, high plaque levels, or poor oral hygiene	A prophylaxis should be performed and a chlorhexidine regimen initiated at least 2 weeks before tooth preparation and continued for 2 weeks after cementation of the definitive prosthesis (see Table 13-2)
Minimal plaque levels, good gingival health, and no bleeding on probing	Minimal benefit would be achieved with chlorhexidine therapy

KEY FACTS

- Although acidulated phosphate fluorides are effective in reducing cariogenic bacteria, their use in the presence of porcelain restorations is contraindicated. Several studies have demonstrated that acidulated fluorides etch porcelain surfaces, thus removing the glazed surface and resulting in poor esthetics, decreased resistance to staining, and increased plaque accumulation.[13]

Chlorhexidine

Research has shown chlorhexidine gluconate mouthrinses to be the most effective agents in reducing supragingival plaque and gingivitis when compared to other antimicrobial agents.[14] A study using 0.12% chlorhexidine gluconate mouthrinse to enhance gingival health during fixed prosthodontic procedures has proven the agent to be highly effective in reducing the Plaque Index, Gingival Index, and number of bleeding sites compared to controls,[15] which makes tooth preparation, gingival retraction, and impression procedures easier and more expedient. Moreover, the frequency of impression remakes in the study was much higher for the control group than for the chlorhexidine-rinsing group. Another important finding was that adjunctive chlorhexidine rinsing significantly reduced the number of putative periodontal pathogens, retarded bacterial colonization of the subgingival/marginal microflora, and favored the establishment of microflora compatible with periodontal health.[16] More than 50% of the subjects in the 7-week study noticed a decrease in the swelling and redness of their gingiva, and 92% of the subjects would recommend chlorhexidine rinsing to a friend.[17] Based on the results of this work, diagnostic and treatment regimens are recommended in Tables 13-1 and 13-2.

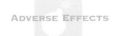

ADVERSE EFFECTS

Long-term daily rinsing with chlorhexidine has not been a problem in terms of development of resistant strains of oral microorganisms[18];

Table 13-2 Chemotherapeutic agents in restorative dentistry

Purpose	Agent	Regimen	Instructions
Gingival enhancement in fixed prosthodontics	0.12% chlorhexidine gluconate	15 mL 2x per day. Rinse for 30 sec; start 2 weeks prior to tooth preparation and continue for 2 weeks following final restoration	Brush and floss teeth. Rinse with chlorhexidine and expectorate; do not rinse, eat, or drink for 30 min
Long-term maintenance of extensive fixed prosthetics	0.4% stannous fluoride gel	Apply gel once a day in stent	Hold both maxillary and mandibular stents in mouth for 4 min, expectorate excess gel; do not rinse, eat, or drink for 30 min
	Over-the-counter sodium fluoride rinse	Daily rinsing	Brush and floss teeth. Rinse with fluoride rinse; do not rinse, eat, or drink for 30 min
Long-term maintenance of periodontally involved teeth/periodontal prosthesis	0.12% chlorhexidine gluconate	Apply rinse with brush or dilute 3:1 and use irrigation device	Daily application with interproximal brush or irrigation device
Denture stomatitis (candidiasis)	Nystatin pastilles	400000–600000 units 4–5x per day	Dissolve pastilles in mouth 4–5x per day; continue 48 h after symptoms have resolved
	Ketoconazole	200–400 mg per day	One tablet daily for 7–14 days
Severe denture stomatitis (systemic candidiasis)	Amphotericin B		Consult patient's physician or specialist for therapy.
Recurrent herpesvirus infection	Topical acyclovir (5% ointment)		Apply ointment as needed to affected area.
	Acyclovir (capsules, oral suspension, or tablets)	200–400 mg 5x per day for 7–10 days	One tablet taken 5x per day for 7–10 days
Severe herpesvirus infection (systemic)	Acyclovir (injection)	250 mg (intravenous) every 8 h for 7 days	Parenteral administration (intravenous) for 7 days

however, twice-daily rinsing with chlorhexidine often results in tooth staining and disagreeable or altered taste sensation. Extended periods (greater than 4 weeks) of rinsing with chlorhexidine can significantly increase the amount of staining; therefore, prophylaxis to control staining should be incorporated into the patient's treatment plan.

Chlorhexidine staining can be a more significant problem for individuals who smoke and/or have long-term provisional restorations in place. Many categories of patients are provisionalized in acrylic resin restorations for an extended period of time, including those who have had periodontal therapy, implant surgery (osseointegration period), endodontics, or orthodontics. This extensive period of provisionalization can be very discouraging for patients if chlorhexidine staining is severe. Several factors can significantly reduce staining when long-term chlorhexidine therapy is desired. The fabrication of well-fitting, non-porous acrylic provisional restorations, for example, is helpful in the reduction of staining. To minimize porosity, the acrylic resin restorations should be fabricated on casts (indirect method) and cured under pressure. Provisional restorations should be well polished with pumice over all aspects, including gingival margins, interproximal surfaces, and gingival embrasures. Localized application of chlorhexidine to the gingival margin area with a brush (rather than rinsing) also can minimize staining of teeth and restorations. One method used to enhance interproximal health employs dipping a small interproximal brush in chlorhexidine gluconate rinse and applying it to specific gingival areas (especially between teeth) as part of the overall daily oral hygiene measures.

Infections Associated with Restorative Dentistry

KEY FACTS

Restorative dental procedures, poor restorations, and removable dental appliances have the potential to irritate intraoral soft tissues and elicit infections in susceptible individuals. This is particularly true for immunocompromised patients. This section describes the signs, symptoms, and management of herpesvirus and candidiasis (fungal) infections. Specific issues relevant to the management of immunocompromised patients are covered in chapter 16.

Recurrent herpesvirus infection

Many factors are associated with recurrent herpes infections. Among them are:

- Respiratory infections
- Sunlight exposure
- Fever
- Trauma
- Exposure to chemicals
- Emotional stress

Dental restorative procedures can cause physiological stress as well as local trauma to soft tissues and thus have the potential to precipitate herpesvirus lesions in individuals whose oral tissues have been previously infected. An initial infection with herpes simplex virus, referred to as the primary herpes infection, cannot be caused by dental treatment. Primary herpesvirus infections can be caused only by contact with live herpesvirus. It is important to note that the severity of an initial infection varies from one individual to another. Some primary infections result in very severe symptoms while others may be quite mild and possibly go unnoticed.

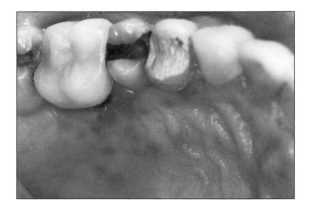

Fig 13-1 Recurrent herpesvirus infection. This patient presented with pain following dental restorative treatment. Small circular ulcerations were observed on the palatal keratinized attached tissue adjacent to the tooth that was treated. Note the classic appearance of ulcerations with erythematous halo that are clustered in the region of the infected sensory nerve.

KEY FACTS

Primary infection with herpes simplex virus in the oral cavity results in a condition known as *acute herpetic gingivostomatitis,* which is a systemic infection with oral lesions. This usually occurs in young individuals, but it can and does occur in adults as well. The virus enters the body through the oral mucosa and causes an acute illness with symptoms such as fever and cervical lymphadenopathy. Vesicles form on the mucosa, then rupture and become ulcerations with erythematous halos. The gingiva is hypertrophic, bright red, and very painful. Often, small (1- to 2-mm) circular lesions can be seen on the affected mucosa. However, in severe infections, these small lesions tend to coalesce into larger, less discrete lesions. After 10 to 14 days, the acute symptoms subside, but the causative virus is not eliminated. Herpes simplex virus infects sensory nerves of the affected tissues and remains latent in the nerve ganglia that supply the site of initial infection (see chapter 5).

In patients with a history of herpesvirus infections, stress induced by dental procedures may precipitate a recurrent herpetic episode. Reactivation of herpesvirus infection occurs in an estimated 40% of those individuals who are infected and harbor a latent virus.[19] The recurrent episode is never as severe as the primary infection. However, similar to a primary infection, recurrent herpetic lesions initially form blisterlike vesicles (commonly referred to as *cold sores* or *fever blisters*) with clear serous fluid. Classically, they are small (1 to 2 mm) circular lesions that cluster in a localized area on the keratinized attached mucosa. Within days, vesicles spontaneously rupture, giving rise to ulcerations with an erythematous halo. Figure 13-1 shows multiple discrete recurrent herpetic ulcerations that are clustered on the attached palatal mucosa adjacent to a tooth that was recently (4 to 5 days earlier) restored with an amalgam buildup. Patients with recurrent herpesvirus infection usually complain of pain in the region of the infected sensory nerve. Ulcerations usually resolve within 10 to 14 days.

Acyclovir Most strains of herpesvirus are susceptible to 5-iodo-2'-deoxyuridine and other nucleoside analogues. Topical application of acyclovir is useful in decreasing the spread and severity of the recurrent infection. For symptomatic relief, especially before meals, topical local anesthetic can be applied to affected areas. Local or systemic application of antibiotics is sometimes advised to prevent opportunistic infection of ulcerations. This is especially true in the immunocompromised individual. In patients with a previous history of herpes infection secondary to dental procedures, pretreatment with acyclovir may be advantageous. A recent clinical report describes the use of acyclovir in a pretreatment protocol to prevent (or lessen the severity of) recurrent herpesvirus infection associated with dental treatment.[20] The protocol consisted of 200 mg acyclovir taken 5 times per day for 5 days starting 2 days before the dental appointment. The patient, who was known to suffer from recurrent infections following dental treatment, did not experience any recurrence.

Candidiasis

Candida albicans is an organism that often opportunistically dominates the microenvironment under a denture. Candidiasis *(Candida* species infection) has several presentations. It can be observed as whitish plaques on the surface of mucosa that can be rubbed off to reveal erythematous and painful underlying tissue or it can be observed as an erosive erythema without plaques.

Candida species are yeastlike fungi that are described as opportunistic because they only cause infections when conditions are altered in favor of their growth. They frequently are present in small numbers in the normal oral microflora. A method to determine the presence of a candidal infection is to examine affected tissue under a microscope. *C albicans* appears as a fine, branching, nonsegmented mycelial net, sometimes with small, oval, budding, thin-walled cells and clusters of microspores.[21] When a diagnosis of candidiasis is confirmed, all contributory factors, including both local and systemic, should be examined. *Candida* frequently becomes infective when host resistance is lowered by antibiotic treatment (see chapters 5 and 7), nutritional deficiency, or immunosuppressive therapy (see chapter 16).

Prosthetic dental appliances that cover tissues are a common local contributory factor associated with candidiasis. Tissues covered by removable prostheses are at risk of becoming irritated, inflamed, and possibly infected if oral hygiene is poor. This is especially true when host immune resistance is compromised. Denture stomatitis (inflammation of oral mucosal tissues adjacent to dentures) can be limited to a localized area of erythema under an appliance or it can be present as a generalized soft tissue inflammation. Plaque accumulation and epithelial denudation can sometimes be seen throughout the mouth. Denture stomatitis is most commonly caused by *C albicans,* but other species may cause or contribute to it as well.

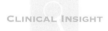
Plaque and debris resulting from poor oral hygiene accumulate on denture surfaces in a manner similar to that which occurs on natural teeth of dentate patients. However, rougher surfaces and porosities in denture acrylic resin facilitate retention of microorganisms. These porosities are difficult to clean or disinfect. As a result, tissues in contact with denture surfaces are constantly exposed to and irritated by bacterial and fungal toxins as well as the rough surfaces themselves. Oral tissues that are covered for extended periods of time may be inhabited by microorganisms other than those that inhabit noncovered tissues due to the altered microenvironment. The changes in pH and oxygen tension favor the growth of virulent microbes that exacerbate denture stomatitis. See chapter 7 for a discussion of adverse microbiological effects.

Minor cases of denture stomatitis may respond well to cleaning and polishing of prostheses and improved oral hygiene. Clean, smooth prosthetic surfaces are more resistant to plaque and debris accumulation and retention than porous surfaces. The following guidelines may help to speed recovery from denture stomatitis:

- It is imperative to replace or reline rough, porous denture surfaces and to professionally clean appliances when infections occur.
- Good oral hygiene should be emphasized.
- Twice-daily oral rinsing with chlorhexidine gluconate also may be considered (see chapter 8).
- Prosthetic appliances should remain out of the mouth as much as possible during the recovery period.

More extensive cases of stomatitis may require specific antimicrobial therapy to be resolved. Consider referral to a specialist. Several antifungal agents are available. Topical agents include:

- Nystatin (oral suspension or pastilles)
- Clotrimazole (lozenges)

These topical agents are applied (rinse or dissolve in mouth) multiple times a day for 2 weeks.

Systemic agents include:

- Ketoconazole (tablets)
- Fluconazole (tablets or injection)
- Amphotericin B (injection)

While all of these agents are useful in treating oral candidiasis, it is the author's experience that topical agents are quite effective in resolving most common infections. The later generation systemic agents such as ketoconazole and fluconazole may have compliance advantages since they are taken orally once a day, but they are also more expensive than the topical agents. More resistant infections, especially those with systemic involvement, may require treatment with amphotericin B.

However, if this level of systemic therapy is deemed necessary, a discussion with a specialist and/or the patient's physician is recommended. Amphotericin B is an extremely toxic agent that is administered parenterally and should be monitored closely.

All measures that enhance the patient's overall general health are useful in treating candidiasis. Consider recommendations to improve nutrition and good oral hygiene habits. It is also important to discontinue any antibiotic therapy, if possible, because this may have precipitated the candidal infection. Consult and work with the patient's physician when more than minor host-related conditions contribute to the problem.

Summary

Optimal periodontal health is essential to the longevity and esthetics of all dental restorations. Establishing and maintaining gingival health prior to and during restorative therapy enhance the precision of final restorations as well as the ease of long-term maintenance. Antimicrobial mouthrinses can enhance gingival health to make fixed prosthodontic procedures easier and more expedient. These mouthrinses improve the quality of the tissue-restoration interface for long-term maintenance of extensive fixed prosthodontics. Future developments in chemotherapeutic agents are sure to offer new and innovative ways to aid in the maintenance of gingival health and in the treatment of such ailments as denture stomatitis and recurrent herpetic infections in conjunction with restorative dental procedures.

References

1. Löe H. Reactions of marginal periodontal tissues to restorative procedures. Int Dent J 1968;18:759–778.

2. Silness J. Periodontal conditions in patients treated with dental bridges. 2. The influence of full and partial crowns on plaque accumulation, development of gingivitis and pocket formation. J Periodontal Res 1970;5:219–224.

3. Sorensen JA. A rationale for comparison of plaque-retaining properties of crown systems. J Prosthet Dent 1989;62:264–269.

4. Segreto VA, Collins EM, Beiswagner BB, de la Rosa M, Isaucs RC, Lang NP, et al. A comparison of mouthrinses containing two concentrations of chlorhexidine. J Periodontal Res 1986;(suppl):23–32.

5. Siegrist AK, Gusberti FA, Brecx ML, Weber HP, Lang NP. Efficacy of supervised rinsing with chlorhexidine di-gluconate in comparison to phenolic and plant alkaloid compounds. J Periodontal Res 1986;(suppl):60-73.

6. Gusberti FA, Sampathkumar P, Siegrist BE, Lang NP. Microbiological and clinical effects of chlorhexidine gluconate and hydrogen peroxide mouthrinses on developing plaque and gingivitis. J Clin Periodontol 1988;15:60–67.

7. Svatun B, Gjermo P, Eriksen HM, Rolla G. A comparison of the plaque-inhibiting effect of stannous fluoride and chlorhexidine. Acta Odontol Scand 1977;35:247–250.

8. Andres CJ, Shaeffer JC, Windeler AS Jr. Comparisons of antibacterial properties of stannous fluoride and sodium fluoride mouthwashes. J Dent Res 1974;53:457–460.

9. Gross A, Tinanoff N. Effect of SnF$_2$ mouthrinse on initial bacterial colonization of tooth enamel. J Dent Res 1977;56:1179–1183.

10. Loesche WJ. Chemotherapy of dental plaque infections. Oral Sci Rev 1976;9:65–107.

11. Yoon NA, Berry CW. The anti-microbial effect of fluorides (acidulated phosphate, sodium and stannous) on *Actinomyces viscosus.* J Dent Res 1979;58:1824–1829.

12. Mazza JE, Newman MG, Sims TN. Clinical and anti-microbial effect of stannous fluoride on periodontitis. J Clin Periodontol 1981;8:203–212.

13. Copps DP, Lacy AM, Curtis T, Carman JE. Effects of topical fluorides on five low-fusing dental porcelains. J Prosthet Dent 1984;52:340–343.

14. Wennström J, Lindhe J. The effect of mouthrinses on parameters characterizing human periodontal disease. J Clin Periodontol 1986;13:86–93.

15. Sorensen JA, Doherty FM, Newman MG, Flemmig TF. Gingival enhancement in fixed prosthodontics. Part I: Clinical findings. J Prosthet Dent 1991;65:100–107.

16. Flemmig TF, Sorensen JA, Newman MG, Nachnani S. Gingival enhancement in fixed prosthodontics. Part II: Microbiologic findings. J Prosthet Dent 1991;65:365–372.

17. Sorensen JA, Newman MG. Gingival enhancement in fixed prosthodontics. Part III: Anamnestic findings. J Prosthet Dent 1991;65:500–504.

18. Briner WW, Grossman E, Bucker RY, Rebitski GE, Sox TE, Setser RE, Ebert MC. Effect of chlorhexidine gluconate mouthrinse on plaque bacterial. J Periodontal Res 1986;(suppl):44–52.

19. Langlais RP, Miller CS. Color Atlas of Common Oral Diseases, ed 2. New York: Williams & Wilkins, 1998.

20. Williamson RT. Diagnosis and management of recurrent herpes simplex induced by fixed prosthodontic tissue management: A clinical report. J Prosthet Dent 1999;82:1–2.

21. Schuster G. Oral Microbiology and Infectious Disease. Baltimore, MD: Williams & Wilkins, 1983.

Thomas Beikler, Dr med
Thomas F. Flemmig, Prof Dr med dent

14

ANTIMICROBIALS IN IMPLANT DENTISTRY

Because of the growing acceptance of dental implants in the treatment of partial and total edentulism,[1] the frequency of implant disorders can be expected to rise, generating a need for a wide variety of antimicrobial therapies.

Recent scientific evidence indicates that implant failures cluster in a small subset of individuals and that a patient who has lost one implant is at an elevated risk for additional implant loss.[2,3] These findings suggest that specific factors may be associated with the outcome of implant therapy.

The purpose of this chapter is to compile the available information about infections in implant dentistry. Suggestions for the prevention and management of implant infections are given.

Implant Disorders

Implant disorders can be divided into two categories (Fig 14-1):

- Implant complications related to the process of primary osseointegration
- Peri-implant diseases that occur after osseointegration has been established

Factors that cause and/or contribute to implant disorders may be:

- Endogenous (systemic or local)
- Exogenous (operator or biomaterial related) (Fig 14-2)[4]

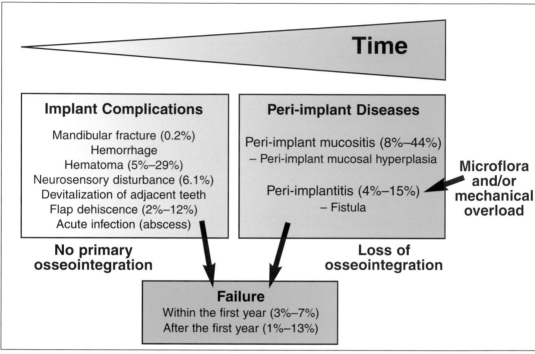

Fig 14-1 Factors contributing to implant disorders.

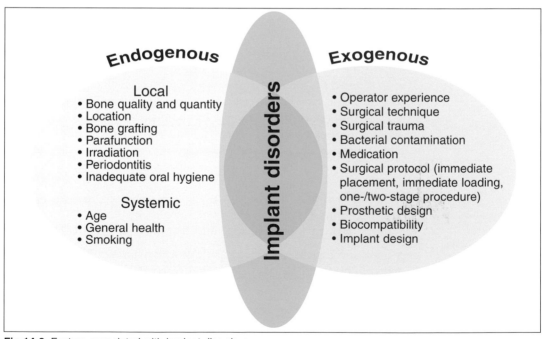

Fig 14-2 Factors associated with implant disorders.

Implant complications

Implant complications can be classified as either intraoperative or early postoperative.

Intraoperative (surgery-related) complications include:

- Injury of anatomic structures
- Excessive bleeding
- Failure to achieve primary implant stability

Early postoperative complications include:

- Wound infections
- Excessive postoperative bleeding
- Flap dehiscence
- Failure to achieve osseointegration (see Fig 14-1)

Of the complications listed above, this chapter discusses only early post-operative wound infections.

Peri-implant diseases

Peri-implant diseases, which primarily occur after osseointegration has been established and the implant has been loaded, are thought to be caused by infections and/or mechanical overload (see Fig 14-1).[5] They include:

- Peri-implant mucositis
- Peri-implant hyperplasia
- Fistula
- Peri-implantitis

Infectious aspects of implant disorders

Infections of the peri-implant tissues have a significant impact on treatment outcome, increasing the implant failure rate up to 5 times.[6] Wound infections may occur in the early postoperative phase (as an implant complication) or during the functional phase, causing peri-implant diseases such as peri-implant mucositis and peri-implantitis.

Peri-implant mucositis is a reversible infection confined to the suprabony peri-implant soft tissues, whereas *peri-implantitis* involves the peri-implant mucosal tissues as well as the peri-implant bone.[7-9] Both forms of implant disease are associated with elevated levels of specific microorganisms that also may have an etiological role in disease progression (Box 14-1).[10-30] Similar subgingival microflora are found in peri-implantitis and periodontitis[15,31-32]; correspondingly, the subgingival microflora found in a healthy peri-implant environment are similar to that of a

---

Box 14-1 Microorganisms associated with peri-implant diseases

Fusobacterium spp[11,12,15,19,25,26,28,29]

Prevotella intermedia[11,12,14,15,28,30]

Porphyromonas gingivalis[12,14,15,19,28,29]

Actinobacillus actinomycetemcomitans[11,12,14,15,25]

Peptostreptococcus micros[15,19,25,26,29,30]

Bacteroides spp[19,25,29]

Capnocytophaga spp[11,12,25]

Prevotella spp[11,15,26]

Spirochetes[28,19,15]

Staphylococcus spp[12,15,25]

Wolinella spp/*Campylobacter rectus*[12,15,25]

Enteric gram-negative bacteria[12,25]

Campylobacter gracilis[29]

Streptococcus intermedius[29]

Streptococcus constellatus[12]

Candida albicans[25]

Eikenella corrodens[15]

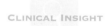

CLINICAL INSIGHT

healthy periodontium.[33–35] In addition, it is important to note that several studies have demonstrated that periodontal pockets may serve as a reservoir for implant infections.[22,32] Therefore, untreated periodontitis seems to be an important risk factor for colonization of the peri-implant pockets by pathogens.

Prevention of Early Postoperative Wound Infections

Presurgical anti-infectious considerations

IMPORTANT PRINCIPLE

Preexisting infections of the oral cavity and its surrounding structures influence the treatment outcome of implant therapy.[36] Infections may originate from and be confined to the oral cavity or they may present as an oral manifestation of systemic diseases,[37,38] in which case they usually are accompanied by an impaired immune response. For example, in patients with periodontitis, cross-infection from diseased periodontal sites to implant sites has been reported.[22,32] Therefore, preexisting periodontitis should be treated prior to implant placement or uncovering.[39,40] To

IMPORTANT PRINCIPLE

obtain optimal results, it is important to treat any intraoral infections or underlying systemic disease before beginning implant therapy.

Peri- and intraoperative anti-infectious considerations

Placement (stage 1) and, for two-stage implant systems, uncovering (stage 2) of dental implants involve the jawbone and the overlying soft tissues. In general, the procedures are performed on an outpatient basis. The invasiveness of implant surgery may be compared to other procedures in oral and periodontal surgery that involve the same tissues. To prevent infection, surgery should take place under aseptic and sterile conditions, and the surgical field should be disinfected with chlorhexidine.[41] Chlorhexidine rinsing significantly reduces the intraoral bacterial load, thereby reducing the potential for infections.[42] Perioperative rinses with 0.12% chlorhexidine have been shown to be effective in reducing or reversing complications associated with intraoral surgical procedures.[43-46]

Stage 2 surgery (exposure of the implants) primarily involves the soft tissues only. Peri-implant pocket probing depth is determined by the thickness of the peri-implant mucosa. Thinning of the mucosal flap during uncovering initially can prevent deep peri-implant pockets.[47] The patient may benefit from the presence of attached keratinized tissue during oral hygiene.[4,48] Existing keratinized mucosa should be preserved by splitting it into two halves and placing one part on the buccal and the other on the lingual side of the implant.[49] However, clinical data acquired via an evidence-based format[50] have failed to show any correlation between the width or mobility of the keratinized mucosa and peri-implant diseases.[51,52]

Twice-daily rinsing with 15 mL of 0.12% chlorhexidine may reduce plaque accumulation, enhance mucosal health, and improve healing.[53-55] A recent report indicates that rinsing with 0.12% chlorhexidine immediately before placement and uncovering surgery and twice daily for 2 weeks following surgery reduces the frequency of early postoperative wound infections in implant surgery from 8.7% to 4.1%.[7] Although in vitro studies reported an inhibitory effect of chlorhexidine on cultured epithelial and HeLa cell growth,[56,57] it does not seem to have an adverse clinical effect on wound healing after mucoperiosteal surgery,[53-55] nor does it alter implant surfaces[58] or inhibit fibroblast attachment to implant surfaces.[59]

When antibiotics are used for prophylaxis of early postoperative wound infections in medically compromised patients, they should be chosen for their effectiveness against the bacteria most likely to cause the infection.[60] In implant surgery, streptococci,[62] anaerobic gram-positive cocci, and anaerobic gram-negative rods are the most likely pathogens to occur. The following guidelines also should be observed when prescribing antibiotics:

- The antibiotic selected for prophylaxis of postsurgical infection should be bactericidal and of low toxicity, eg, penicillin or amoxicillin.[28,62]
- In case of penicillin allergy, clindamycin, metronidazole, or a first-generation cephalosporin may be an alternative choice.[62,63] However, a first-generation cephalosporin is recommended only if the allergic reaction to penicillin is not anaphylactic.[63]

CLINICAL INSIGHT

KEY FACTS

INFORMATION ABOUT
SPECIFIC DRUG

IMPORTANT PRINCIPLE

- When antibiotics are given for the prophylaxis of postoperative wound infection, it is highly recommended that the first dosage should be administered preoperatively (eg, an oral dose of penicillin V should be administered 1 hour before surgery)[64,65] to achieve sufficient antibiotic tissue concentrations during surgery. Although the duration of most antibiotic regimens recommended for implant placement surgery extends over 3 to 10 days,[42,66] prolonging prophylaxis beyond the first postoperative day does not appear to provide additional benefit.[67–70]

Although it has been demonstrated that the prophylactic use of antibiotics in implant surgery (stage 1 and stage 2) may somewhat increase the survival rate and reduce the risk of failure,[61] it also carries an increase in cost and an elevated risk for side effects, including anaphylaxis and the induction of resistant bacterial strains.

Since the incidence of postoperative wound infections after oral or periodontal surgery is generally low following 0.12% chlorhexidine perioperative rinsing,[47–50] a prophylactic antibiotic regimen is warranted only when complications frequently occur and/or the complications have severe sequellae. Thus, perioperative antibiotics may be indicated[68] only when:

- The patient's host response is impaired
- A massive bacterial contamination of noncontaminated tissues is expected, ie, surgery in inflamed sites or the immediate insertion of implants after tooth loss by trauma where contamination usually occurs[71]
- The surgical procedure extends over 3 hours.[63]

The surgical protocols of implant systems available in North America and Europe do not always recommend routine prophylactic perioperative systemic antibiotics.[72–75] For some implant systems, topical antibiotics, such as bacitracin, are recommended for placement in the cover screw hole during implant placement.[66] However, there is no scientific evidence for the benefit of this regimen.

For one-stage and two-stage implant systems, the same considerations regarding systemic antibiotics apply. Because a one-stage implant is immediately exposed to the oral environment, bacterial colonization will begin during the crucial bone-healing phase. During this time it is imperative that loading of the implant is prevented to allow osseointegration to occur. In most cases a health-associated microflora colonizes one-stage implants immediately after insertion.[21] It appears prudent to aid oral hygiene with adjunctive antimicrobial rinsing (15 mL 0.12% chlorhexidine twice daily) during the time of bone healing for 3 to 6 months to prevent bacterial colonization and premature implant loading induced by mechanical oral hygiene (Table 14-1).

If patients with immunodeficiencies, metabolic diseases, risks for metastatic infections secondary to transient bacteremia, or irradiation in the head and neck area are selected for implant therapy, the same principles for prophylactic antibiotic coverage apply as for other oral surgery procedures.

Table 14-1 Prevention of infection-related implant complications

Timing	Local application	Systemic administration
Preoperative	Supragingival debridement; if periodontitis is present, supra- and subgingival debridement; adequate oral hygiene treatment of local infections	Treatment of systemic diseases that may favor local infections
Peri/intraoperative	Rinses with 0.12% chlorhexidine preoperatively	According to surgical protocol of implant system, or if surgery lasts more than 3 h or is extensive, 2 g penicillin V by mouth (1 h preoperatively)
Postoperative	Rinses with 15 mL 0.12% chlor-hexidine twice daily, up to 3–6 months	
Maintenance	Supportive implant therapy (3-month recall intervals)	

Treatment of Early Postoperative Wound Infections

CLINICAL INSIGHT

Acute postoperative infections after placement usually occur on the third or fourth day following surgery.[76] When they occur, the following steps should be taken:

- Surgical drainage should be established immediately.
- A culture should be taken for identification of pathogens and antibiotic susceptibility testing.
- Empiric antibiotic therapy with penicillin V (administered orally) should be initiated.

CLINICAL INSIGHT

CLINICAL INSIGHT

If the patient is allergic to penicillin, available alternatives include clindamycin, metronidazole, or a first-generation cephalosporin (if there is no immediate-type hypersensitivity to penicillins). The antibiotics should be administered 3 days beyond the occurrence of marked clinical improvement (usually at the fourth day), hence for a minimum of 7 days. However, if no clinical improvement occurs within the first 2 days, the antibiotic should be changed according to the identified pathogens and susceptibility-test results. If there is no improvement after specific systemic antibiotic therapy, removal of the implants should be considered. In serious cases of fulminant and spreading infections, the patient may need to be admitted to a hospital for specific high-dose, intravenous antibiotic treatment. The survival of an implant in cases of early infection is always questionable.

If flap dehiscences develop over the implant during the healing phase (3 to 6 months postoperative), the possible causes (eg, pressure of a denture on the implant) should be eliminated and the soft tissue around the dehiscence should eventually be excised. Whether flap coverage should be attempted or the implant should be left exposed remains controversial.[72] If the implant is left exposed, topical antimicrobials (chlorhexidine) should be administered to prevent plaque accumulation.

The first clinical signs of osseointegration are usually assessed during the two-stage procedure or after a one-stage implant has been loaded. If osseointegration has not occurred, the implant, including the connective tissue lining the socket, should be removed. If an infection occurs, the tissues should be allowed to heal before another implant is placed in the same site.

Acute infections following uncovering should be treated with debridement and local antimicrobials. If fluctuation is present, drainage should be established. If no clinical improvement occurs within the first 24 hours, systemic penicillin therapy is recommended. Simultaneously, identification of pathogens and antibiotic susceptibility testing should be carried out followed by specific systemic antibiotic therapy. Mobile implants may be removed.

Prevention of Peri-implant Diseases

An increasing number of studies point to the detrimental effect of microbial colonization around dental implants.[77–79] Infection of the peri-implant tissues can cause peri-implant bone destruction[18] and may result in implant failure.[79] Good oral hygiene is an important step in preventing infection. The following measures will facilitate patient compliance with oral hygiene:

- Instruct the implant patient on proper oral hygiene and repeat these instructions regularly at maintenance visits.
- A prosthesis design that facilitates cleaning will increase patient compliance.
- The mode of oral hygiene—that is, manual toothbrush, rotary electric toothbrush,[80,81] dental floss, and/or supragingival irrigation with water—should be adjusted to the specific anatomic and prosthetic situation of each patient.

Implant maintenance also is important in the prevention of infection and should include:

- Supra- and subgingival debridement with air-abrasive systems
- Specially designed plastic or titanium scaler
- Floss and/or rubber cup polishing with fine abrasive paste.

Instruments that may injure the implant and abutment surface such as stainless steel curettes should be avoided since the resulting roughening of the surface may enhance bacterial adhesion.

Due to the potential for cross-contamination from teeth to implants, implants in partially edentulous patients are at greater risk for peri-implantitis than implants in completetly edentulous patients.[14] Thus, a 3-month maintenance interval appears to be advisable in partially edentulous patients, especially since supportive periodontal therapy has been shown to maintain peri-implant health and to prevent subgingival colonization of microorganisms associated with peri-implant complications.[82,83] For fully edentulous patients, the regimen outlined above should be followed and, if necessary, the recall should be customized to the patient's needs.

Treatment of Peri-implant Diseases

Peri-implant mucositis

Peri-implant mucositis, which is characterized by a bleeding tendency with peri-implant pockets of less than 4 mm deep, develops[79] when plaque is allowed to accumulate around implants. The prevalence of peri-implant mucositis increases the longer implants are in place.[17,84] Peri-implant mucositis is treated by plaque removal through the following methods:

- Patient should be instructed on oral hygiene measures adapted to the specific anatomic situation.
- Regular professional cleanings should be initiated.
- The time interval between the maintenance visits should be shortened.
- Adjunctive to mechanical home care, the use of antimicrobial rinses[85,86] and supragingival irrigation with antimicrobials or water may be beneficial.

Despite the safety of long-term use of some antimicrobial agents, their side effects, such as staining and taste alteration, may be a nuisance. However, adjunctive supragingival irrigation with water, a beneficial oral hygiene adjunct for periodontitis patients, may be similarly helpful for implant patients.[87,88]

Local application of antimicrobial agents that release a sustained high dose into the affected site over a course of several days also might provide beneficial effects in peri-implant mucositis treatment. Recommended agents are tetracycline HCl fibers (Actisite, Alza, Mountain View, CA)[89] or 25% metronidazol dental gel (Elyzol, Dumex, Copenhagen, Denmark).[90,91] Similar to periodontal therapy, tetracycline HCl fibers are placed into the peri-implant sulcus/pocket and are removed after 10 days. The 25% metronidazole dental gel is applied in the peri-implant sulcus/pocket and/or in the internal spaces of the fixture-abutment assembly. If peri-implant mucositis is refractory to mechanical and antimicrobial therapy and is associated with lack of keratinized and/or attached mucosa, gingiva extension surgery to ease oral hygiene may be indicated. However, most studies did not find a positive correlation between the width of attached or keratinized mucosa and peri-implant health.[15,17,51,92]

Peri-implant mucosal hyperplasia

Peri-implant mucosal hyperplasia is a rare peri-implant–associated condition that appears to be associated mostly with unfavorable conditions for local oral hygiene, such as insufficient space below the implant-borne fixed partial denture or under overdentures.[93] Improperly seated implant components also may lead to peri-implant mucosal hyperplasia. Mechanical debridement followed by a home-care regimen with adjunctive irrigation or rinsing with antimicrobials (as described for the treatment of peri-implant mucositis) should be attempted first.

If its design does not permit proper oral hygiene, the fixed partial denture should be removed temporarily or a provisionary fixed partial denture with wide-open embrasures should be made. After the lesion has been resolved, a new fixed partial denture that permits proper cleaning should be manufactured. In refractory cases, identification of bacterial pathogens and susceptibility tests may be performed and specific topical[89–91] or systemic antibiotics administered (Tables 14-2 and 14-3). In some cases, flap procedures or gingivectomy followed by a stringent maintenance regimen may resolve the lesion.[94]

Peri-implant fistula

Peri-implant fistula occurs very rarely, usually at the level of the implant-abutment connection. It may be associated with a loose or fractured abutment screw or plaque formation along the central abutment screw.[2] Microorganisms may penetrate the capillary space around the microgap between implant and abutment,[95,96] thus establishing a granulation tissue at the fixture-abutment junction that may propagate toward the mucosal surface and appear as a fistula. Recommended treatment steps[51] include:

- Excision of the fistula and mechanical debridement
- Cleaning and disinfection of the abutment and abutment screw
- Application of sealing agents between abutment and prosthesis
- Improvement of oral hygiene
- Surgical soft tissue corrections, if necessary.

Systemic antibiotics may be given in refractory cases after identification of the putative pathogens.

Table 14-2 Recommended therapies for the treatment of peri-implant mucositis and peri-implantitis[79]

Diagnosis	Clinical parameters*				Recommended therapy†
	Plaque Index	Bleeding on probing	Suppuration	Radiological defect	
Peri-implant mucositis	+/−	−	−	−	(A)
	+	+	−	−	A
Peri-implantitis	+	+	+/−	+/−	A + B
	+	+	+/−	++	A + B + C
	+	+	+/−	+++	A + B + C + D
	+	+	+/−	++++	E

*Clinical parameters: + designates present; − designates not present; +/− designates may be present.
†Recommended therapy codes:
   A. Mechanical debridement (plastic scalers, rubber cup, air-abrasive systems) and oral hygiene reinstruction.
   B. Antiseptic therapy: Rinsing with 0.1–0.12% chlorhexidine digluconate, pocket irrigation with 0.2% chlorhexidine, oral application of chlorhexidine gel.
   C. Antibiotic therapy: Systemic agent selected on the basis of microbiological testing or treatment with topical antimicrobial agents.
   D. Surgical therapy to change tissue morphology: Gingivectomy, apically repositioned flap, or guided bone regeneration procedure.
   E. Explantation (removal of implant).

Peri-implantitis

Diagnosis Peri-implantitis is associated with radiological signs of bone loss, suppuration, bleeding on probing, and increased pocket probing depths (see Table 14-2).

For peri-implantitis around implants that are progressively losing bone, treatment should be aimed toward eliminating bacterial infection, occlusal overload, and any other possible etiological factors. The affected implant should be decontaminated before repair is attempted. Air-abrasive systems, which cause little or no surface damage and possibly support stabilization by favoring cell adhesions,[97] have been found to be effective in decontaminating implant surfaces.[98] Care should be taken to prevent an air-emphysema when using high-pressure air-spray instrumentation at the surgical site.[99] Residual osseous defects may be treated with osseous graft materials and/or periodontal regenerative techniques.[100]

An increasing number of reports document clinical or radiological evidence of bone fill following regenerative treatment of peri-implant lesions[44,101–103]; however, true reosseointegration is rarely achieved.[104] Adjunctive irrigation or rinsing with antimicrobials as previously described for the treatment of peri-implant mucositis also should be initiated. In the treatment of peri-implantitis refractory to mechanical and topical antimicrobial therapy (see Table 14-3), appropriate microbiological analyses and antibiotic susceptibility testing should be initiated.

IMPORTANT PRINCIPLE

CLINICAL INSIGHT

IMPORTANT PRINCIPLE

Table 14-3 Antibiotic treatment of peri-implant infections

Agent	Local or systemic	Instructions for administration
Tetracycline fiber (Actisite)	Local	Apply to peri-implant sulcus/pocket and keep in place for 10 days
Metronidazole gel (Elyzol)	Local	Apply to the internal space of abutment-fixture assembly
Ornidazole	Systemic	2 x 500 mg by mouth every 12 h for 10 days
Metronidazole	Systemic	3 x 400 mg by mouth every 8 h for 8 days

Experimental and clinical studies have reported systemic administration of imidazole compounds such as ornidazole (1,000 mg per day for 10 days) or metronidazole[79,105] to be successful in resolving peri-implantitis. If an implant that has lost most of its bony support does not serve its function, it should be removed to prevent further bone loss or severe infection.

IMPORTANT PRINCIPLE For all recommended antimicrobials, it is imperative to rule out allergies and interferences with other drugs the patient may be taking. If necessary, alternative drugs need to be administered. Due to limited data in implant dentistry, the indications for antimicrobial therapy are still vague and mostly empirical. Further investigations regarding the management of peri-implant infections must be made to determine the optimal therapy for the various peri-implant complications.

References

1. Fiorellini JP, Martuscelli G, Weber HP. Longitudinal studies of implant systems. Periodontol 2000 1998;17:125–131.

2. Weyant RJ, Burt BA. An assessment of survival rates and within-patient clustering of failures for endosseous oral implants. J Dent Res 1993;72:2–8.

3. Hutton JE, Heath MR, Chai JY, Harnett J, Jemt T, Johns RB, et al. Factors related to success and failure rates at 3-year follow-up in a multicenter study of overdentures supported by Brånemark implants. Int J Oral Maxillofac Implants 1995;10:33–42.

4. Esposito M, Hirsch JM, Lekholm U, Thomsen P. Biological factors contributing to failures of osseointegrated oral implants. I. Success criteria and epidemiology. Eur J Oral Sci 1998;106:527–551.

5. Goodacre CJ, Kan JY, Rungcharassaeng K. Clinical complications of osseointegrated implants. J Prosthet Dent 1999;81:537–552.

6. Tonetti MS. Risk factors for osseodisintegration. Periodontol 2000 1998;17:55–62.

7. Lambert PM, Morris HF, Ochi S. The influence of 0.12% chlorhexidine digluconate rinses on the incidence of infectious complications and implant success. J Oral Maxillofac Surg 1997;55(12,suppl 5):25–30.

8. Flemmig TF. Antimikrobielle Therapie infektionsbedingter Peri-implantopathien. Parodontologie 1995;6:231–241.

9. Lang NP, Mombelli A, Tonetti MS, Brägger U, Hämmerle CH. Clinical trials on therapies for peri-implant infections. Ann Periodontol 1997;2:343–356.

10. Pontoriero R, Tonelli MP, Carnevale G, Mombelli A, Nyman SR, Lang NP. Experimentally induced peri-implant mucositis. A clinical study in humans. Clin Oral Implants Res 1994;5:254–259.

11. Augthun M, Conrads G. Microbial findings of deep peri-implant bone defects. Int J Oral Maxillofac Implants 1997;12:106–112.

12. Rosenberg ES, Torosian JP, Slots J. Microbial differences in 2 clinically distinct types of failure of osseointegrated implants. Clin Oral Implants Res 1991;2:135–144.

13. Flemmig TF, Höltje WJ. Peri-implantäre Mukosa und Knochen bei Titan-Implantaten: Die Rolle von Plaque, Zahnstein, befestigter Gingiva und Suprakonstruktion. Z Zahnärztl Implantol 1988;4:153–157.

14. Kalykakis G, Gregory-George KZ, Yildirim M, Spiekermann H, Russell JN. Clinical and microbiological status of osseointegrated implants. J Periodontol 1994;65:766–770.

15. Ellen RP. Microbial colonization of the peri-implant environment and its relevance to long-term success of osseointegrated implants. Int J Prosthodont 1998;11:433–441.

16. Lekholm U, Ericsson I, Adell R, Slots J. The condition of the soft tissues at tooth and fixture abutments supporting fixed bridges. A microbiological and histological study. J Clin Periodontol 1986;13:558–562.

17. Lekholm U, Adell R, Lindhe J, Brånemark PI, Ericsson B, Rocker B et al. Marginal tissue reactions at osseointegrated titanium fixtures. II. A cross-sectional retrospective study. Int J Oral Maxillofac Surg 1986;15:53–61.

18. Lindquist LW, Rockler B, Carlsson GE. Bone resorption around fixtures in edentulous patients treated with mandibular fixed tissue-integrated prostheses. J Prosthet Dent 1988;59:59–63.

19. Listgarten MA, Lai CH. Comparative microbiological characteristics of failing implants and periodontally diseased teeth. J Periodontol 1999;70:431–437.

20. Mombelli A, Van Oosten MA, Schürch E Jr, Lang NP. The microbiota associated with successful or failing osseointegrated titanium implants. Oral Microbiol Immunol 1987;2:145–151.

21. Mombelli A. Microbiology of the dental implant. Adv Dent Res 1993;7:202–206.

22. Mombelli A, Marxer M, Gaberthüel T, Grunder U, Lang NP. The microbiota of osseointegrated implants in patients with a history of periodontal disease. J Clin Periodontol 1995;22:124–130.

23. Nakou M, Mikx FH, Oosterwaal PJ, Kruijsen JC. Early microbial colonization of permucosal implants in edentulous patients. J Dent Res 1987;66:1654–1657.

24. Rams TE, Roberts TW, Tatum H Jr, Keyes PH. The subgingival microflora associated with human dental implants. J Prosthet Dent 1984;51:529–534.

25. Alcoforado GA, Rams TE, Feik D, Slots J. Microbial aspects of failing osseointegrated dental implants in humans. J Parodontol 1991;10:11–18.

26. Salcetti JM, Moriarty JD, Cooper LF, Smith FW, Collins JG, Socransky SS, Offenbacher S. The clinical, microbial, and host response characteristics of the failing implant. Int J Oral Maxillofac Implants 1997;12:32–42.

27. Sanz M, Newman MG, Nachnani S, Holt R, Stewart R, Flemmig T. Characterization of the subgingival microbial flora around endosteal sapphire dental implants in partially edentulous patients. Int J Maxillofac Implants 1990;5:247–253.

28. Sbordone L, Barone A, Ramaglia L, Ciaglia RN, Iacono VJ. Antimicrobial susceptibility of periodontopathic bacteria associated with failing implants. J Periodontol 1995;66:69–74.

29. Tanner A, Maiden MF, Lee K, Shulman LB, Weber HP. Dental implant infections. Clin Infect Dis 1997;25(suppl 2):S213–S217.

30. Danser MM, van Winkelhoff AJ, van der Velden U. Periodontal bacteria colonizing oral mucous membranes in edentulous patients wearing dental implants. J Periodontol 1997;68:209–216.

31. Bauman GR, Mills M, Rapley JW, Hallmon WW. Plaque-induced inflammation around implants. Int J Oral Maxillofac Implants 1992;7:330–337.

32. Gouvoussis J, Sindhusake D, Yeung S. Cross-infection from periodontitis sites to failing implant sites in the same mouth. Int J Oral Maxillofac Implants 1997; 12:666–673.

33. Apse P, Ellen RP, Overall CM, Zarb GA. Microbiota and crevicular fluid collagenase activity in the osseointegrated dental implant sulcus: A comparison of sites in edentulous and partially edentulous patients. J Periodontol Res 1989;24:96–105.

34. Lee KH, Maiden MF, Tanner AC, Weber HP. Microbiota of successful osseointegrated dental implants. J Periodontol 1999;70:131–138.

35. Quirynen M, Listgarten MA. Distribution of bacterial morphotypes around natural teeth and titanium implants ad modum Brånemark. Clin Oral Implant Res 1990; 1:8–12.

36. Wang IC, Reddy MS, Geurs NC, Jeffcoat MK. Risk factors in dental implant failure. J Long Term Eff Med Implants 1996;6:103–117.

37. Rivera-Hidalgo F, Stanford TW. Oral mucosal lesions caused by infective microorganisms. I. Viruses and bacteria. Periodontol 2000 1999;21:106–124.

38. Stanford TW, Rivera-Hidalgo F. Oral mucosal lesions caused by infective microorganisms. II. Fungi and parasites. Periodontol 2000 1999;21:125–144.

39. Brägger U, Burgin WB, Hämmerle CH, Lang NP. Associations between clinical parameters assessed around implants and teeth. Clin Oral Implant Res 1997;8:412–421.

40. Silverstein LH, Kurtzman D, Garnick JJ, Schuster GS, Steflik DE, Moskowitz ME. The microbiota of the peri-implant region in health and disease. Implant Dent 1994;3:170–174.

41. Adell R, Lekholm U, Brånemark PI. Surgical procedures. In: Brånemark PI, Zarb GA, Albrektsson T. Tissue-Integrated Prostheses. Osseointegration in Clinical Dentistry. Chicago: Quintessence, 1985:211–232.

42. Veksler AE, Kayrouz GA, Newman MG. Reduction of salivary bacteria by pre-procedural rinses with chlorhexidine 0.12%. J Periodontol 1991;62:649–651.

43. Bonine FL. Effect of chlorhexidine rinse on the incidence of dry socket in impacted mandibular third molar extraction sites. Oral Surg Oral Med Oral Pathol Oral Radiol Endod 1995;79:154–157.

44. Hämmerle CH, Fourmousis I, Winkler JR, Weigel C, Brägger U, Lang NP. Successful bone fill in late peri-implant defects using guided tissue regeneration. J Periodontol 1995;66:303–308.

45. Lang NP, Schild U, Brägger U. Effect of chlorhexidine (0.12%) rinses on periodontal tissue healing after tooth extraction. I. Clinical parameters. J Clin Peridontol 1994;21:415–421.

46. Larsen PE. The effect of a chlorhexidine rinse on the incidence of alveolar ostitis following the surgical removal of impacted mandibular third molars. J Oral Maxillofac Surg 1991;49:932–937.

47. Adell R, Lekholm U, Rocker B, Brånemark PI. A 15-year study of osseointegrated implants in the treatment of the edentulous jaw. Int J Oral Surg 1981;10:387–416.

48. Proceedings of the 1996 World Workshop in Periodontics. Consensus report implant therapy II. Ann Periodontol 1996;1:816–820.

49. Kenney EB, Weinlander M. Uncovering implants. J Calif Dent Assoc 1989;17:18–21.

50. Newman MG. Improved clinical decision making using the evidence-based approach. Ann Periodontol 1996;1:I–IX.

51. Weber HP, Cochran DL. The soft tissue response to osseointegrated dental implants. J Prosthet Dent 1998;79:79–89.

52. Wennström JL, Bengazi F, Lekholm U. The influence of the masticatory mucosa on the peri-implant soft tissue condition. Clin Oral Implants Res 1994;5:1–8.

53. Langebaek J, Bay L. The effect of chlorhexidine mouthrinse on healing after gingivectomy. Scand J Dent Res 1976;84:224–228.

54. Newman MG, Sanz M, Nachnani S, Saltini C, Anderson L. Effect of 0.12% chlorhexidine on bacterial recolonization following periodontal surgery. J Periodontol 1989;60:577–581.

55. Sanz M, Newman MG, Anderson L, Matoska W, Otomo-Corgel J, Saltini C. Clinical enhancement of post-periodontal surgical therapy by a 0.12% chlorhexidine gluconate mouthrinse. J Periodontol 1989;60:570–576.

56. Helgeland K, Heyden G, Rölla G. Effect of chlorhexidine on animal cells in vitro. Scand J Dent Res 1971;79:209–215.

57. Goldschmidt P, Cogen R, Taubman S. Cytopathologic effects of chlorhexidine on human cells. J Periodontol 1977;48:212–215.

58. Thomson-Neal D, Evans GH, Meffert RM. Effects of various prophylactic treatments on titanium, sapphire, and hydroxyapatite-coated implants: An SEM study. Int J Periodontics Restorative Dent 1989;9:300–311.

59. Burchardt WB. The Effect of Chlorhexidine and Stannous Fluoride on Fibroblast Attachment to Three Different Implant Surfaces [thesis]. Kansas City: University of Kansas City, 1990.

60. Paluzzi RG. Antimicrobial prophylaxis for surgery. Med Clin North Am 1993; 77:427–441.

61. Dent CD, Olson JW, Farish SE, Bellome J, Casino AJ, Morris HF, Ochi S. The influence of preoperative antibiotics on success of endosseous implants up to and including stage II surgery: A study of 2,641 implants. J Oral Maxillofac Surg 1997;55(12,suppl 5):19–24.

62. Garg A, Reiche O. Pharmacological agents used in implant dentistry. Part III. Antibiotics. Implant Soc 1992;3:7–8.

63. Peterson LJ. Antibiotic prophylaxis against wound infections in oral and maxillofacial surgery. J Oral Maxillofac Surg 1990;48:617–620.

64. Burke JF. The effective period of preventive antibiotic action in experimental incisions and dermal lesions. Surgery 1961;124:268–276.

65. Dajani AS, Taubert KA, Wilson W, Bolger AF, Bayer A, Ferrieri P, et al. Prevention of bacterial endocarditis. Recommendations by the American Heart Association. JAMA 1997;277:1794–1801.

66. Interpore IMZ Technique Manual, rev 3. Irvine, CA: Interpore International, 1987.

67. Conte JE Jr, Cohen SN, Roe BB, Elashoff RM. Antibiotic prophylaxis and cardiac surgery: A prospective double-blind comparison of single-dose versus multiple-dose regimen. Ann Intern Med 1972;76:943–949.

68. Kaiser AB. Antimicrobial prophylaxis in surgery. N Engl J Med 1986;315:1129–1138.

69. Nelson CL, Green TG, Porter RA, Warren RD. One day versus seven days of preventive antibiotic therapy in orthopedic surgery. Clin Orthop 1983;176:258–263.

70. Stone HH, Hanney BB, Kolb LD, Geheber CE, Hooper CA. Prophylactic and preventive antibiotic therapy: Timing, duration and ecomomics. Ann Surg 1979;189:691–699.

71. Lekholm U, Adell R, Brånemark PI. Possible complications. In: Brånemark PI, Zarb GA, Albrektsson T. Tissue-Integrated Prostheses. Osseointegration in Clinical Dentistry. Chicago: Quintessence, 1985:233–240.

72. Patrick D, Zosky J, Lubar R, Buchs A. Longitudinal clinical efficacy of Core-Vent dental implants: A five-year report. J Oral Implantol 1989;15:95–103.

73. Calcitek Inc. Integral biointegrated dental implants. Instructions for use phase 1: implant placement for Integral (4.0mm Diameter). 1988.

74. Schulte W. Das enossale Tübinger Implantat aus Al2O3 (Frialit). Der Entwicklungsstand nach 6 Jahren. Zahnärztl Mitt 1981;71:1181–1192.

75. Maeglin B. Allgemeine chirurgische Prinzipien. In: Schroeder A, Sutter F, Krekeler G. Orale Implantologie. Allgemeine Grundlagen und ITI-Hohlzylindersystem. Stuttgart: Thieme, 1988:256–264.

76. Schilli W, Krekeler G. Der verlagerte Zahn. Berlin: Quintessenz, 1984.

77. Pontoriero R, Tonelli MP, Carnevale G, Mombelli A, Nyman SR, Lang NP. Experimentally induced peri-implant mucositis. A clinical study in humans. Clin Oral Implants Res 1994;5:254–259.

78. Berglundh T, Lindhe J, Marinello C, Ericsson I, Liljenberg B. Soft tissues reaction to de novo plaque formation on implants and teeth. An experimental study in the dog. Clin Oral Implants Res 1992;3:1–8.

79. Mombelli A, Lang NP. The diagnosis and treatment of peri-implantitis. Periodontol 2000 1998;17:63–76.

80. Boyd RL, Murray PA, Robertson PB. Effect on periodontal status of rotary electric toothbrushes versus manual toothbrushes during periodontal maintenance. I. Clinical results. J Periodontol 1989;60:390–395.

81. Murray PA, Boyd RL, Robertson PB. Effect on periodontal status of rotary electric toothbrushes versus manual toothbrushes during periodontal maintenance. II. Microbiological results. J Periodontol 1989;60:396–401.

82. Flemmig TF, Berwick RHF, Newman MG, Kenney EB, Beumer J, Nachnani S, et al. Effekt von recall auf die subgingivale mikroflora von osseointegrierten implantaten. Z Zahnärztl Implantol 1990;6:45–51.

83. Berwick RHF, Flemmig TF, Kenney EB, Beumer J, Newman MG, Nep R, et al. Maintenance of gingival health around Brånemark fixtures with UCLA abutment [abstract 365]. J Dent Res 1989;68:912.

84. Adell R, Lekholm U, Rockler B, Brånemark PI, Lindhe J, Eriksson B, Sbordone L. Marginal tissue reactions at osseointegrated titanium fixtures. I. A three-year longitudinal prospective study. Int J Oral Maxillofac Surg 1986;15:39–52.

85. Lamster IB, Alfano MC, Seiger MC, Gordon JM. The effect of Listerine Antiseptic on reduction of existing plaque and gingivitis. Clin Prev Dent 1983;5:12–16.

86. Löe H, Schiött CR, Karring G, Karring T. Two years oral use of chlorhexidine in man. I. General design and clinical effects. J Periodontal Res 1976;11:135–144.

87. Flemmig TF, Epp B, Newman MG, Kornman KS, Haubitz I, Klaiber B. Adjunctive supragingival irrigation with acetylsalicylic acid in periodontal supportive therapy. J Clin Periodontol 1995;22:427–433.

88. Newman MG, Cattabriga M, Etienne D, Flemmig TF, Sanz M, Kornman KS, et al. Effectiveness of adjunctive irrigation in early periodontitis: Multi-center evaluation. J Periodontol 1994;65:224–229.

89. Schenk G, Flemmig TF, Betz T, Reuther J, Klaiber B. Controlled local delivery of tetracycline HCl in the treatment of peri-implant mucosal hyperplasia and mucositis. A controlled case series. Clin Oral Implants Res 1997;8:427–433.

90. Kleisner J, Kundert E, Geiser E, Andreoni C, Marinello CP. Effects of Elyzol dental gel on the submarginal microflora at implants [abstract]. [From the program of the annual meeting of the Swiss Society of Periodontology, 1994:48.]

91. Kleisner J, Marinello CP, Kundert E, Lüthy H. Prevention of bacterial colonization on implant components in vivo by a topical metronidazol gel. Acta Med Dent Helv 1996;1:250–257.

92. Krekeler G, Schilli W, Diemer J. Should the exit of the artificial abutment tooth be positioned in the region of the attached gingiva? Int J Oral Surg 1985;14:504–508.

93. Johns RB, Jemt T, Heath MR, Hutton JE, McKenna S, McNamara DC, et al. A multicenter study of overdentures supported by Brånemark implants. Int J Oral Maxillofac Implants 1992;7:513–522.

94. Rapley JW, Mills MP, Wylam J. Soft tissue management during implant maintenance. Int J Periodontics Restorative Dent 1992;12:373–381.

95. Persson LG, Lekholm U, Leonhardt A, Dahlen G, Lindhe J. Bacterial colonization on internal surfaces of Brånemark system implant components. Clin Oral Implants Res 1996;7:90–95.

96. Quirynen M, van Steenberghe D. Bacterial colonization of the internal part of two-stage implants. An in vivo study. Clin Oral Implants Res 1993; 4:158–161.

97. Augthun M, Tinschert J, Huber A. In vitro studies on the effect of cleaning methods on different implant surfaces. J Periodontol 1998;69:857–864.

98. Dennison DK, Hüerzeler MB, Quinones C, Caffesse RG. Contaminated implant surfaces: An in vitro comparison of implant surface coating and treatment modalities for decontamination. J Periodontol 1994;65:942–948.

99. Brown FH, Ogletree RC, Houston GD. Pneumoparotitis associated with the use of an air-powder prophylaxis unit. J Periodontol 1992;63:642–644.

100. Dahlin C, Sennerby L, Lekholm U, Linde A, Nyman S. Generation of new bone around titanium implants using a membrane technique: An experimental study in rabbits. Int J Oral Maxillofac Implants 1989;4:19–25.

101. Mattout P, Nowzari H, Mattout C. Clinical evaluation of guided bone regeneration at exposed parts of Brånemark dental implants with and without bone allograft. Clin Oral Implants Res 1995;6:189–195.

102. Jovanovic SA. The management of peri-implant breakdown around functioning osseointegrated dental implants. J Periodontol 1993;64(11,suppl):1176–1183.

103. von Arx T, Kurt B, Hardt N. Treatment of severe peri-implant bone loss using autogenous bone and a resorbable membrane. Case report and literature review. Clin Oral Implants Res 1997;8:517–526.

104. Wetzel AC, Vlassis J, Caffesse RG, Hämmerle CH, Lang NP. Attempts to obtain reosseointegration following experimental peri-implantitis in dogs. Clin Oral Implants Res 1999;10:111–119.

105. Persson LG, Araujo MG, Berglundh T, Grondahl K, Lindhe J. Resolution of peri-implantitis following treatment. An experimental study in the dog. Clin Oral Implants Res 1999;10:195–203.

Section 5

Special Considerations

Joan Otomo-Corgel, DDS, MPH
Stephen T. Sonis, DMD, DMSc

PROPHYLACTIC ANTIBIOTIC USE

Important Notice Regarding the Use of Antibiotic Prophylaxis

IMPORTANT PRINCIPLE

It is not possible to make recommendations regarding antibiotic prophylaxis for all clinical situations. Practitioners should consult the patient's attending physician(s) prior to providing dental care if questions arise regarding antibiotic prophylaxis. Any unusual clinical event should be noted and corrected immediately.[1]

Antibiotic prophylaxis is the administration of antibiotics to patients who have no known infection for the purpose of preventing microbial colonization and reducing the potential for postoperative complications. The principles guiding the selection of a regimen of antibiotic prophylaxis are listed in Box 15-1.

Box 15-1 Principles of antibiotic prophylaxis

- Benefits from prophylaxis outweigh the risks of antibiotic-related allergy, toxicity, superinfection, and the development of drug-resistant microbial strains[2]
- An antibiotic loading dose should be used
- The antibiotic should be selected based on the organism most likely to cause an infection[3]
- Before spread of microorganisms, the antibiotic should be present in blood and target tissues[4]
- Antibiotic prophylaxis should be continued as long as contamination from the operative site persists[5]

Bacteremia Leading to Colonization

Dental causes of bacteremia

It is well established that any procedure resulting in gingival bleeding may produce significant bacteremia.[6] Bacteremias have been documented after routine examination procedures, periodontal probing, prophylactics, brushing, flossing, and the use of pulsating-pressure irrigating devices. Both the degree of tissue manipulation and the status of oral health influence the magnitude of the bacteremia. Patients with gingival inflammation and periodontal disease develop significantly greater bacteremias, both in spectra and in amount of bacteria released, than do patients with clean, healthy mouths.

Colonization

In the healthy patient, bacteremias appear to be of little clinical importance. In the patient predisposed to localized bacterial colonization following bacteremia, however, a potentially life-threatening situation can develop.[7]

Infective Endocarditis

Etiology

KEY FACTS

In infective endocarditis (IE), bacteria, *Mycoplasma,* fungi, *Rickettsia,* or *Chlamydia* that are introduced into the blood colonize and multiply on the defective part or roughened surface of the heart. Areas of low blood flow and high turbulence are especially susceptible. An endocarditis results, with subsequent stenosis of the mitral valve. The oral cavity is the most frequently documented source of bacteremia leading to this condition. Streptococci of the viridans type are most often implicated; *Streptococcus sanguis* is generally regarded as the most common causative microorganism of infective endocarditis.[8] Some studies, however, have detected a decline in streptococcal IE[9–11] and an increase in IE caused by *Staphylococcus aureus, Staphylococcus epidermidis,* and HACEK (*Haemophilus influenzae, Actinobacillus actinomycetemcomitans, Cardiobacterium hominis, Eikenella corrodens, Kingella kingae*) microorganisms.[9]

Susceptibility

Experts on the subject of IE and patient susceptibility have not reached a consensus on risk categorization. Pallasch[12] has developed a risk table with categories based on potential for bacteremia and risk-benefit ratios for antibiotic efficacy versus toxicity (Box 15-2). The American Heart

Antibiotic prophylaxis recommended

Very high risk
Previous episode of infective endocarditis
Heart valve prosthesis
Coarctation of the aorta
Indwelling catheter left side of the heart

High risk
Rheumatic heart disease
Other acquired valvular heart disease
Congenital heart disease
    Ventricular septal defect
    Patent ductus arteriosus
    Tetralogy of Fallot
    Complex cyanotic heart disease
    Systemic pulmonary artery shunt
    Indwelling catheter right side of heart
    Mitral valve surgery
    Mitral valve prolapse with murmur
    Ventriculoatrial shunts for hydrocephalus
    Idiopathic hypertrophic subaortic stenosis

Intermediate risk
Tricuspid valve disease
Assymetric septal hypertrophy

Other possible risks
Orthopedic prosthetic devices
Immunosuppression
Hemodialysis

Antibiotic prophylaxis usually not recommended

Low risk
Mitral valve prolapse without murmur
Coronary artery disease
Atherosclerotic plaque
Previous myocardial infarction
Coronary bypass
Indwelling cardiac pacemaker
Congenital pulmonary stenosis
Uncomplicated secundum septal atrial defect
Ligated ductus arteriosus (> 6 months after surgery)
Autogenous vascular grafts (> 6 months after surgery)
Surgically closed atrial or septal defects, without Dacron patches (> 6 months
    after surgery)

*Very high-risk, high-risk, and intermediate-risk patients should receive antibiotic prophylaxis. No chemoprophylaxis is normally required for low-risk patients; check with patient's physician. Other indications may include orthopedic prosthetic appliances, hemodialysis, and impaired host defenses. Reprinted with permission of California Dental Association.[12]

Box 15-3 Risk categorization for cardiac conditions associated with endocarditis according to the American Heart Association[13]

Endocarditis prophylaxis recommended

High-risk category

Prosthetic cardiac valves, including bioprosthetic and homograft valves

Previous bacterial endocarditis

Complex cyanotic congenital heart disease (eg, single ventricle states, transposition of the great arteries, tetralogy of Fallot)

Surgically constructed systemic pulmonary shunts or conduits

Moderate-risk category

Most congenital cardiac malformations (other than above and below)

Acquired valvar dysfunction (eg, rheumatic heart disease)

Hypertrophic cardiomyopathy

Mitral valve prolapse with valvar regurgitation and/or thickened leaflets*

Endocarditis prophylaxis not recommended

Negligible-risk category+

Isolated secundum atrial septal defect

Surgical repair of atrial septal defect, ventricular septal defect, or patent ductus arteriosus (without residua beyond 6 months)

Previous coronary artery bypass graft surgery

Mitral valve prolapse without valvar regurgitation*

Physiologic, functional, or innocent heart murmurs*

Previous Kawasaki disease without valvar dysfunction

Previous rheumatic fever without valvar dysfunction

Cardiac pacemakers (intravascular and epicardial) and implanted defibrillators

*See text for further details.
+At no greater risk than the general population.

Association (AHA) revised its recommendations in 1997, stratifying risk into categories of high, moderate, and negligible (Box 15-3).

Premedication

Fortunately, most of the organisms implicated in IE are generally susceptible to the penicillins, with some notable exceptions. The current recommendations by the AHA, originally formulated in 1984, are penicillin-based. The advisory board of the *Medical Letter,* an authoritative and timely publication, changed their recommendation to an amoxicillin-based regimen because of its favorable uptake and spectrum properties. (Amoxicillin has been successfully used for IE prophylaxis for some time in the United Kingdom.) In 1997, a committee of the AHA updated its

Table 15-1 Prophylactic regimens for dental, oral, respiratory tract, or esophageal procedures[13]

Situation	Agent	Regimen*		Timing
		Adult	Child[†]	
Standard general prophylaxis	Amoxicillin	2 g orally	50 mg/kg orally	1 h before procedure
Unable to take oral medicines	Ampicillin	2 g IM/IV	50 mg/kg IM/IV	Within 30 min before procedure
Allergic to penicillin	Clindamycin	600 mg orally	20 mg/kg orally	1 h before procedure
	Cephalexin[‡] or cephadroxil[‡]	2 g orally	50 mg/kg orally	1 h before procedure
	Azithromycin or clarithromycin	500 mg orally	15 mg/kg orally	1 h before procedure
Allergic to penicillin and unable to take oral medicines	Clindamycin	600 mg IV	20 mg/kg IV	30 min before procedure
	Cefazolin[‡]	1 g IM/IV	25 mg/kg IM/IV	30 min before procedure

*IM—intramuscular; IV—intravenous.
[†]Total child's dose is based on child's body weight and should not exceed adult dose.
[‡]Cephalosporins should not be used in individuals with immediate-type hypersensitivity reaction (urticaria, angioedema, or anaphylaxis to penicillins).

KEY FACTS

recommendations for the prevention of bacterial endocarditis in individuals at risk for this disease.[13] These guidelines are meant to aid practitioners but are not intended as the standard of care or as a substitute for clinical judgment (see Table 15-1).

Major changes in the guidelines include:

1. Emphasis of the fact that most cases of endocarditis are not attributable to an invasive procedure
2. Stratification of cardiac condition into high, moderate, and negligible risk categories (Box 15-3)
3. Clearer specification of procedures that may cause bacteremia and for which prophylaxis is recommended
4. An algorithm that clearly defines when antibiotic prophylaxis is recommended for mitral valve prolapse (Fig 15-1)
5. Reduction of preoperative dose of amoxicillin to 2 g; follow-up dose no longer recommended
6. Changes in the types of antibiotics recommended in cases of penicillin allergy and patients unable to take oral medications
7. Recommendations for dental procedures and endocarditis prophylaxis (Box 15-4).

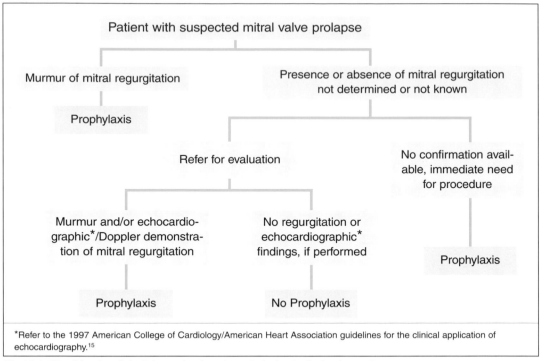

Fig 15-1 Algorithm for clinical determination of prophylaxis of mitral valve prolapse.

Patients with special considerations

Three groups of patients require alteration of antibiotic prophylaxis for IE:

1. Patients who are on antibiotics for dental or medical purposes
2. Patients who require a series of dental procedures over a 9- to 14-day period
3. Susceptible patients with aggressive periodontitis.[14]

IMPORTANT PRINCIPLE

Patients already on an antibiotic recommended by the American Heart Association regimen for another medical or dental reason should be given a different antibiotic premedication agent. For example, data suggest that penicillin-resistant organisms may develop in patients taking ampicillin; therefore, prophylaxis with clindamycin should be considered. Patients should continue their nonpremedication antibiotic as prescribed.

For patients who require a series of dental procedures within a 9- to 14-day period, condensing therapy should be considered to maximize use of the prophylaxis. If the time between procedures is less than 9 to 14 days, it may be more effective to alternate antibiotic agents to reduce the potential for developing resistant strains of bacteria.

Box 15-4 Dental procedures and endocarditis[13]

Endocarditis prophylaxis recommended*

Dental extractions

Periodontal procedures including surgery, scaling and root planing, probing, and recall maintenance

Dental implant placement and reimplantation of avulsed teeth

Endodontic (root canal) instrumentation or surgery only beyond the apex

Subgingival placement of antibiotic fibers or strips

Initial placement of orthodontic bands, but not brackets

Intraligamentary local anesthetic injections

Prophylactic cleaning of teeth or implants where bleeding is anticipated

Endocarditis prophylaxis not recommended

Restorative dentistry[†] (operative and prosthodontic) with or without retraction cord[‡]

Local anesthetic injections (nonintraligamentary)

Intracanal endodontic treatment; postplacement and post-buildup

Placement of rubber dams

Postoperatitve suture removal

Placement of removable prosthodontic or orthodontic appliances

Taking of oral impressions

Fluoride treatments

Taking of oral radiographs

Orthodontic appliance adjustment

Shedding of primary teeth

---

*Prophylaxis is recommended for patients with high- and moderate-risk cardiac conditions.
[†]Includes restoration of decayed teeth and replacement of missing teeth.
[‡]Clinical judgment may indicate antibiotic use in selected circumstances that may cause significant bleeding.

Actinobacillus actinomycetemcomitans is associated with localized aggressive periodontitis[14] and occurs in approximately one third of advanced cases of adult periodontitis. *A actinomycetemcomitans* may be resistant to penicillin; therefore, it is recommended that a pretreatment antibiotic regimen be provided first if cultures indicate high levels of *A actinomycetemcomitans* in an endocarditis-susceptible patient. Systemic tetracycline (250 mg 4 times a day for 21 days) or metronidazole and amoxicillin (250 mg of each 3 times daily for 8 days) may be used to eradicate organisms prior to the dental procedure. One day after completion of one of these regimens, dental treatment can be carried out with the AHA-recommended premedication.[16] Another regimen of metronidazole plus augmentin (250 mg each twice a day for 3 days) was shown to be effective against *A actinomycetemcomitans*[17] and may be considered a preparation for premedication; however, consultation with the patient's physician is advised.

Other Systemic Disorders

There are no data validating the use of the AHA's recommendations for antibiotic prophylaxis for the disorders described below; the clinician should base the potential for bacteremia and potential sequelae on an individual patient's risk-benefit ratio.

Hemodialysis patients

Hemodialysis removes impurities from the blood of patients with chronic renal failure. Blood is channeled from an artery to a dialysis machine, where it is cleaned and sent back through a vein. An indwelling arteriovenous shunt is surgically created to provide repeated access for the procedure. The associated risk for postoperative infection and infection of the catheter varies with each patient. If the patient is a cardiac risk and a hemodialysis patient, appropriate AHA premedication should be provided; however, any form of antibiotic prophylaxis should be provided only after consultation with the patient's nephrologist.

IMPORTANT PRINCIPLE

Transplant patients

To maximize the chances of graft survival, immunosuppression of organ transplant recipients is required. Transplant patients receive chronic doses of corticosteroids, usually prednisone, and possibly short courses of cytotoxic drugs such as Cytoxan. As a consequence of chronic immunosuppression, transplant recipients are susceptible to infection and therefore may require antibiotic prophylaxis before dental treatment and aggressive treatment of dental infection. The course of antibiotics recommended by the AHA may be adequate for most organ transplant patients; however, it is crucial that the dentist and physician communicate prior to dental treatment.

Immunocompromised patients

Cancer chemotherapy, bone marrow transplantation, other immunocompromising procedures, and leukemia place patients at risk for bacteremia-induced infections (see chapter 16). Again, consultation with the patient's physician is necessary to determine if the AHA premedication regimen or an alternate regimen is needed based on the patient's recent lab results and oral health status.

Antibiotic prophylaxis has been recommended when the granulocyte count falls to 1,000 to 3,500 per mm.[18–20] In these cases, dental procedures should be provided only on an emergency basis. Recent evidence indicates that immunocompromised patients have an increased mortality from gram-negative bacteria; therefore, meticulous oral hygiene and removal of sources of oral and periodontal bacteria need to be provided continually during surgical procedures.

> **Box 15-5** Patients at increased risk of hematogenous total joint infection[21]
>
> ***Immunocompromised/immunosuppressed patients***
> Inflammatory arthropathies: rheumatoid arthritis, systemic lupus erythematosus
> Disease-, drug-, or radiation-induced immunosuppression
>
> ***Other patients***
> Insulin-dependent (Type I) diabetes
> First 2 years following joint placement
> Previous prosthetic joint infections
> Malnourishment
> Hemophilia

Patients with joint prostheses

KEY FACTS

It has been suggested that a correlation exists between dental manipulation and late, nonoperation-associated infection of joint prostheses used in total hip replacement.[21] It is speculated that the bacteremia resulting from dental treatment seeds the prosthesis and produces infection. In July 1997, the American Dental Association and the American Academy of Orthopaedic Surgeons published the following advisory statement: "Antibiotic prophylaxis is not indicated for dental patients with pins, plates, and screws, nor is it routinely indicated for most dental patients with total joint replacements. However, it is advisable to consider premedication in a small number of patients who may be at potential risk of hematogenous total joint infection."[20] For a list of patients potentially at risk, see Box 15-5.

Patients with other diseases

Diminished capacity to fight infection Patients with a variety of other systemic disorders, as well as the very young or very old, may have a diminished capacity to deal with infection (see chapter 18). Antibiotic prophylaxis before dental manipulation may be desirable for patients with poorly controlled diabetes mellitus,[22] leukemia, Down syndrome, or cirrhosis of the liver; patients receiving steroids; splenectomized individuals; and patients with impaired host defenses.

To allow for varying medical status and degree of oral infection, these patients require individual consultation with their physicians. In particular, patients with acquired immunodeficiency virus should not receive antibiotic prophylaxis without first consulting with a physician due to potential development of antibiotic-resistant organisms that could create serious bacterial, viral, or fungal infections.

In each of these cases, communication with the patient's physician is imperative to determine the status of the patient's systemic disease and to assess the patient's current individual ability to deal with potentially infectious organisms.

Conclusions

Further research and evaluation of the use of antibiotics before dental procedures for the purpose of prophylaxis are greatly needed. When there is minimal inflammation, there is minimal to indiscernible bacteremia. Preoperative disinfection (eg, with chlorhexidine gluconate) may reduce bacteremia and is recommended by the 1997 AHA guidelines. A high level of oral hygiene reduces bacteremia, a fact that should be consistently reiterated to the patient. The dental profession should recognize the implications and indications of antibiotic prophylaxis, and attempts should be made to continually reduce inflammation in the oral tissues and to minimize the use of antibiotics during dental therapy.

References

1. Ciancio SG. Clinical Pharmacology for Dental Professionals. New York: McGraw-Hill, 1980.

2. Polk HC Jr, Lopez-Mayor JF. Postoperative wound infection: A prospective study of determinant factors and prevention. Surgery 1969;66:97–103.

3. Weinstein L. The chemoprophylaxis of infection. Ann Intern Med 1954;42:287.

4. Ryan DM, Cars O, Hoffstedt B. The use of antibiotic serum levels to predict concentrations in tissue. Scand J Infect Dis 1986;18:381–388.

5. Pallasch TJ. Pharmacokinetic principles of antimicrobial therapy. Periodont 2000 1996;10:5–11

6. Crawford JJ, Sconyers JR, Moriarty JD, King RC, West JF. Bacteremia after tooth extraction studied with the aid of prereduced anaerobically sterilized culture media. Appl Microbiol 1974;27:927–932.

7. Sipes JN, Thompson RI, Hook EW. Prophylaxis of infective endocarditis. A reevaluation. Annu Rev Med 1977;28:371–391.

8. Durack DT. Infective and noninfective endocarditis. In: Hurst JW, Schlant EC, Rackley CE, Sonnenblick EH, Wenger NK (eds). The Heart, ed 7. New York: McGraw-Hill, 1990:1230–1252.

9. Brandenburg RO, Giuliani ER, Wilson WR, et al. Infective endocarditis—A 25 year overview of diagnosis and therapy. J Am Coll Cardiol 1983;1:280–291.

10. Hessen MT, Abrutyn E. Gram-negative bacterial endocarditis. In: Kaye D (ed). Infective Endocarditis, ed 2. New York: Rave, 1992:251–264.

11. Gossius G, Gunnes P, Rasmussen K. Ten years of infective endocarditis: A clinicopathologic study. Acta Med Scand 1985;217:171–179.

12. Pallasch TJ. Antibiotic prophylaxis: Theory and reality. J Calif Dent Assoc 1989;17(6):27–39.

13. Dajani AS, Taubert KA, Wilson W, Bolger AF, Bayer A, Ferrieri P, et al. Prevention of bacterial endocarditis. Recommendations by the American Heart Association. JAMA 1997;227:1794–1801.

14. Armitage GC. Development of a classification system for periodontal diseases and conditions. Ann Periodontol 1999;4:1–6.

15. Cheitlin MD, Alpert JS, Armstrong WF, Aurigemma GP, Beller GA, Bierman FZ, et al. ACC/AHA guidelines for the clinical application of echocardiography. A report of the American College of Cardiology/American Heart Association Task Force on Practice Guidelines (Committee on Clinical Application of Echocardiography). Developed in collaboration with the American Society of Echocardiograpy. Circulation, 1997;95:1686–1744.

16. Slots J, Rosling BG, Genco RJ. Suppression of penicillin-resistant oral *Actinobacillus actinomycetemcomitans* with tetracycline. Considerations in endocarditis prophylaxis. J Periodontol 1983;54(4):193–196.

17. van Winkelhoff AJ, Rodenburg JP, Goené RJ, Abbas F, Winkel EG, de Graaff J. Metronidazole plus amoxicillin in the treatment of *Actinobacillus actinomycetem-comitans*–associated periodontitis. J Clin Periodontol 1989;16(2):128–131.

18. Antimicrobial prophylaxis and treatment in patients with granulocytopenia. Med Lett Drugs Ther 1981;23(12):55–56.

19. DePaola LG, Peterson DE, Overholser CD Jr, Suzuki JB, Minah GE, Williams LT, et al. Dental care for patients receiving chemotherapy. J Am Dent Assoc 1986;112:198–203.

20. Sonis ST, Fazio RC, Fang I. Principles and Practice of Oral Medicine. Philadelphia: WB Saunders, 1984.

21. Advisory Statement. Antibiotic prophylaxis for dental patients with total joint replacements. American Dental Association; American Academy of Orthopaedic Surgeons. J Am Dent Assoc 1997;128:1004–1008.

22. Alexander RE. Routine prophylactic antibiotic use in diabetic dental patients. J Calif Dent Assoc 1999;27:611–618.

Joan Otomo-Corgel, DDS, MPH

16

Antimicrobial Therapy for Immunocompromised Patients

Oral infections can seriously affect morbidity and mortality in immuno-compromised patients, and the number of these patients who present for care in the dental office continues to increase. This chapter covers antimicrobial treatment for prophylaxis and secondary infections in human immunodeficiency virus (HIV), cancer chemotherapy, and bone marrow/organ transplant patients.

HIV-Infected Patients

Although the death rate among those infected with HIV is declining in the United States and Europe, an estimated 34 million people have been infected with the virus.[1] Therefore, increasing numbers of people living with HIV—people whose immunologic repertoire predisposes them to increased susceptibility to opportunistic infections—will be presenting for treatment. The World Health Organization Clearinghouse on Oral Problems Related to HIV Infection and the World Health Organization Collaborating Center on Oral Manifestations of the Immunodeficiency Virus have an internationally accepted classification of oral manifestations of HIV (Box 16-1).[2]

Periodontal lesions

Periodontal lesions of linear gingival erythema (LGE), necrotizing ulcerative gingivitis (NUG), and necrotizing ulcerative periodontitis (NUP) have been associated with HIV-infected patients.

Box 16-1 Revised classification of oral lesions associated with HIV[2]

Group 1: Lesions strongly associated with HIV infection

Candidiasis
　Erythematous
　Pseudomembranous
Hairy leukoplakia
Kaposi sarcoma
Non-Hodgkin lymphoma
Periodontal disease
　Linear gingival erythema (LGE)
　Necrotizing ulcerative gingivitis (NUG)
　Necrotizing ulcerative periodontitis (NUP)

Group 2: Lesions less commonly associated with HIV infection

Bacterial infections
　Mycobacterium avium-intracellulare
　Mycobacterium tuberculosis
Melanotic hyperpigmentation
Necrotizing (ulcerative) stomatitis (NS)
Salivary gland disease
　Dry mouth due to decreased salivary flow rate
　Unilateral or bilateral swelling of major salivary glands
Thrombocytopenia purpura
Ulceration not otherwise specified (NOS)
Viral infections
　Herpes simplex virus
　Human papillomavirus (wartlike lesions)
　　Condyloma acuminatum
　　Focal epithelial hyperplasia
　　Verruca vulgaris
　Varicella-zoster virus
　　Herpes zoster
　　Varicella

Group 3: Lesions seen in HIV infections

Bacterial infections
　Actinomyces israelii
　Escherichia coli
　Klebsiella pneumoniae
Cat-scratch disease
Drug reactions (ulcerative, erythema, multiform, lichenoid, toxic spidermolysis)
Epithelioid (bacillary)
Fungal infection other than candidiasis
　Cryptococcus neoformans
　Geotrichum candidum
　Histoplasma capsulatum
　Aspergillus flavus
　Mucoraceae (mucormycosis/zygomycosis)
Neurologic disturbances
　Facial palsy
　Trigeminal neuralgia
Recurrent aphthous stomatitis
Viral infections
　Cytomegalovirus
　Molluscum contagiosum

LGE is described as a distinctive erythema of the marginal gingiva extending 2 to 3 mm apical from the free gingival margin.[3] Plaque does not appear to be directly associated with the condition and there is no bleeding on probing.[4] Candidal infection has been suggested to be etiologic in some cases of LGE,[5] but other studies have indicated both *Candida albicans* and periodontopathic flora consistent with adult periodontitis (*Poryphyromonas gingivalis, Prevotella intermedia, Actinobacillus actinomycetemcomitans, Fusobacterium nucleatum,* and *Campylobacter rectus*).[6,7]

Treatment recommendations include a culture or smear to identify the possible fungal infection and, in positive cases, follow-up antimycotic treatment in the form of twice-daily rinsing with chlorhexidine gluconate 0.12%. (See chapter 5 for more information.) Scaling and root planing are not recommended because erythematous tissue has been reported to be unresponsive to the treatment.[1]

Necrotizing periodontal diseases appear to be caused by bacteria. NUG is associated with gingival tissues only; there is no apparent clinical attachment loss. NUP develops rapidly from NUG. It may lead to a local, acutely painful ulceronecrotic lesion of the oral mucosa that exposes bone and may extend into contiguous tissues.[1]

Treatment involves encouraging patients to engage in meticulous home care, frequent periodontal debridement and monitoring, and adjunctive use of metronidazole and simultaneous antimycotic therapy.[8,9] Routine antibiotic prophylaxis is not recommended because it may lead to the development of resistant bacterial strains and candidal overgrowth; moreover, studies have shown that it makes no difference in wound healing.[10]

KEY FACTS

Oral candidiasis

Lamster et al[5] have found that distinctly different *Candida* species from those isolated from tongue and buccal mucosa appear to have a role in HIV-associated periodontal disease. There is a probable association between *Candida* and LGE as well as increased subgingival colonization of *Candida* in the presence of HIV infection.[5,11,12] In addition, unusual subgingival pathogens, including *Enterobacter cloacae, Klebsiella pneumoniae,* and *Clostridium* species, have been detected.[13,14] Further research is warranted in this area to determine etiology; in the meantime, oral candidiasis and other periodontal diseases are considered symptoms of HIV disease.

Odontogenic infection

IMPORTANT PRINCIPLE

Odontogenic infection can be a significant problem in HIV-infected patients. Periapical and pericoronal infection should be treated aggressively with root canal therapy or extraction. An HIV-positive patient whose immune system is adequate may be treated routinely if dental/periodontal infections occur. However, if the immune system changes—that is, if

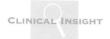

AIDS develops—adjunctive prophylatic antimicrobial therapy should be considered. Consultation with the patient's physician is essential to determine the need for prophylaxis, the type of antibiotic to be used, and the duration of therapy. These decisions should be based on the degree to which the patient's immmune system is compromised and the severity of the oral infection.

Cancer Chemotherapy

The dental patient undergoing chemotherapy may be myelosuppressed or immunosuppressed or may present with direct cytotoxic effects on oral tissues. Chemotherapy alone or in combination with radiation therapy destroys, suppresses, or prevents the spread of rapidly dividing (mitotically active) cells; therefore, normal cells as well as malignant cells may be altered. Gastrointestinal, reproductive, skin/hair, and hematopoietic (bone marrow) cells often are destroyed or adversely affected.

Oral changes

KEY FACTS

Odontogenic and periodontal infections are more prevalent in patients who become neutropenic during chemotherapy, which can occur 7 to 10 days after it is initiated. Odontogenic infections that would be limited to the oral cavity in an otherwise healthy patient can undergo systemic spread in the patient on cancer chemotherapy. If possible, sources of dental/periodontal infection should therefore be eliminated prior to initiation of cancer chemotherapy.

Gingivitis is common among patients undergoing cancer chemotherapy (see Box 16-2). Myelosuppression may necessitate the control of gingival hemorrhage by pressure dressing and/or topical hemostatic agents. The clinician should be aware of the patient's platelet count, which can affect gingival bleeding. When counts decrease to less than 40,000 per mm, thrombocytopenic bleeding is possible and is increasingly likely when counts drop below 20,000 per mm.[15] Note that periodontal manifestations may occur prior to diagnosis of the systemic condition.

KEY FACTS

Patients with a white blood cell count of less than 2,000 cells per mm or an absolute granulocyte count less than 1,500 per mm, and patients who will shortly develop neutropenia should be considered for antibiotic prophylaxis prior to emergency dental procedures. Selection of appropriate antibiotic therapy requires consultation with the patient's physician. Routine dental/periodontal therapy should be avoided. Some protocols even call for elimination of oral home care procedures due to the potential for septicemia.[16] Others recommend gentle debridement with gauzes and soft swabs dipped in chlorhexidine gluconate or povidone iodine, warm saltwater rinses, or chlorhexidine rinses.

Mucositis of the soft tissues of the oral cavity during cancer chemotherapy is also common. This is caused by the toxic effects of

> **Box 16-2** Oral changes associated with chemotherapy
>
> Mucositis
> Xerostomia
> Dysphagia
> Dysgeusia
> Gingivitis
> Soft tissue infection
> Candidiasis
> Sialadenitis
> Periodontal abscesses
> Pericoronitis
> Acute necrotizing ulcerative gingivitis (ANUG)
> Viral infections (herpes simplex virus)
> Neurologic effects

chemotherapy on the oral epithelium, but it can be secondarily infected by bacteria, candidal organisms, and/or herpes simplex virus. If a patient presenting with mucositis is undergoing combination drug therapy or chemoradiation therapy, lesions may last longer. Patients with mucositis should have frequent, gentle, professional debridements; practice meticulous home care; and use antimicrobial mouthrinses (Table 16-1).

Reactivation of herpes simplex virus in a severe and disseminated form also may occur in patients undergoing chemotherapy. Herpes simplex virus should be treated with antiviral medications such as acyclovir.[17] Fifty-four percent of adult patients with leukemia develop oral lesions during chemotherapy. Candidiasis also may be present and should be treated with appropriate antifungal agents (Table 16-1). See chapter 5 for more details.

Bone marrow transplantation

Bone marrow transplantation provides an option for patients with cancer and bone marrow disorders. It involves high-dose chemotherapy and/or total body irradiation to destroy cancer cells and suppress the immune system, which reduces the risk of host rejection of the grafted material.[18] The high doses of radiation increase the severity of the aforementioned complications associated with chemotherapy. Because of the incidence or reactivation of herpes simplex virus (over 80% in some studies), acyclovir prophylaxis commonly is used (see note in Table 16-1). Patients are evaluated before transplant, and those found to have positive antibodies to herpes simplex virus receive acyclovir prophylaxis throughout their therapy.

KEY FACTS

Table 16-1 Antimicrobial therapy for secondary infections

Type of infection	Treatment	Administration
Candidiasis	Nystatin suspension	Swish in mouth for 2 min, then swallow, 4 times/day for 14 days
	Clotrimazole troches	Dissolve 1 troche in mouth 5 times/day for 14 days
	Ketoconazole tablets	Take 1 tablet/day for 14 days
Odontogenic	Discuss antibiotic/antimicrobial Rx with MD; should be premedicated, especially if neutropenic	
Viral*	Acyclovir (intravenous)	5 mg/kg given over 1 hour 3 times/day for 5–7 days
	Acyclovir capsules	1 capsule 5 times/day for 7–10 days
Mucositis	0.12% chlorhexidine rinse	7 mL for 30 sec 3 times/day, starting the day before therapy and continuing until mucositis resolves
	Lukewarm saline or sodium bicarbonate solution (5%) rinse[20]	Apply topically before bedtime; no rinsing or drinking afterward
	Povidone iodine solution (5%) rinse	Apply topically before bedtime; no rinsing or drinking afterward

*Acyclovir prophylaxis for bone marrow transplant: Begin regimen of 1 acyclovir capsule 3 times/day 1 day before treatment and continue for 6 weeks. If during this period patient develops severe mucositis, administer 5 mg/kg 3 times/day of intravenous form of acyclovir until mucositis resolves, then resume therapy with the capsule form.

IMPORTANT PRINCIPLE Patients undergoing the transplant process need to be followed meticulously by the dental team. Prophylactic daily rinses of chlorhexidine gluconate have been recommended to reduce plaque, gingivitis, and candidiasis.[19] Delicate but thorough home care is imperative. Oral side effects of mucositis and painful ulcerations lead to an inability to eat or even talk comfortably. Because oral infections may lead to sepsis, frequent debridement and monitoring are necessary.

KEY FACTS If xerostomia occurs, the patient is more susceptible to caries, periodontal disease, *Candida*, and mucositis. Consequently, the patient may require daily fluoride therapy and a bland diet low in fermentable carbohydrates. The fluoride should not be administered within 4 hours of a chlorhexidine gluconate rinse because the latter bonds to fluoride, thereby reducing its effectiveness.

References

1. WHO end of the year annual report on HIV and AIDS. Geneva: WHO, 1998.
2. Classification and diagnostic criteria for oral lesions in HIV infection. EC Clearinghouse on Oral Problems Related to HIV Infection and WHO Collaborating Center on Oral Manifestations of the Immunodeficiency Virus. J Oral Pathol Med 1993;22:289–291.

3. Winkler JR, Grassi M, Murray PA. Clinical description and etiology of HIV-associated periodontal disease. In: Robertson PB, Greenspan JS (eds). Oral Manifestations of AIDS. Proceedings of the First International Symposium on Oral Manifestations of AIDS. Littlehouse: PSG, 1988:49.

4. Robinson PG, Winkler JR, Palmer G, Westenhouse J, Hilton JF, Greenspan JS. The diagnosis of periodontal conditions associated with HIV infection. J Periodontol 1994;65:236–243.

5. Lamster IB, Grbic JT, Mitchell-Lewis DA, Begg MD, Mitchell A. New concepts regarding the pathogenesis of periodontal disease in HIV infection. Ann Periodontol 1998;3:62–75.

6. Murray PA, Grassi M, Winkler JR. The microbiology of HIV-associated periodontal lesions. J Clin Periodontol 1989;16:636–642.

7. Murray PA, Winkler JR, Peros JW, French CK, Lippke JA. DNA probe detection of periodontal pathogens in HIV-associated periodontal lesions. Oral Microbiol Immunol 1991;6:34–40.

8. Glick M, Muzyka BC, Slakin LM, Lurie D. Necrotizing ulcerative periodontitis: A marker for immune deterioration and a predictor for the diagnosis of AIDS. J Periodontol 1994;65:393–397.

9. Robinson PG, Cooper H, Hatt J. Healing after dental extractions in men with HIV infection. Oral Surg Oral Med Oral Pathol 1992;74:426–430.

10. Glick M, Abel SN, Muzyka BC, LeLorenzo M. Dental complications after treating patients with AIDS. J Am Dent Assoc 1994;125:296–301.

11. Lucht E, Heimdahl A, Nord CE. Periodontal disease in HIV-infected patients in relation to lymphocyte subsets and specific microorganisms. J Clin Periodontol 1991;18:252–256.

12. Moore LV, Moore WE, Riley C, Brooks CN, Burmeister JA, Smibert RM. Periodontal microflora of HIV positive subjects with gingivitis or adult periodontitis. J Periodontol 1993;64:48–56.

13. Zambon JJ, Reynolds HS, Genco RJ. Studies of the subgingival microflora in patients with acquired immunodeficiency syndrome. J Periodontol 1990;61:699–704.

14. Rams TE, Andriolo M Jr, Feik, D, Abel SN, McGivern TM, Slots J. Microbiological study of HIV-related periodontitis. J Periodontol 1991;62:74–81.

15. Periodontal considerations in the management of the cancer patient. Committee on Research, Science and Therapy of the American Academy of Periodontology. J Periodontol 1997;68:791–801.

16. Mealey BL, Semba SE, Hallmon WW. Dentistry and the cancer patient. Part I. Oral manifestations and complications of chemotherapy. Compendium 1994;15: 1252,1254,1256.

17. Borowski B, Benhamou E, Pico JL, Laplanche A, Margainaud JP, Hayat M. Prevention of oral mucositis in patients treated with high-dose chemotherapy and bone marrow transplantation: A randomized controlled trial comparing two protocols of dental care. Eur J Cancer B Oral Oncol 1994;30B:93–97.

18. DeBiase CB. Oral care for the bone marrow transplant patient. Periodont Mgt 1996;3:1–7.

19. Epstein JB, Vickars L, Spinelli J, Reece D. Efficacy of chlorhexidine and nystatin rinses in prevention of oral complications in leukemia and bone marrow transplantation. Oral Surg Oral Med Oral Pathol 1992;73:682–689.

20. Semba SE, Mealey BL, Hallmon WW. Dentistry and the cancer patient. Part 2. Oral health management of the chemotherapy patient. Compend Contin Educ Dent 1994;15:1378, 1380–1387.

Joan Otomo-Corgel, DDS, MPH

17

CONSIDERATIONS FOR FEMALE PATIENTS

IMPORTANT PRINCIPLE

Approximately 12 million women take oral contraceptives, 18 million are on hormone replacement therapy, and every woman is at one time affected by puberty, menstruation, pregnancy, and/or all phases of menopause.[1] Each of these conditions or phases is associated with fluctuations in the production and utilization of estrogen and progesterone, which have the ability to alter concentration of systemic medications and produce changes in oral tissues. For example, 30% to 75% of pregnant women suffer from mild to severe gingivitis.[2] Therefore, it is essential to keep the medical histories of female patients up to date and to consider fluctuations in hormone levels before prescribing systemic antimicrobial/antibiotic therapy. This chapter discusses side effects and risks associated with the use of antibiotics and antimicrobials in women, with an emphasis on the effects of such treatment on pregnant and lactating women.

Considerations for Antibiotic Prescriptions

ADVERSE EFFECTS

Vaginitis

A common side effect of antibiotic use is vaginitis. When the vaginal mixed flora is depressed by the presence of an antibiotic, an overgrowth of *Candida* species can result. Recently, studies have indicated a possible association of vaginitis with preterm low-birth-weight deliveries. A postmenopausal patient is less likely to develop *Candida* infections because the vaginal flora have already been altered by an absence of estrogen.[3] Other bacterial vaginal infections can occur in these patients, however.

The older patient's symptoms could be caused by atrophic changes in the vagina that require hormone replacement therapy in addition to antibiotic treatment.

Although many women are aware of the likelihood of vaginitis when they are placed on antibiotics, it is important to remind a female patient of the risks and consult with her gynecologist about the feasibility of prophylactic vaginal suppositories (eg, nystatin) if the antibiotic is deemed necessary for the proposed dental therapy. If yeast infection or vaginitis occurs, it is best to refer a patient to her gynecologist rather than to risk inappropriate treatment.

Contraceptive failure

Antibiotic use in women has been implicated in the failure of oral contraceptives.[4,5] The effect of antibiotics on the enterohepatic circulation in relation to contraceptive steroids is proven in animals, but only rifampin, an antituberculosis agent, has been shown to cause contraceptive failure in humans by this mechanism.[6] Recently, studies have questioned the re-

lationship of antibiotics to oral contraceptive failure,[7–12] but until further research clarifies this issue, it is prudent to alert patients using birth control pills to the possibility of contraceptive failure and advise them to use alternative methods of birth control.

The Pregnant or Nursing Patient

Selection of an antibiotic for pregnant or nursing women must be made with equal consideration for mother and child. Antibiotics with systemic effects cross the placenta and reach the fetus. Note that the effect of a particular medication on the fetus depends on the type of antimicrobial, dosage, trimester, and duration of the course of therapy. The US Federal Drug Administration established a classification system to rate fetal risk levels associated with many prescription drugs (Box 17-1). Although drug concentrations in breast milk are usually low, a neonate's ability to metabolize drugs is underdeveloped, especially in infants born prematurely.[13–15] Tables 17-1 and 17-2 summarize the risks of antibiotic use in pregnant and nursing women.

When prescribing approved antibiotics to pregnant women, it is important to remember that the overall physiological changes that accompany pregnancy, particularly in the third trimester, reduce the serum concentration of antibiotics. Consequently, an adaptation—often a doubling—of the therapeutic dose is recommended.[16]

Box 17-1 FDA classification system*

A. Controlled studies in women fail to demonstrate a risk to the fetus in the first trimester (and there is no evidence of a risk in later trimesters) and the possibility of fetal harm appears remote

B. (1) Animal-reproduction studies have not demonstrated a fetal risk, but there are no controlled studies in pregnant women

   (2) Animal-reproduction studies have shown an adverse effect (other than a decrease in fertility) that was not confirmed in controlled studies in women in the first trimester (and there is no evidence of a risk in later trimesters)

C. (1) Studies in animals have revealed adverse effects on the fetus (teratogenic, embryocidal, or other) and there are no controlled studies in women

   (2) Studies in women and animals are not available; drugs should be given only if the potential benefit justifies the potential risk to the fetus

D. There is positive evidence of human fetal risk, but the benefits from use in pregnant women may be acceptable despite the risk (eg, if the drug is needed in a life-threatening situation or for a serious disease for which safer drugs cannot be used or are ineffective)

X. Studies in animals or human beings have demonstrated fetal abnormalities, there is evidence of fetal risk based on human experience, or both, and the risk of the use of the drug in pregnant women clearly outweighs any possible benefit. The drug is contraindicated in women who are or may become pregnant.

*A five-category system used by the FDA to classify drugs based on their potential for causing birth defects.

Table 17-1 Risks of antibiotic use in pregnant women

Drug	FDA category (prescription drug)	Safe to use during pregnancy?	Risks
Penicillins	B	Yes	Diarrhea
Erythromycin	B	Yes, avoid estolate form	Intrahepatic jaundice in mother
Clindamycin	B	Yes, with caution	Drug concentration in fetal bones, spleen, lung, and liver
Cephalosporins	B	Yes	Limited information
Tetracycline	D	Avoid	Depression of bone growth, enamel hypoplasia, grey-brown tooth discoloration in primary dentition
Ciprofloxacin	C	Avoid	Possible development of cartilage erosion in fetus
Metronidazole	B	Avoid (controversial)	Theoretical carcinogenic data in animals
Gentamicin	C	Caution, consult physician	Limited information, ototoxicity possible in fetus
Vancomycin hydrochloride	C	Caution, consult physician	Limited information
Clarithromycin	D	Avoid, use only if the potential benefit justifies the risk to the fetus	Limited information, adverse effects on pregnancy, outcome, and embryofetal development in animals

Table 17-2 Dental drug administration during breast-feeding

Drug	Safe to use while breast-feeding?*
Penicillins	Yes
Erythromycin	Yes
Clindamycin	Yes (with caution)
Cephalosporins	Yes
Tetracycline	Avoid
Ciprofloxacin	Avoid
Metronidazole	Avoid
Gentamicin	Avoid
Vancomycin hydrochloride	Avoid

*All antibiotics carry a risk of diarrhea and sensitization in the mother and infant.

Antibiotics and their effects in pregnant and lactating women

INFORMATION ABOUT SPECIFIC DRUG

Penicillins Penicillins (amoxicillin, augmentin, ampicillin) can be used in pregnancy without any known teratogenic effects.[13–16] Some controversy exists over whether breast-feeding causes the infant to become sensitized to penicillin. Parents should inform their children's pediatricians if their children were nursed when the mother was taking penicillins. Ampicillin is excreted in breast milk, though not in therapeutic doses. Also, an infant may develop candidiasis or diarrhea while the mother is on penicillins and breast-feeding.

INFORMATION ABOUT SPECIFIC DRUG

Tetracycline Tetracycline should not be prescribed to a pregnant or lactating patient.[16] It accumulates in bones and chelates calcium, inhibiting bone growth and discoloring teeth in the fetus, especially in the last half of pregnancy. Severe hepatoxicity also might occur in the mother. Infants exposed to tetracycline in breast milk have not shown bone and teeth changes, probably because the tetracycline is chelated by calcium in the breast milk. It is nevertheless contraindicated in lactating women because of the high concentration of the drug in breast milk.

INFORMATION ABOUT SPECIFIC DRUG

Cephalosporins Cephalosporins cross the placenta but are not associated with teratogenic effects or with concentrations of the drug in the fetus. Cephalexin is not believed to be excreted in breast milk in significant amounts.

INFORMATION ABOUT SPECIFIC DRUG

Erythromycin Erythromycin is often given to penicillin-sensitive patients; however, erythromycin estolates can cause intrahepatic cholestatic jaundice in the mother and is contraindicated in pregnancy and lactation. One recent study showed drug concentration in breast milk to be 100% of maternal serum levels.[17]

Clindamycin Clindamycin will cross the placenta and appear in the breast milk. It concentrates in fetal liver, kidney, bone, spleen, and lung tissues. Although no bone-growth changes have been reported from the drug, newborns should be examined closely if they were exposed in utero.

Metronidazole Metronidazole crosses the placenta and reaches high concentrations in breast milk. Although there has been no documented fetal damage from its use, data from animal studies have suggested that metronidazole could be carcinogenic.[18] Consult the patient's physician when this agent is considered in cases of severe or refractory oral infection.

Azithromycin This macrolide antibiotic, used to treat orofacial and respiratory tract infections, is believed to be safe for use by pregnant patients.[16]

Aminoglycosides Aminoglycosides frequently are used to treat urinary tract infections during pregnancy and are associated with ototoxicity and nephrotoxicity in the mother. When aminoglycosides have been taken during the last trimester, the infant should be evaluated for hearing loss. Aminoglycosides will enter breast milk and, although not absorbed by the infant's gut, may disturb intestinal flora.

Sulfonamides Sulfonamides are safe to administer in the first and second trimesters of pregnancy, but use during the third trimester or when breast-feeding can lead to kernicterus in premature infants. Glucose-6-phosphate dehydrogenase (G6PD) deficiency can result in hemolysis in infants who receive sulfonamides or nitrofurantoins. A family history of G6PD deficiency would contraindicate use of sulfonamides and trimethoprim sulfonamide combinations.

Chloramphenicol Chloramphenicol will cross the placenta and is excreted in breast milk in significant amounts. It cannot be metabolized by an infant's liver or kidney, and if used near term can cause "gray syndrome," which has a high death rate. Chloramphenicol should not be given to nursing mothers because of the underdeveloped enzyme systems of infants. A G6PD-deficient infant could contract neonatal hemolysis if his or her nursing mother uses chloramphenicol.[13,19]

Periodontal considerations

An increase in gingival inflammation and gingival exudate is a common oral manifestation of increased levels of ovarian hormones (estrogen and progesterone).[20,21] Pregnancy, oral contraceptives, menstruation, and puberty have been documented in relation to transient periods of gingivitis. As pregnancy progresses, there is a significant increase in gingival inflammation and proportions of *Prevotella intermedia, Porphyromonas gingivalis,* and *Prevotella melaninogenica* followed by a return to prepregnancy levels at parturition.[22,23]

It has been shown that estrogen increases cellular proliferation in blood vessels. Progesterone increases vascular dilation, thus increasing permeability,[24] which results in edema and accumulation of inflammatory cells. Progesterone also increases proliferation of newly formed capillaries in gingival tissues, alters the rate and pattern of collagen production, increases the metabolic breakdown of folate, and decreases plasminogen activator inhibitor factor type 2, which increases proteolysis.[25] Pregnancy also produces a maternal immunosuppression that renders the patient more susceptible to gingival inflammation.[26–28]

Most clinicians and researchers agree that if the pregnant woman institutes excellent home care, the incidence of gingivitis is reduced.[29] Antibiotics are not the treatment of choice at initial notice of gingival inflammation and should be reserved for use only when their benefits outweigh the risks. The safest times to treat the pregnant patient with antibiotics is during the second trimester and the first half of the third trimester.[30] Expanding infection with systemic involvement may require systemic antibiotics. It is important to recognize that the total blood volume of the pregnant woman will increase 40% to 55%; therefore, medication is more likely to be cleared and dosages may need to be increased.

Meticulous removal of irritants and good oral hygiene will reduce the need for systemic medications. Supportive periodontal maintenance visits should be made no less often than every 3 months during pregnancy and titrated according to the individual patient's needs. A patient on oral contraceptives is also more likely to have gingival inflammation and should be monitored and debrided at closer intervals as well.

Special note on pain medication associated with oral infection

A frequent question is whether oral pain medications should be given to pregnant or lactating women undergoing dental treatment. Postoperative dental pain, when severe, can be treated with analgesics with caution. Codeine, although it crosses the placental barrier and appears in small amounts in breast milk, can be given in therapeutic doses when needed for acute pain. Acetaminophen can be used safely as a nonnarcotic pain medication, but aspirin should be avoided during pregnancy and lactation because of its possible effects on the infant's platelets. Local anesthetics can be used with no ill effects to a fetus.

Summary: Benefits outweigh risks

It would be illogical to ignore or delay treatment of a dental infection during pregnancy since systemic effects of infection can be harmful to mother and fetus. For example, recent evidence associates periodontitis with preterm low birth weight.[31–33] Moreover, bacteremia and septicemia carry greater potential risk to the fetus than an antibiotic that crosses the

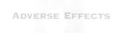

placental barrier. When antibiotics are given during pregnancy or breast-feeding, it is best to coordinate care with an obstetrician or pediatrician.

References

1. Wyeth Ayerst, 2000.

2. Raber-Durlacher JE. Pregnnang Gingivitis [thesis]. Amsterdam: Proefschrift Universiteit van Amsterdam, 1993.

3. Friedrich E. Vulvar Disease. Philadelphia: Saunders, 1976:17–25.

4. Gibson J, McGowan DA. Oral contraceptives and antibiotics: Important considerations for dental practice. Br Dent J 1994;177:419–422.

5. Zachariasen RD. Loss of oral contraceptive efficacy by concurrent antibiotic administration. Women Health 1994;22:17–26.

6. Gupta KC, Ali MY. Failure of oral contraceptive with rifampicin. Med J Zambia 1980–1981;15:23.

7. Helms SE, Bredle DL, Zajic J, Jarjoura D, Brodell RT, Krishnarao I. Oral contraceptive failure rates and oral antibiotics. J Am Acad Dermatol 1997;36:705–710.

8. Back DJ, Orme ML. Pharmacokinetic drug interactions with oral contraceptives. Clin Pharmacokinet 1990;18:472–484.

9. Fraser IS, Jansen RP. Why do inadvertent pregnancies occur in oral contraceptive users? Effectiveness of oral contraceptive regimens and interfering factors. Contraception 1983;27:531–551.

10. Murphy AA, Zacur HA, Charache P, Burkman RT. The effect of tetracycline on levels of oral contraceptives. Am J Obstet Gynecol 1991;164:28–33.

11. Antibiotic intereference with oral contraceptives. ADA Health Foundation Research Institute, Department of Toxicology. J Am Dent Assoc 1991;122:79.

12. Neely JL, Abate M, Swinker M, et al. The effect of doxycycline on serum levels of ethinyl estradiol, norethindrone, and endogenous progesterone. Obstet Gynecol 1991;77:416–420.

13. Beeley L. Adverse effects of drugs in later pregnancy. Clin Obstet Gynaecol 1986; 13:197–214.

14. Beeley L. Adverse effects of drugs in the first trimester of pregnancy. Clin Obstet Gynaecol 1986;13:177–195.

15. Bowes W. The effect of medications on the lactating mother and her infant. Clin Obstet Gynecol 1980;23:1073–1080.

16. Leophonte P. Antibiotics during pregnancy and breast feeding: Consequences for the treatment of respiratory infections [in French]. Rev Mal Respir 1988;5:293–298.

17. Zhang Y, Zhang Q, Xu Z. Tissue and body fluid distribution of antibacterial agents in pregnant and lactating women [in Chinese]. Chung Hua Fu Chan Ko Tsa Chih 1997;32:288–-292.

18. Giacoia GP, Catz CS. Drugs and pollutants in breast milk. Clin Perinatol 1979;6: 181–196.

19. O'Brien TE. Excretion of drugs in human milk. Am J Hosp Pharm 1974;31:844–854.

20. Löe H, Silness J. Periodontal disease in pregnancy. 1. Prevalence and severity. Acta Odontol Scand 1984;21:533–551.

21. Raber-Durlacher JE, van Steenbergen TJM, van der Velden U, de Graaf J, Abraham-Inpijn L. Experimental gingivitis during pregnancy and post-partum: Clinical, endocrinological and microbiological aspects. J Clin Periodontol 1994;21:549–558.

22. Kornman KS, Loesche WJ. The subgingival flora during pregnancy. J Periodontal Res 1980;15:111–122.

23. Offenbacher S, Jared HL, O'Reilly PG, Wills SR, Salvi GE, Lawrence HP, et al. Potential pathogenic mechanisms of periodontitis associated pregnancy complications. Ann Periodontol 1998;3:233–250

24. Lindhe J, Brånemark PI. Changes in vascular permeability after local application of sex hormones. J Periodontal Res 1967;2:259–265.

25. Kinnby B, Matsson L, Astedt B. Aggravation of gingival inflammatory symptoms during pregnancy associated with the concentration of plasminogen activator inhibitor type 2 (PAI-2) in gingival fluid. J Periodontal Res 1996;31:271–277.

26. Raber-Durlacher JE, Leene W, Palmer-Bouva CC, Raber J, Abraham-Impijn L. Experiomental gingivitits during pregnancy and post partum: Immunohistochemical aspects. J Periodontol 1993;64:211–218.

27. O'Neil TC. Maternal T-lymphocyte response and gingivitis in pregnancy. J Periodontol 1979;50:178–184.

28. Lopatin DE, Kornman KS, Loesche WJ. Modulation of immunoreactivity to periodontal disease-associated microorganisms during pregnancy. Infect Immun 1980;28:713–718.

29. Littner MM, Kaffe I, Tamse A, Moskona D. Management of the pregnant patient. Quintessence Int 1984;15:253–257.

30. Steinberg BJ, Rose LF. Introduction to the diseases of the endocrine system and the mechanism of action of hormones: Dental considerations. In: Rose LF, Kaye D (eds). Internal Medicine for Dentistry. St. Louis: Mosby, 1983:1210–1214.

31. Dasanayake AP. Poor periodontal health of the pregnant woman as a risk factor for low birth weight. Ann Periodontol 1998;3:206–212.

32. Offenbacher S, Katz V, Fertik G, Collins J, Boyd D, Maynor G, et al. Periodontal infection as a possible risk factor for preterm low birth weight. J Periodontol 1996;67(10 Suppl):1103–1113.

33. Gibbs RS, Romero R, Hillier SL, Eschenbach DA, Sweet RL. A review of premature birth and subclinical infection. Am J Obstet Gynecol 1992;166:1515–1528.

Mark J. Redd, DDS
Stefan A. Hienz, PhD, DMD

18

PATIENTS WITH COMMON SYSTEMIC DISEASES

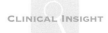

CLINICAL INSIGHT

As a result of advances in medical science, people are living with disorders that only a few years ago were fatal. Patients being treated for these chronic systemic disorders are often on multiple drug regimens; it is therefore essential that clinicians obtain a complete medical history and consider possible drug interactions before prescribing any medications. Because dental procedures may produce considerable bacteremia, it is particularly important that dentists have an understanding of a patient's underlying pathophysiology before making appropriate treatment-planning decisions. Consequently, clinicians also should consult with the physicians of patients at increased risk of infection before prescribing an antibiotic regimen (Fig 18-1).

KEY FACTS

To achieve maximum benefits from antimicrobial therapy, antibiotics must be administered prior to treatment.[1] Although they were not intended for such use, the guidelines issued by the American Heart Association for antibiotic prophylaxis can be used in the management of patients who are at increased risk of infection or delayed healing. Common systemic conditions requiring special consideration for antimicrobial therapy are discussed in this chapter and summarized in Table 18-1. Specific antimicrobial regimens for dentistry are presented in Table 18-2.

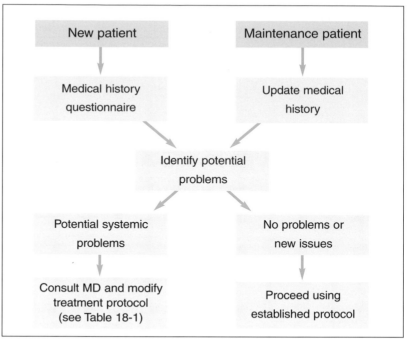

Fig 18-1 Identification of potential systemic problems.

Diabetes Mellitus

Background Diabetes mellitus (DM) refers to a group of disorders marked by hyperglycemia. Although each disorder in this group has its own unique pathogenesis, patients with DM share an inability to produce insulin in amounts necessary to meet their metabolic needs. They are prone to complications that are related to the severity of their insulin deficiency and an inability to achieve glycemic control.[2] The prevalence rate for diabetes has increased sixfold over the last 40 years[3]; it is estimated that 15 to 20 million individuals in the United States have diabetes, although only half of the affected individuals have been diagnosed.

Specific considerations Infection occurs frequently in diabetic patients, and the coexistence of infection and diabetes affects the management of both. Patients with uncontrolled DM have decreased host resistance, impaired granulocyte function, and delayed wound healing, which may increase their risk of infection. Control of blood glucose often leads to an improvement in resistance to infection. The need for antibiotics may vary depending on the patient's metabolic control, but for the treatment of acute dental infections, the choice of antibiotic, dosage, and route of

Table 18-1 Antibiotic considerations for patients with common systemic diseases

Systemic disease	Potential problems	Treatment modifications
Diabetes	Increased risk of infection in individuals with poor glycemic control	Antibiotic prophylaxis with postoperative regimen
	Increased incidence of candidiasis	Use of antifungal agents
	Sulfonylurea hypoglycemic agents used in treatment increase hypoglycemic effect with sulfonamides	Avoid use of sulfonamides
Sickle cell disease	Increased risk of infection	Antibiotic prophylaxis with postoperative regimen
Glucose-6-phosphate dehydrogenase deficiency	Hemolysis of erythrocytes with administration of certain antibiotics	Avoid use of sulfonamides, penicillin, and streptomycin
	Hemolysis of erythrocytes with dental infection	Antibiotic use taking drug sensitivity into account
White blood cell disorders (leukemia, lymphoma, multiple myeloma)	Increased risk of infection	Antibiotic prophylaxis with postoperative regimen
Rheumatoid arthritis	Corticosteroids, penicillamine, gold compounds, antimalarials, sulfasalazine, and immunosuppressive agents used in treatment increase risk of infection and delayed healing	Antibiotic prophylaxis
Systemic lupus erythematosus	Corticosteroids used in treatment increase risk of infection	Antibiotic prophylaxis with postoperative regimen
	Increased risk of infective endocarditis	Antibiotic prophylaxis
	Increased incidence of candidiasis	Use of antifungal agents
Sjögren syndrome	Increased incidence of candidiasis (caused by xerostomia)	Use of antifungal agents
Renal disease	Infection of vascular access site or transplanted organ	Antibiotic prophylaxis
	Altered renal metabolism of drugs	Avoid nephrotoxic antibiotics (tetracylcine and streptomycin)
Liver disease	Increased risk of infection	Antibiotic prophylaxis
Congenital heart diseases	Increased risk of infective endocarditis	Antibiotic prophylaxis
Congestive heart failure	Digoxin used in treatment	Avoid use of erythromycin
Chronic obstructive pulmonary disease	Theophylline used in treatment; theophylline toxicity can develop with certain antibiotics	Avoid use of macrolide antibiotics
Asthma	Theophylline used in treatment; theophylline toxicity can develop with certain antibiotics	Avoid use of macrolide antibiotics
Tuberculosis	Rifampin used in treatment increases liver toxicity with use of macrolide antibiotics, zidovudine, fluconazole, ketoconazole, and itraconazole	Avoid use of macrolide antibiotics, zidovudine, fluconazole, ketoconazole, and itraconazole
Bleeding and coagulation disorders	Decreased platelet function with β-lactam antibiotics	Avoid use of β-lactam antibiotics
	Increased bleeding problems with infection	Antibiotic prophylaxis
Organ transplantation	Tacrolimus used in treatment increases nephrotoxicity with erythromycin, clarithromycin, amphotericin B, clotrimazole, fluconazole, itraconazole, and ketoconazole	Avoid use of erythromycin, clarithromycin, amphotericin B, clotrimazole, fluconazole, itraconazole, and ketoconazole
	Decreased tacrolimus plasma concentration with rifampin and rifabutin	Avoid use of rifampin and rifabutin

Table 18-2 Common antimicrobial regimens in dentistry*

Clinical situation	Antimicrobial regimen
Antibiotic prophylaxis	Guidelines of the American Heart Association (1997)
	Erythromycin base 250 mg, #4, 4 tabs 1 h prior to treatment
	Chlorhexidine gluconate 0.12%, rinse 20 mL for 30 sec
Postoperative antibiotics	Amoxicillin 500 mg, #21, 1 tab every 8 h
	Cephalexin 250 mg, #28, 1 tab every 6 h
	Clindamycin 300 mg, #14, 1 cap every 6 h
	Erythromycin base 250 mg, #28, 1 tab every 6 h
	Chlorhexidine gluconate 0.12%, 1 bottle, rinse 20 mL for 30 sec every 8 h
Antibiotic treatment for acute infections	Penicillin V potassium 500 mg, #28, 1 tab every 6 h
	Amoxicillin 500 mg with clavulanate potassium 125 mg, #28, 1 tab every 6 h
	Erythromycin base 250 mg, #28, 1 tab every 6 h
	Cephalexin 250 mg, #28, 1 cap every 6 h
	Dicloxacillin sodium 250 mg, #28, 2 caps every 6 h
	Clindamycin 300 mg, #14, 1 cap every 6 h
	Metronidazole 250 mg, #40, 1 tab every 6 h
	Chlorhexidine gluconate 0.12%, 1 bottle, rinse 20 mL for 30 sec every 8 h
Antifungals (topical)	Nystatin 200000 units, #70, dissolve 1 pastille every 5 h
	Clotrimazole 10 mg, #70, dissolve 1 troche every 5 h
Antifungals (systemic)	Ketoconazole 200 mg, #10, 1 tab every 24 h
	Fluconazole 100 mg, #15, 2 tabs first day then 1 tab every 24 h

*Adapted from Wynn et al.[25]

administration is usually the same as for nondiabetic individuals.[2] Patients for whom glycemic control is in question should be considered for antibiotic prophylaxis before surgical procedures and tooth extractions, followed by an appropriate postoperative antibiotic regimen.[4,5]

In addition to a compromised immune system, these individuals often suffer from xerostomia. This can facilitate the emergence of opportunistic infections, including candidiasis, which is often treated with antifungal agents such as nystatin and clotrimazole.[4,6]

Bleeding and Coagulation Disorders

Background Most bleeding disorders are iatrogenic. Patients receiving coumarin to prevent recurrent thrombosis have the potential for bleeding problems. Most of these patients are receiving anticoagulant medication because they have had a recent myocardial infarction, a cerebrovascular accident, or thrombophlebitis.[7]

Von Willebrand disease is the most common inherited coagulation disorder, affecting 1 of every 800 to 1,000 persons in the United States. Hemophilia A, factor VIII deficiency, affects 1 of every 10,000 persons in the United States. Hemophilia B, factor IX deficiency, affects 1 of every 100,000 persons in the United States.[7]

Specific considerations Infection is known to complicate bleeding problems through alteration of the vascular wall. Antibiotic prophylaxis is suggested to prevent postoperative infections in patients with active periodontal disease and/or conditions that might render the patient susceptible. However, β-lactam antibiotics should be avoided because of their ability to interfere with platelet function.[3]

Anemias

Sickle cell disease

Background Sickle cell disease is a genetically derived disorder characterized by the presence of an abnormal hemoglobin molecule designated hemoglobin S. It is estimated that 8% to 10% of black Americans and up to 30% of black Africans are heterozygous for hemoglobin S. Sickled red blood cells are the cause of end-organ pathology in sickle cell disease; the spleen is the first and most common organ involved. This is a direct consequence of microvascular occlusion at the level of the capillaries and small venules. The net result is total vaso-occlusion with subsequent tissue infarction. The reduction in size or loss of the spleen may be a contributing factor to the likelihood of widespread bacterial infections.[8]

Specific considerations Infections as well as surgical procedures will invariably require antibiotic coverage.[9] Prophylactic antibiotics are recommended for surgical procedures to prevent wound infection or osteomyelitis. Intramuscular or intravenous antibiotics should be considered for use in sickle cell disease patients who have acute dental infections.

Glucose-6-phosphate dehydrogenase deficiency

Background Glucose-6-phosphate dehydrogenase (G6PD) is an enzyme needed for the hexose monophosphate shunt pathway. Blockage of this pathway in individuals with G6PD deficiency leads to the accumulation of oxidants in the red blood cells and their hemolysis. Glucose-6-phosphate dehydrogenase A deficiency, the most common form of the condition, is found in 11% of black Americans. Glucose-6-phosphate dehydrogenase MED deficiency, the second most common form, is found in ethnic groups of Mediterranean descent.[2,10]

Specific considerations While infection is the most common event that triggers hemolysis in G6PD A deficiency, drugs, including sulfonamides, aspirin, and chloramphenicol, are the most common trigger for hemolysis in G6PD MED deficiency. Penicillin, streptomycin, and isoniazid also have been linked to hemolysis in the latter group of patients. Dental infections may accelerate the rate of hemolysis; therefore, steps should be taken to avoid dental infections, and if they occur they must be dealt with effectively, taking drug sensitivity into account.

White Blood Cell Disorders

Leukemia, lymphoma, and multiple myeloma

Background Leukemia, neoplasm of the white blood cells, can involve myeloid or lymphoid cell proliferation and can occur in both an acute and a chronic form. Leukemia occurs in all races and at any age. There are approximately 27,000 new cases per year in the United States. Lymphoma, cancer of the lymphoid organs, is the seventh most common malignancy worldwide. Multiple myeloma is a lymphoproliferative disorder characterized by multiply cloned malignant plasma cells. Incidence is equal among men and women, and mean survival is only 2 years. Most cases occur in persons older than 65 years.[3]

IMPORTANT PRINCIPLE

Specific considerations Prophylactic antibiotics are used in leukemia patients and often are also recommended to prevent infection following a surgical procedure performed on patients with lymphoma or multiple myeloma. The need for prophylaxis depends on the type of medical treatment the patient is receiving and the status of the disease. For example, patients in remission usually do not require prophylaxis; however, prophylaxis is recommended for those receiving treatment for most acute oral infections because such infections are associated with profound granulocytopenia (less than 100 granular leukocytes per microliter of blood). In such cases, antibiotic prophylaxis should be continued for up to 1 week.[3] As a result of a compromised immune system, individuals with leukemia, lymphoma, or multiple myeloma often suffer from candidiasis, which often is treated with antifungal agents.

Disorders of Immune-Mediated Injury

Rheumatoid arthritis

Background Rheumatoid arthritis, an autoimmune disease of unknown etiology, is characterized by a symmetric inflammation of joints. Estimates of prevalence range from 1% to 2% of the population. Disease onset usually occurs in individuals between 35 and 50 years of age and is more prevalent in women than in men by a 3:1 ratio. Severe rheumatoid arthritis reduces a person's life expectancy by 10 to 15 years. This increased mortality rate usually is attributed to infection, pulmonary and renal disease, and gastrointestinal bleeding.[3]

Specific considerations The treatment of rheumatiod arthritis is palliative, utilizing pharmacological agents to reduce inflammation and swelling and relieve pain and stiffness of the joints. Many of these drugs, such as corticosteroids, penicillamine, gold compounds, antimalarials, sulfasalazine, and immunosuppressive agents, can cause blood dyscrasias that can lead to increased infections, delayed healing, and prolonged bleeding. It is recommended that patients with rheumatoid arthritis or patients taking the previously mentioned drugs receive prophylactic antibiotics for dental procedures likely to cause bleeding.[3]

Systemic lupus erythematosus

Background Systemic lupus erythematosus (SLE) is a multisystem, autoimmune disease of unknown etiology that primarily affects women of childbearing age (the female-to-male ratio is 5:1) and is more common and severe in blacks and Hispanics than in whites.[3] The course of the disease is highly variable and unpredictable. In SLE, the immune system attacks the host yet is unable to mount an effective attack against outside agents. Infection is a major source of morbidity and mortality in SLE patients worldwide.[11] Infections may mimic SLE flares, leading to delay in diagnosis or inappropriate increases in immunosuppressive treatment.

Specific considerations Corticosteroid therapy is common in the management of the SLE patient. Unfortunately, corticosteroids are immunosuppressive, affecting polymorphonuclear leukocytes and immunoglobin, and predispose the patient to infection.[12] Although any prednisone dose doubles the infection rate, doses greater than 20 mg daily have the most profound effect.[13] Therefore, the use of prophylactic antibiotics for periodontal and oral surgical procedures may be considered for leukopenic patients taking corticosteroids or cytotoxinc; however, it is highly recommended that the clinician consult with the patient's physician before prescribing any medication.

Infective endocarditis also is a potential problem in SLE patients. Libman-Sacks endocarditis (nonbacterial verrucous endocarditis) is found in 50% of patients at autopsy. The risk of infective endocarditis in SLE patients is similar to that in patients with rheumatic heart disease and prosthetic heart valves.[14] Following the guidelines set by the American Heart Association, antibiotic prophylaxis should be prescribed for dental procedures likely to cause bleeding.[3] (See chapter 15.)

Candidiasis occurs frequently in SLE patients. Constant inspection of the mouth and pharynx for signs of thrush and early institution of treatment (fluconazole for severe cases and clotrimazole troches for mild cases) might prevent many cases of systemic candidal infections.[11] (See chapter 5.)

CLINICAL INSIGHT

KEY FACTS

IMPORTANT PRINCIPLE

KEY FACTS

Sjögren syndrome

Background Sjögren syndrome, the second most common connective tissue disease, is characterized by a clinical triad of keratoconjunctivitis sicca, a salivary component (xerostomia), and another connective tissue disease, usually rheumatoid arthritis.[15]

Specific considerations Studies have suggested an increased incidence of oral candidiasis among patients with Sjögren syndrome, attributable to the reduction in salivary output in patients with the disorder.[16] Treatment of chronic oral candidiasis may employ topical drugs such as nystatin or clotrimazole or a systemic drug such as ketoconazole. Although systemic administration is convenient and not unpleasant, ketoconazole does not seem to be effective in patients with severe xerostomia.[15]

Renal Disease

Background There are approximately 8 million people in the United States who currently suffer from some form of renal disease. Chronic renal failure (CRF) is a progressive deterioration of nephrons that may be caused by a variety of factors. It manifests when 50% to 75% of the 2 million total nephrons lose function. It is a bilateral, progressive, and chronic deterioration of nephrons that results in uremia and ultimately leads to death—approximately 60,000 patients die annually as a result of CRF.[3,17] Signs and symptoms of uremia caused by CRF are manifested in a number of organ systems, including the cardiovascular, gastrointestinal, neuromuscular, endocrine, hematologic, neurologic, and dermatologic systems. Uremia may lead to anemia, bleeding problems, hypertension, electrolyte and fluid disturbances, and altered drug metabolism.[3,7] As disease progresses, conservative management of patients becomes inadequate and peritoneal dialysis or hemodialysis is required. An alternative to lifelong dialysis is renal transplantation.[3,18]

Specific considerations Patients receiving hemodialysis and those with transplants should be considered for antimicrobial prophylaxis before dental treatment that induces bleeding to protect the function and patency of the vascular access site and the transplant. Drug therapy may need to be adjusted depending on the degree of CRF, the patient's dialysis schedule, or the presence of a transplant. Because the metabolism of many drugs is altered in CRF patients as well as in those undergoing dialysis, antimicrobials that are nephrotoxic, such as tetracycline and streptomycin, should be avoided. Dosages of acyclovir, penicillin V, cephalexin, and ketoconazole should be reduced in patients with CRF.[3,17] The risks and potential problems, such as bacterial and fungal infections caused by poor oral health and gingival overgrowth secondary to cyclosporine therapy, should be explained to patients, as should the requirements for establishing and maintaining a healthy oral cavity.[19]

Liver Diseases

Background Liver diseases can lead to abnormalities in the metabolism of amino acids, ammonia, protein, carbohydrates, and lipids. Many biological functions performed by the liver, such as synthesis of coagulation factors and drug metabolism, can be adversely affected.[3] The most common liver disorders include viral hepatitis and alcoholic cirrhosis. Hepatitis might lead to cirrhosis, which is characterized by irreversible chronic injury of the hepatic parenchyma and includes extensive fibrosis in association with the formation of regenerative nodules.[3,17,18]

Specific considerations In addition to a deficiency of coagulation factors, cirrhotic patients have an impaired immune response caused by a diminished T-cell response and ethanol bathing of the sinusoids, which impairs Kupffer cells.[20,21] (Kupffer cells represent over 60% of the body's total reticuloendothelial capacity.) Consequently, antibiotic prophylaxis might be indicated, especially in patients with end-stage liver disease and those who have undergone liver transplantation.[3,19,20] A patient who has chronic active hepatitis or is a carrier of hepatitis B surface antigen (HBsAg) and has impaired liver function should avoid drugs metabolized by the liver, such as ampicillin and tetracycline.[3,12,19] However, no special drug considerations are necessary in the treatment of a completely recovered hepatitis patient.

Cardiovascular Diseases

Congenital heart diseases

Background Congenital heart diseases are alterations in the structure of the developing heart that cause changes in blood flow. These lesions constitute 1% to 3% of all cases of heart disease after infancy.

Specific considerations The primary concern in the treatment of this patient population, as well as patients with cardiac valvular abnormalities and surgically corrected cardiac and vascular malformations, is the prevention of infective endocarditis or endarteritis following dental procedures that produce transient bacteremiae.[22] Antibiotic prophylaxis should be prescribed (following American Heart Association recommendations) for dental procedures likely to cause bleeding. (See chapter 15 for more information.)

Cardiac arrhythmias

Background Cardiac arrhythmias may be disturbances of rhythm, rate, or conduction of the heart. They are found in healthy individuals as well as in those with various forms of other cardiovascular disease. The overall prevalence in the US has been estimated to be approximately 10% of the population.

Specific considerations The clinician should consider antibiotic prophylaxis when the underlying cardiac problem indicates need and/or when the patient has a pacemaker.[3,7,22,23]

Ischemic heart disease

Background Atherosclerosis is the underlying cause of ischemic heart disease, which affects more than 6 million Americans.[7]

Specific considerations Antibiotic prophylaxis generally is not indicated in these patients. However, patients who have undergone surgery to correct cardiac and vascular disease should receive antibiotic prophylaxis to prevent infective endocarditis or endarteritis following dental procedures that produce transient bacteremiae.

Congestive heart failure

Background Congestive heart failure (CHF), most commonly caused by coronary artery disease, hypertension, and valvular disease, affects between 1 and 2 million people in the United States.[3,7]

Specific considerations Patients with treated or poorly managed CHF are at risk for infection during dental treatment and should be considered for antibiotic prophylaxis. However, note that erythromycin should not be used in conjunction with digitalis glycosides because of digoxin toxicity.[3,12,24]

IMPORTANT PRINCIPLE

A note concerning cardiovascular diseases

Interestingly, some recent opinion holds that while certain dental treatments do not seem to be a risk factor for infective endocarditis, cardiac valvular abnormalities are strong risk factors for the disease.[25,26] Reliable quantitative data on the importance of oral bacteremia in the etiology of infective endocarditis are lacking, a fact that leaves the clinician with unproven assumptions regarding prophylaxis, fostering a standard of care that is well intentioned but possibly inappropriate.[27,28] Therefore, it is important for the dentist to keep up with the changes in recommendations for antibiotic coverage in these patients.

Diseases of the Respiratory System

Chronic obstructive pulmonary disease

Background Chronic obstructive pulmonary disease (COPD) is one of the principal causes of pulmonary disability in the United States. COPD is a condition in which there is chronic obstruction to air flow caused by chronic bronchitis and/or emphysema. It affects 13.5 million Americans, is primarily associated with smoking, and causes significant morbidity in the United States.[3,7] The management of COPD is based on the degree of obstruction, the extent of disability, and the relative reversability of the patient's illness.

Specific considerations Theophylline, although not a first-line agent in the treatment of COPD, has a narrow therapeutic range. Numerous factors and medications can replace the protein-bound fraction of the drug in the bloodstream and cause theophylline toxicity. Therefore, in patients taking theophylline, macrolide antibiotics and ciprofloxacin hydrochloride should be avoided because these drugs can result in an increase in serum concentrations and rapidly lead to theophylline toxicity.[3,29,30] Patients with COPD are at greater risk for recurrent infections with *Streptococcus pneumoniae* and *Haemophilus influenza* and are sometimes given continuous antibiotic therapy to prevent micropurulent relapses.[7,29] To avoid possible drug resistance, a different antibiotic regimen should be implemented in the treatment of dental infections in those patients.

Asthma

Background Asthma is a disease of airways that is characterized by increased responsiveness of the tracheobronchial tree to a multiplicity of stimuli. It is manifested physiologically by a widespread narrowing of the air passages and clinically by paroxysms of dyspnea, cough, and wheezing. It has been suggested that approximately 5% of adults and 7% to 10% of children in the United States and Australia have the disorder.

Specific considerations Drugs used in asthma therapy include beta-adrenergic agonists, methylxanthines (theophylline), glucocorticoids, chromones, and anticholinergics. Clearance of theophylline is reduced in the elderly and those with hepatic dysfunction and with the concurrent use of macrolides, ciprofloxacin, allopurinol, cimetidine, and propanolol. Dosage requirements should be adjusted accordingly; therefore, it is important to consult with an asthmatic patient's physician before prescribing antibiotics.[3,7,29,30]

Tuberculosis

Background Tuberculosis (TB), a chronic bacterial infection caused by *Mycobacterium tuberculosis,* is characterized by the formation of granulomas in infected tissues by cell-mediated hypersensitivity. Tuberculosis, which has made a resurgence in the last few years, continues to be a major problem in the United States, especially with the emergence of multiple drug-resistant strains of TB. Lack of compliance is suggested to be the most important cause of treatment failure.[29]

ADVERSE EFFECTS

Specific considerations Daily therapy with isoniazid and rifampin for 9 to 12 months is the most effective regimen available,[7] but it has serious side effects and drug interactions. Side effects include liver toxicity and hepatitis and are more pronounced in patients older than 35. Isoniazid and rifampin also can cause leukopenia and thrombocytopenia, increasing the risk for infection and bleeding[3,31–33]; therefore, antibiotic prophylaxis should be considered in these patients. However, it is important to note that rifampin increases the metabolism of zidovudine, clarithromycin, ketoconazole, itraconazole, and fluconazole, requiring clinicians to adjust dosages of these antimicrobials accordingly.

References

1. Classen DC, Evans RS, Pestotnik SL, Horn SD, Menlove RL, Burke JP. The timing of prophylactic administration of antibiotics and the risk of surgical-wound infection. N Engl J Med 1992;326(5):281–286.

2. Mealey B. Diabetes and periodontal diseases. J Periodontol 1999;70:935–949.

3. Little JW, Falace DA, Miller CS, Rhodus NL. Dental Management of the Medically Compromised Patient, ed 5. St. Louis: Mosby, 1997.

4. Rees TD. The diabetic dental patient. Dent Clin North Am 1994;38:447–463.

5. Alexander RE. Routine prophylactic antibiotic use in diabetic dental patients. J Calif Dent Assoc 1999;27:611–618.

6. Skoczylas L, Terezhalmy GT, Langlais RP, Glass BJ. Dental management of the diabetic patient. Compendium 1988;9:390,392–395,398–399.

7. Fauci AS, Braunwald E, Isselbacher KJ, Wilson JD, Martin JB, Kasper DL, Hauser SL, Longo DL (eds). Harrison's Principles of Internal Medicine, ed 14. New York: McGraw-Hill, 1998.

8. Sansevere JJ, Milles M. Management of the oral and maxillofacial surgery patient with sickle cell disease and related hemoglobinopathies. J Oral Maxillofac Surg 1993;51: 912–916.

9. Sams DR, Thornton JB, Amamoo PA. Managing the dental patient with sickle cell anemia: A review of the literature. Pediatr Dent 1990;12(5):316–320.

10. Beck WS, Tepper RI. Hemolytic anemias. IV. Metabolic disorders. In: Beck WS (ed). Hematology, ed 5. Cambridge, MA: MIT Press, 1991:283–299.

11. Petri M. Infection in systemic lupus erythematosus. Rheum Dis Clin North Am 1998;24:423–456.

12. Yagiela JA, Neidle EA, Dowd FJ (eds). Pharmacology and Therapeutics for Dentistry. St. Louis: Mosby, 1998.

13. Staples PJ, Gerding DN, Decker JL, Gordon RS Jr. Incidence of infection in systemic lupus erythematosus. Arthritis Rheum 1974;17:1–10.

14. Mills JA. Systemic lupus erythematosus. N Engl J Med 1994;330:1871–1879.

15. Hernandez YL, Daniels TE. Oral candidiasis in Sjogren's syndrome: Prevalence, clinical correlations, and treatment. Oral Surg Oral Med Oral Pathol 1989;68:324–329.

16. Navazesh M, Wood GJ, Brightman VJ. Relationship between salivary flow rates and *Candida albicans* counts. Oral Surg Oral Med Oral Pathol Oral Radiol Endod 1995;80:284–288.

17. Naylor GD, Fredericks MR. Pharmacologic considerations in the dental management of the patient with disorders of the renal system. Dent Clin North Am 1996;40:665–683.

18. Little JW, Falace DA. Therapeutic considerations in special patients. Dent Clin North Am 1984;28:455–469.

19. Douglas LR, Douglass JB, Sieck JO, Smith PJ. Oral management of the patient with end-stage liver disease and the liver transplant patient. Oral Surg Oral Med Oral Pathol Oral Radiol Endod 1998;86:55–64.

20. Watson RR, Borgs P, Witte M, McCuskey RS, Lantz C, Johnson MI, et al. Alcohol, immunomodulation, and disease. Alcohol Alcohol 1994;29:131–139.

21. Witte MH, Borgs P, Way DL, Ramirez G Jr, Witte CL, Bernas MJ. AIDS, alcohol, endothelium, and immunity. Alcohol 1994;11(2):91–97.

22. Dajani AS, Taubert KA, Wilson W, Bolger AF, Bayer A, Ferrieri P, et al. Prevention of bacterial endocarditis. Recommendations by the American Heart Association. JAMA 1997;277:1794–1801.

23. Lockhart PB, Schmidtke MA. Antibiotic considerations in medically compromised patients. Dent Clin North Am 1994;38:381–402.

24. Wynn RL, Meiller TF, Crossley HL, eds. Drug Information Handbook for Dentistry, ed 6. Cleveland: Lexi-Comp, 2000.

25. Strom BL, Abrutyn E, Berlin JA, Kinman JL, Feldman RS, Stolley PD, et al. Dental and cardiac risk factors for infective endocarditis. A population-based, case-control study. Ann Intern Med 1998;129:761–769.

26. Lacassin F, Hoen B, Leport C, Selton-Suty C, Delahaye F, Goulet V, et al. Procedures associated with infective endocarditis in adults. A case control study. Eur Heart J 1995;16:1968–1974.

27. Hall G, Heimdahl A, Nord CE. Bacteremia after oral surgery and antibiotic prophylaxis for endocarditis. Clin Infect Dis 1999;29:1–10.

28. Lockhart PB, Durack DT. Oral microflora as a cause of endocarditis and other distant site infections. Infect Dis Clin North Am 1999;13:833–850.

29. Hatch CL, Canaan T, Anderson G. Pharmacology of the pulmonary diseases. Dent Clin North Am 1996;40:521–541.

30. Levin JA, Glick M. Dental management of patients with asthma. Compend Contin Educ Dent 1996;17:284,287–288,290.

31. George DK, Crawford DH. Antibacterial-induced hepatotoxicity. Incidence, prevention and management. Drug Saf 1996;15:79–85.

32. Heathcote J, Wanless IR. Hepatotoxicity: Newer aspects of pathogenesis and treatment. Gastroenterologist 1995;3:119–129.

33. Westphal JF, Vetter D, Brogard JM. Hepatic side-effects of antibiotics. J Antimicrob Chemother 1994;33:387–401.

Edwin J. Zinman, DDS, JD

LEGAL CONSIDERATIONS

Infectious disease is the third leading cause of death in the United States, after cardiac disease and cancer, and the leading cause in the Third World.[1] The sixth leading cause of death in the United States is adverse drug reactions, which account for the deaths of 137,000 and the serious illness of 2,711,000 hospitalized Americans annually.[2] Fatal medication errors among outpatients doubled between 1983 and 1993.[3]

The standard of care of antibiotic chemotherapy limitation for preventive treatment of dental microbial infections is prudent usage. Imprudent or indiscriminate prescribing of antimicrobials places the patient at increased risk for adverse reactions, which in turn subjects the practitioner to liability. In addition, the overprescription of antibiotics propagates acquired drug resistance, reducing antimicrobial efficacy in the general population.

Antibiotics should not be regarded as the absolute panacea for infection control. Drainage and debridement of a localized abscess to remove infected purulent exudate may be necessary to promote antibiotic effectiveness. A patient's innate immune defenses may be ineffective if copious amounts of pus prevent antibiotics from walling off the infection.

Fiduciary Responsibility

IMPORTANT PRINCIPLE

Every dentist is bound by duty to act with fiduciary responsibility—that is, with the responsibility of a guardian—toward his or her patients to minimize the risk of injury and promote dental health. It is the same duty of reasonable and prudent practice that other fiduciaries such as accountants, lawyers, or banks owe to their clients. In short, a dentist is expected to act as a trustee for the best interest of the patient irrespective of the

257

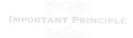

dentist's own best financial interest. Good documentation and record keeping are an essential part of a dentist's responsibilities.

Prudent vs Customary Practice

Prudent practice

As a general guideline, prudent practice in dentistry is an accumulation of methods taught in dental schools and continuing education courses and suggested in competent scientific articles, treatises, and textbooks. Prudent guidelines regarding the appropriate standard of treatment care have been promulgated by such organizations as the California Dental Association[4] and the American Academy of Periodontology.[5]

Customary practice

Customary practice, an arithmetic computation of what the majority of practitioners do under a given set of clinical circumstances, may constitute evidence of what a reasonable and prudent practitioner would do under the same circumstances[6]; however, it cannot be the only determinant of what a careful and prudent practitioner should do. For instance, some oral surgeons customarily rely on panographic radiography alone for the diagnosis of fractures. Yet it is well known and taught that such tomographic films as the Panorex do not have the diagnostic accuracy of static-beam periapical radiographs.[7-12] Consequently, a radiographically diagnosable fracture could be misdiagnosed as normal. Therefore, a practitioner who follows the customary practice of some practitioners, or even a majority of practitioners, does not necessarily meet the legal standard of care required of a prudent practitioner.

Patients should not dictate the standard of care if it is contrary to their dental and medical interests. For example, if a patient with an existing heart valve arrives at the dentist's office without taking the prescribed dosage of antibiotics 1 hour before the appointment in accordance with American Heart Association guidelines, the dentist should refuse to treat that patient (see chapter 15). A practitioner must not acquiesce if a patient promises to take the prophylactic medication immediately after the appointment and to remember to follow the dentist's directions at the next scheduled maintenance appointment. A patient cannot legally and validly consent to negligent care. A dentist who permits a patient to override his or her best judgment and recommendations violates the standard of care pursuant to the circumstances. Examples of customary dental practices that violate the standard of care are included in Box 19-1.

In summary, no matter how many dentists engage in them, negligent practices are never right. A customarily negligent practice does not equate with the standard of care of prudent practitioners.

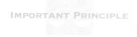

Box 19-1 Customary dental practices that violate the standard of care

1. Failure to take diagnostic-quality radiographs for caries or periodontal disease
2. Improper angulation or development of radiographs[14–16]
3. Diagnosis of pathology solely on a wet reading rather than waiting for the image to be finally fixed on the film[17–19]
4. Failure to use a calibrated periodontal probe for the diagnosis of periodontal disease
5. Incomplete charting of pathology on dental records[20]
6. Failure to diagnose major oral lesions associated with AIDS (only 22% of dentists routinely used gloves for all patients)[21]
7. Use of experimental drugs, such as Sargenti paraformaldehyde endodontic paste or N2
8. Failure to prescribe antibiotics in accordance with recommendations of the American Heart Association[22]
9. Failure to acquire adequate informed consent[23]
10. Use of inadequate sterilization techniques[24]

Causation

IMPORTANT PRINCIPLE

Legal causation is measured by either the proximate cause or the substantial factor test. Under the proximate cause test, the proof of legal causation is that "but for" the actions of the tort-feasor (wrongdoer), the damage or injury would not have occurred. Many states, such as California, have eliminated proximate cause in favor of the substantial factor test, which requires the plaintiff to prove only that the tort-feasor's conduct or omissions constituted a substantial factor in causing injury.[13] Thus, the wrongdoing need not be the only factor which contributed to the cause of the plaintiff's injuries; so long as its contribution to the injury was significant, the wrongdoer is still liable. Consequently, when a negligent factor and an innocent factor combine to cause injury, the wrongdoing tort-feasor is subject to liability. For instance, postoperative antibiotics may not entirely eliminate the potential for postoperative infection, but omitting to prescribe them may constitute a substantial factor in increasing the incidence or severity of postoperative infection and thereby render the dentist liable.

By way of defense, evidence may be introduced suggesting that infection would have occurred in any event, regardless of whether the dentist had followed recommended prophylactic administration. However, following the recommended regimen reduces the risk of adverse consequences; therefore, the standard of care should always be followed to reduce the risk, regardless of whether such risk is completely avoidable. While the causal link—that the harm was more likely than not a factual result of the dentist's negligence—must be established by expert testimony, the issue of causation remains a jury question.[25]

Alternative Methods of Treatment

Majority vs minority methods

There can be more than one acceptable treatment for a given dental infection. It is not negligent to follow a school of thought different from that of the majority of practitioners, provided that the minority method of treatment is adhered to by respected members of the profession.[6] For example, while many practitioners do not believe an antibiotic is prophylactically required following tooth extraction if there is no pronounced swelling or fever,[26] some practitioners prescribe prophylactic antibiotic therapy for any residual infection or to prevent secondary infection.[27,28] Either course of action is acceptable; however, where a substantial risk of infection exists, antibiotics are required by all prudent practitioners, irrespective of how many practitioners customarily meet that standard. Prudent practice also dictates prophylactic antibiotics when there is a sinus exposure and a risk of oroantral fistula develops.[29]

Foreseeable risk

The legal test is not whether a given method of treatment has resulted in injury in the past, but whether injury is a foreseeable risk, or the likelihood of injury is increased, by imprudent practice.[30] Unlike a dog, which is legally entitled to one free bite before it is determined to have vicious propensities, dentists are responsible for the "first bite" if such negligent conduct creates a foreseeable, unreasonable risk of harm to the patient.[31]

Duty to Refer to a Specialist

If immediate blood levels of an antibiotic are required because of life-threatening acute infections, oral antibiotics may be insufficient.[32] Moreover, studies have shown that approximately one half of all prescriptions are not filled or followed by the patient.[33,34] Consequently, to obtain an adequate blood level of an antibiotic, intramuscular or intravenous antibiotic therapy may be required.[35] If the dentist does not have the antibiotic available in parenteral form, then immediate referral to an oral surgeon or physician for parenteral administration is recommended.

Antibiotics alone may be inadequate therapy for a fulminating space infection with purulence because adequate blood levels of the drug may not reach the site effectively. Accordingly, when fluctuance occurs, surgical incision and drainage procedures along with bacterial culture/susceptibility tests should supplement antibiotic therapy (see chapter 2). An untrained generalist should refer such procedures to an oral surgeon; otherwise, the generalist will be held to the standard of care of an oral surgeon who ordinarily performs incision and drainage.

Duty to Obtain Medical History

Every patient, whether for emergency treatment or complete examination, can be treated adequately only after a complete medical history is taken.[36] Examples of such histories have been published in the American Dental Association's *Accepted Dental Therapeutics*.[37] Updating a patient's medical history is required at each recall visit since appropriate treatment for an individual patient can change from one year to the next. Frequently litigated examples are the occurrence of rheumatic fever between dental visits and newly acquired drug allergies. A signed medical history is not legally required; however, in the event that the patient disputes that a medical history was taken, a signed and dated history is more credible to a jury than a dentist's memory.

Locality Rule

Under former laws and the minority rules of some states, a dentist could be judged only by the standards of other dentists practicing in that locality.[38] This antiquated rule existed because access to current methodology was not equal between rural and urban practitioners. Modern communication and transportation have eliminated the need for the rule. In abolishing it, the Massachusetts Supreme Court held, "The time has come when the medical profession should no longer be balkanized by the application of varying geographical standards in malpractice cases."[39]

The changing standard of care regarding antibiotic prophylaxis in patients with rheumatic valvular defects with regurgitation, intracardiac prostheses, and prosthetic joint replacements is an example of knowledge with a national scope. Thus, a dentist who prescribed the 1992 recommended dosage level[40–42] instead of the dosage recommended in 1997[43–45] would be liable for not increasing the frequency or dosage of prophylactic antibiotics if it could be proven that the onset or severity of subacute bacterial endocarditis was causally related to the insufficient blood level of the prescribed antibiotic.

Consultation with a Physician

A dentist is legally regarded as an expert on the pathophysiology of structures of the maxillofacial area. It is therefore important that the dentist be alert to oral implications such as diminished resistance to infections and resultant poor healing, autoimmune and immunosuppressive diseases, diabetes, and other systemic diseases.

Neoplastic and autoimmune diseases

Because disease severity or degree of patient control of a disease can affect the decision for antibiotic coverage in surgical or dental procedures involving the gingiva, physician consultation is suggested for patients suffering from neoplastic or selected autoimmune diseases.

Diabetes

Although diabetes is a risk factor for periodontitis, treatment of a well-controlled diabetic should not vary from that of a systemically healthy patient with the same periodontal diagnosis. Antibiotics are required only if an otherwise healthy patient also would be prescribed antibiotics—for example, in the therapeutic treatment of acute or postoperative infections.

Diabetes can affect the patient adversely during and after surgery by increasing the risk of onset and severity of infection. Consequently, the regulation of a patient's insulin during surgery is a medical decision obtained through consultation with the patient's physician. On the other hand, the decision to prescribe postoperative therapeutic doses of antibiotics is usually determined by the treating dentist, who is more familiar with the nature of the dental surgical procedure than the patient's physician.

AIDS

Antibiotics for an AIDS patient may interfere with the patient's existing medication and may result in superinfection because of the patient's immunosuppressed status. Accordingly, consultation with the patient's primary physician is required.

Yeast is the main cause of fungal infections in the oral cavity, and *Candida albicans* is the most prevalent species. Dentists should therefore be alert to diagnosing and treating fungal infections with antifungicides in those immunocompromised patients whose yeast flora increase as a result of lowered resistance. In HIV-seropositive patients whose AIDS symptoms have not manifested, the oral cavity can be the first body site affected by *Candida* infections, which represent the premonitor sign of the syndrome.[42]

Failure to consult

A dentist who fails to consult with a dental specialist or a patient's physician when the presenting infection is not controllable initially or postoperatively with oral antibiotics may be negligent. For instance, if a patient who received appropriate prophylactic antibiotics such as oral penicillin for periodontic, endodontic, or impaction surgery complains of pain or dysphagia and exhibits submandibular or infraorbital swelling 48 hours or more after surgery, a consultation with an oral surgeon is mandatory since oral antibiotics most likely would be inadequate to control the spreading infection. The fulminating infection could potentially impair the airway, cause blindness, or precipitate a cavernous sinus thrombosis or brain abscess. In such a situation, incision, drainage, and culturing for susceptible microorganisms would be required by the standard of care.

Necessity for Culture

Routine treatment

Cultures are not currently used during routine dental treatment. Although previously recommended, they are no longer used to verify the sterility of root canal systems after endodontic cleaning and shaping. Proper biomechanical debridement of the root canal is considered sufficient.[46]

Oral infection

Cultures are used for cellulitis in which initial antibiotic dosage and selection have failed to prevent the infection from invading adjacent tissue spaces or for the immunocompromised patient whose clinical course cannot be predicted. The spreading infection may be caused by a resistant or arcane microorganism that a culture and susceptibility test, including blood culture, can isolate and identify. Although penicillin is the drug of choice for oral infections, penicillinase-producing organisms present in an infection may reduce its effectiveness. Culturing can pinpoint the appropriate antimicrobial drug and dosage to be administered under such circumstances.

Although a dentist need not identify the specific etiologic organism before prescribing an antimicrobial drug, he or she is duty-bound to identify the causative organisms if initial antibiotic therapy proves ineffective. Only by identifying the principal pathogenic organisms can selective antibiotic therapy control otherwise resistant microorganisms.

Dosage

Antibiotics must be prescribed in adequate dosages. Patients should be advised to complete all prescribed antibiotic regimens to protect against the development of resistant strains. Prevalence of increasingly resistant strains has resulted in concomitant increases in duration, dosage, and strength of drug prescribed. For instance, 250 mg of penicillin taken four times per day as a therapeutic or prophylactic dose is now outmoded; a minimum of 500 mg four times per day plus the appropriate loading dose of up to 2,000 mg should be prescribed. When a dentist fails to prescribe an adequate dosage of antimicrobial, the legal burden of proof that the cause of the infection or its spread was not the lower than acceptable prescribed levels may fall upon the dentist.[47]

Informed Consent

The legal doctrine of requiring informed consent to inherent and collateral risks of a procedure applies primarily to elective procedures where the therapeutic risks are usually not appreciated by the patient. Specifically, the patient should be told of the benefits and likely risks associated with a drug and the consequences of not taking the prescribed medication. Patient information for several drugs, including tetracycline, penicillin, and erythromycin, is available from the American Dental Association and the American Medical Association in the form of tear-out pads.

Reasonable risk

When informed consent is not given, many states permit the jury to consider as a defense whether a reasonable person would have refused antibiotics if informed of the reasonably foreseeable material risks. Therefore, even if the dentist did not advise the patient of the significant risks associated with the antibiotic, if a reasonable person would have taken such risks, then the dentist's nondisclosure to the litigating patient would be exculpated.[48]

Elective vs nonelective antibiotic use

Once an infection occurs, the prescribing of antibiotics is nonelective—that is, it is principally the doctor's decision rather than a decision of both doctor and patient. The dentist should stress the risks of spreading infection if the drugs are not taken as prescribed or to completion.

Conversely, prophylactic antibiotic coverage may be considered elective in certain instances; the risks and benefits are weighed by the patient before prophylaxis proceeds. No discussion of rare or remote risks is generally required, but the predictable short-term risks and serious side effects should be reviewed. If antibiotics are refused, the dentist should record the reason on the patient's chart. If prophylactic antibiotics are mandated—for example, for mitral valve prolapse with regurgitation—treatment should be refused if the patient refuses antibiotics because a patient cannot legally consent to negligent care.

Gastrointestinal disturbances are usually self-limiting and short term. Neuropathies, such as the auditory eighth nerve injury caused by strep-

IMPORTANT PRINCIPLE

IMPORTANT PRINCIPLE

IMPORTANT PRINCIPLE

tomycin, should be considered and discussed before prescribing since alternative antibiotics with less serious sequellae may offer therapeutically equivalent effectiveness with greater safety.

Oral contraceptives

It is theoretically possible that antibiotics may reduce the effectiveness of oral contraceptives. Although the risk is small, the magnitude of responsibility is great, particularly in the event of a malformed baby requiring lifetime medical care. At least two cases of dental negligence involving a dentist's failure to warn of the antibiotic inhibition of oral contraceptive effectiveness in pregnancy prevention have been settled out of court.[49] Therefore, in an abundance of caution, a prescribing dentist should provide the warning to women of childbearing years who have indicated their use of oral contraception in their medical history. A dentist also may wish to write a warning on the prescription itself so that the pharmacist may include it on the warning label as an extra precaution and also as additional evidence that the patient was adequately warned.[50]

Case Histories

Duty to obtain medical history

Scandalis v Kaiser[51] A periodontist was protected from an adverse jury verdict because his records contained a signed medical history in which the patient denied ever having diabetes. After undergoing one quadrant of periodontal surgery without antibiotics, the patient developed cellulitis and Ludwig's angina. Following hospitalization, the patient died because of the incorrect use of insulin by the hospital staff. Although the case was settled in the middle of trial for $525,000, the periodontist was dismissed from the lawsuit before the trial began since the patient's signed history denying diabetes proved he had acted with due care. In the absence of a signed medical history form, the jury would have had to resolve whether they believed that the doctor took a medical history.

Failure to prescribe antibiotics

Snow v Xavier[52] A Massachusetts case involving antibiotic coverage resulted in one of the largest dental malpractice verdicts ever. A general dentist extracted a third molar from a patient who later returned with postoperative complications, including signs of infection. The dentist did not prescribe antibiotics and the patient subsequently developed spinal meningitis and was comatose for several months. At trial, the plaintiff was 20 years old and suffering the painful and crippling effects of meningitis. The jury awarded the plaintiff $2.75 million. (A medical negligence verdict also was handed down for $29 million for failure to promptly administer antibiotics for bacterial meningitis.[53])

Improving Quality of Care with Computerization

Quality in dental health care is the application of evidence-based dental science to the individual patient's particular needs. Upholding the standard of care maintains this quality of health care for patient protection. The Institute of Medicine defines quality as "the degree to which health services for individuals and populations increase the likelihood of desired health outcomes and are consistent with current professional knowledge."[54]

The National Roundtable on Health Care Quality, funded by the US federal government and private sources, concluded in its 1998 report that "serious and widespread quality problems exist throughout American medicine."[55] Computer programs and reminder systems that assist health care providers in prescribing antibiotics have helped remedy this problem and reduced mortality among patients treated with antibiotics by 27%.[3]

A study by a committee of the Institute of Medicine on the quality of health care in America suggests that health care errors are a leading cause of death and injury in the US. The report estimates between 48,000 and 98,000 Americans die annually from preventable medical-care errors.[56,57]

Prescription Drugs

Prescription drugs are the fastest growing component of personal health expenditures in the US, amounting to $78.9 billion in 1997. Spending for prescription drugs has increased at double-digit rates: 10.6% in 1995, 13.2% in 1996, and 14.1% in 1997. Contributing to this rise are increased FDA approvals of expensive new drugs and direct advertising to consumers by pharmaceutical products manufacturers. Such advertising is likely to increase further following a US district judge's decision that the FDA cannot limit prescription drug advertising to FDA-approved usages because pharmaceutical manufacturers are guaranteed the right to advertise off-label usage under their constitutional right to free speech.[58]

The learned intermediary doctrine is premised upon the notion that the prescribing doctor is in the best position to make a balanced and individualized assessment as to whether a particular drug is appropriate for a particular patient and to advise the patient about the drug's benefits and risks. This does not apply to a situation in which a manufacturer deliberately encourages patients to take an active role in selecting a prescription medication. When a manufacturer advertises a prescription drug directly to the public, it is the manufacturer's duty to warn the patient/consumer of the drug's risks.[59]

Overprescribing

Antibiotics should be prescribed judiciously rather than zealously. Excessive prescribing or overprescribing unnecessarily exposes the patient to increased financial costs as well as substantial risk of antibiotic complications. Overprescribing also increases the number of antibiotic-resistant organisms in the general population. Ordinarily, a practitioner is legally protected if foreseeably inherent risk complications such as allergic reactions occur since a prudent practitioner does not warrant or guarantee a perfect result. Thus, if antibiotic prescribing is reasonably necessary therapy and the patient is warned of reasonably foreseeable risks, an antibiotic complication is considered an acceptable risk. On the other hand, an antibiotic complication is considered the result of negligent care if use of the antibiotic was reasonably avoidable and therefore unnecessary.

For instance, a severe anaphylactic reaction to an antibiotic may occur in a previously sensitized allergic patient. A clinician therefore should not prescribe an antibiotic to a patient with a known medical history of allergic reaction to that particular antibiotic. For healthy patients, prophylactic antibiotics for routine periodontal surgery or extractions are contraindicated. Routine utilization of antibiotics as a prophylactic against postsurgical infections in medicine or dentistry is not the standard of care since it exposes the patient to reasonably avoidable antibiotic complications. Prudent practice dictates discreet prescribing of antibiotics. Following are examples of imprudent practice.

Unnecessary prescribing

Judicious use of antimicrobial therapy mandates restrained rather than indiscriminate prescribing. For example, simple surgical procedures with little chance of postsurgical infection contraindicate prophylactic antibiotics. Clinical infection signs such as facial space swelling, lymphadenopathy, or febrility, on the other hand, are indications. It is estimated that half of prescribed antibiotics, including those administered to hospitalized patients, are unnecessary or injudiciously selected.[60] Prevention of antibiotic complications requires the prudent practitioner not to prescribe prophylactic antibiotics when the risks exceed the benefits.

Wrong antibiotic choice

Prescribing a broad-spectrum antibiotic when a narrow-spectrum one would be sufficient or prescribing unnecessarily long courses of antibiotic therapy increases the risk of resistant bacterial strain development.

Failure to monitor

Bacterial resistance to a single antibiotic group or to multiple groups (multidrug resistance) frequently results from the genetic transfer abilities of bacteria, which allow them to create pathogens with antibiotic-resistant genes.[61] It is therefore important that clinicians monitor the effectiveness of prescribed antibiotics and consider changing the antibiotic or the method of therapeutic management if the antibiotic proves ineffective.

Manufacturer's Guidelines

FDA-approved manufacturer's guidelines for the use of prescription drugs, which are based on the knowledge gained by competent scientists in the product development stage, generally should be followed. However, as a legal defense, an expert may question the necessity of adhering to a product manufacturer's guidelines if such guidelines were established in the absence of well-controlled research data justifying the recommendation. For instance, guided tissue regeneration (GTR) manufacturers recommend antibiotic prophylaxis since the efficacy of membranes to promote osseous regeneration may be lost if postoperative infection occurs. Although postoperative membrane infection manifests infrequently, virtually all surgical procedures entail some degree of risk of postoperative infection. Neither systemic antibiotics nor local antimicrobial rinses are proven effective in preventing bacterial colonization of GTR membranes. Although local antibiotic administration is more effective than systemic use in preventing membrane contamination, clinical outcomes are not improved.[62] Moreover, the rationale for antimicrobial therapy in GTR has not been proven.

Package Inserts

A dentist is legally required to be familiar with current drug package inserts usually replicated in the *Physicians' Desk Reference* (PDR) or the *Dentists' Desk Reference* for prescribed or dispensed drugs. Standard dental practice also requires dentists to be aware of changes in such information as new knowledge of deleterious side effects becomes known.

Physicians' Desk Reference

New York state's highest court has held that the PDR alone may not be used to establish the standard of care.[63,64] The court reasoned that drug manufacturers compose the information contained in the PDR for a variety of reasons, including compliance with FDA regulations, advertising needs, and communication with the medical and dental professions. If the PDR were allowed to establish the standard of care, then drug manufacturers, rather than medical or dental professionals, would set the standard.

The New York court also concluded that the PDR may have some significance in identifying the standard of care but that expert testimony is required to interpret whether the drug in question was properly prescribed and monitored for a particular patient. The patient/plaintiff may be permitted to present expert testimony that the PDR represents the standard of care. However, the patient is barred from entering the PDR's actual contents into evidence as stand-alone proof of the standard of care.

Manufacturers' warnings are not intended to serve as a professional standard of practice. Dentists and physicians must be allowed to exercise independent, individualized professional judgment in prescribing medications for particular patients. PDR and package insert recommendations can be considered evidence of the standard of care only when offered in conjunction with expert testimony that a defendant violated the applicable standard of care in prescribing a drug.[65] In sum, when a dentist prescribes a drug, he or she is obligated to possess knowledge of the drug's risks.[66]

Infective Endocarditis Prophylaxis

Although a few articles[67,68] question the efficacy of antibiotic prophylaxis in preventing bacterial endocarditis, until the American Heart Association changes its 1997 position, the prudent practice is to follow the AHA prophylactic guidelines.[43]

Conclusion

Careful and prudent practice in prescribing antibiotics is the best prophylaxis for the prevention of malpractice. To paraphrase Alexander Pope: To err is human; to err in the use of antibiotics may be harmful, but it is preventable with due care.

References

1. Beierle JW. A viewpoint on the coming impact of emerging diseases. J Calif Dent Assoc 1999;27(5):369–375.

2. Moore, TJ. Time to act on drug safety. JAMA 1998;279:1571–1573.

3. Bodenheimer T. The American health care system—the movement for improved quality in health care. N Engl J Med 1999;340:488–492.

4. California Dental Association. General Guidelines for the Assessment of Clinical Qualities and Professional Performance [monograph]. Sacramento: CDA, 1977.

5. American Academy of Periodontology. Guidelines for Periodontal Therapy. Chicago: AAP, 1983.

6. *Barton v Owen*, 71 Cal App3d 484, 139 Cal Rptr 494 (1977). Restatement Second of Torts section 299A(E). (See also Kruger G. Textbook of Oral Surgery, ed 5. St. Louis: Mosby, 1979:173.)

7. Advantages and disadvantages of the use of dental tomographic radiology. Council on Dental Materials and Devices. J Am Dent Assoc 1977;94:147.

8. Christen AG, Segreto VA. Distortion and artifacts encountered in Panorex radiography. J Am Dent Assoc 1968;77:1096–1101.

9. Mitchel LD Jr. Panoramic roentgenography. J Am Dent Assoc 1963;66:777–786.

10. Brueggemann IA. Evaluation of the Panorex unit. Oral Surg Oral Med Oral Pathol 1967;24:348–358.

11. Updegrave WJ. Panoramic dental radiography. Dent Radiogr Photogr 1963;36(4):76–78.

12. Appelbaum M. Differential diagnosis of cervical radiolucencies. Dent Radiogr Photogr 1983;56(1):15–18.

13. Book of Approved California Jury Instructions [BAJI], BAJI No. 3.75 (1999); Restatement (Second) of Torts § 431(2); *Rutherford v. Owens-Illinois*, Inc. 16 Cal.4th 953 (1997).

14. Beideman RW, Johnson ON, Alcox RW. A study to develop a rating system and evaluate dental radiographs submitted to a third party carrier. J Am Dent Assoc 1976;93:1010–1013.

15. Accuracy required for proper perio diagnosis. ADA News 17 November 1995;26:8.

16. Abstract of 1990 IADR meeting. J Dent Res 1990;69(special issue).

17. Glavind C, Löe H. Errors in the clinical assessment of periodontal destruction. J Periodontal Res 1967;2:180–184.

18. Glazer SA. Reliability of x-ray scores in the Navy Periodontal Disease Index. US Navy Med 1972;60(4):34–37.

19. Morgulis JR, Oliver RC. Developing a periodontal screening evaluation. J Calif Dent Assoc 1979;7:59–64.

20. Harney D. Medical Malpractice. Indianapolis: Allen Smith, 1973:286.

21. Zinman EJ. Usual and customary versus prudent practice. TIC 1981;40:4–6, 13–14.

22. Sadowsky D, Kunzel C. "Usual and customary" practice versus the recommendations of experts: Clinical noncompliance in the prevention of bacterial endocarditis. J Am Dent Assoc 1989;118:175–180.

23. Zinman EJ. Informed consent to periodontal surgery—advise before you incise. J West Soc Periodontol Abstr 1976;24(3):101–115.

24. Cuny E, Fredekind RE, Budenz AW. Dental safety needles' effectiveness: Results of a one-year evaluation. J Am Dent Assoc 2000;131:1443–1448. OSHA revised bloodborne pathogens compliance directive [news release]. Washington DC: US Department of Labor; November 5, 1999.

25. *Harlow v Chin*, 405 Mass 697, 545 NE2d 602 (1989). Harper F, James F, Gray O. Law of Torts 89-113 (1986).

26. Alexander RE. Eleven myths of dentoalveolar surgery. J Am Dent Assoc 1998;129: 1271–1279.

27. Kruger G. Textbook of Oral Surgery, ed 3. St. Louis: Mosby, 1968:187.

28. Morse DR, Furst ML, Belott RM, Lefkowitz RD, Spritzer IB, Sideman, BH. Prophylactic penicillin versus penicillin taken at the first sign of swelling in cases of asymptomatic pulpal-periapical lesions: A comparative analysis. Oral Surg Oral Med Oral Pathol 1988;65:228–232.

29. Kruger G. Textbook of Oral Surgery, ed 5. St. Louis: Mosby, 1979:284. (See also: Principles of antibiotic therapy v. Indications for antibiotic usage. 1982. Dent. Drug Serv Newsl 3(4):1.)

30. *Crane v Smith*, 23 Cal2d 288, 144 P2d 356 (1944). 4 Witkin 496 (1974) Summary of California Law (8th ed.). Torts, p. 496; Restatement Second of Torts, pp. 289, 291-293; Prosser on Torts (4th ed.) pp. 145-149 (1971).

31. *Donathan v McConnell*, 121 Mont 230, 193 P2d 819 (1945).

32. Gilman AG, Goodman LS, Gilman A. The Pharmacological Basis of Therapeutics, ed 6. New York: Macmillan, 1980:5.

33. Boyd JR, Covington TR, Stanaszek WF, Coussons RT. Drug defaulting. I. Determinants of compliance. Am J Hosp Pharm 1974;31:362–367.

34. Stewart RB, Cluff LE. A review of medication errors and compliance in ambulant patients. Clin Pharmacol Ther 1972;13:463–468.

35. Principles of antibiotic therapy. Oral versus parenteral routes. Dent Drug Serv Newsl 1982;3(6):1–3.

36. Wood L. A Handbook of Dental Malpractice. Springfield, IL: Thomas, 1967:33.

37. American Dental Association. Guide to Dental Therapeutics, ed 2. Chicago: ADA, 2000.

38. *Sanderson v Moline*, 7 Wash App 439, 499 P2d 1281 (1972).

39. *Brune v Belinkoff*, 235 NE2d 793 (Mass 1968).

40. Beeson P, Cecil RL, McDermott W, Wyngaarden JB (eds). Textbook of Medicine, ed 15. Philadelphia: Saunders, 1979:396.

41. Updated antibiotic labeling for prevention of bacterial endocarditis. FDA Drug Bull 1980;10(2):12–13.

42. Stenderup A. Oral mycology. Acta Odontol Scand 1990;48:3–10.

43. Dajani AS, Taubert KA, Wilson W, Bolger AF, Bayer A, Ferrieri P, et al. Prevention of bacterial endocarditis. Recommendations by the American Heart Association, JAMA 1997;277:1794–1801.

44. Updated antibiotic labeling for prevention of bacterial endocarditis. J Am Dent Assoc 1980;101:597.

45. Owen R. Erythromycin problems. J Am Dent Assoc 1983;106:590.

46. Cohen S, Burns R. Pathways of the Pulp, ed 2. St. Louis: Mosby, 1980:713.

47. *Stone v Foster*, 106 Cal App3d 334, 164 Cal Rptr 901 (1980).

48. *Cobbs v Grant*, 8 Cal3d 228, 194 Cal Rptr 505 (1973).

49. Antibiotics may interfere with oral contraceptives. ADA News 5 March 1990;21:1.

50. Morse DR. Serious sequellae and malpractice in endodontics. Ann Dent 1988;47:33–37.

51. *Scandalis v Kaiser Permanente*, Sacramento Superior Court of Calif. (1972).

52. *Snow v Xavier*, Somerville Journal Mass (1981).

53. *Marcelin v St. John's Episcopal Hospital*, N.Y. Sup. No. 24450 (1982).

54. Associated Press, Nursing errors cited in many patient deaths, Sept. 10, 2000.

55. Tort Reform in the States. Trial 2000;Aug:28.

56. Kohn, Corrigan, Donaldson. To Err Is Human: Building a Safer Health System. Washington DC: National Academy Press, 1999.

57. Brienza J. Medical mistakes study highlights need for systemwide improvements. Trial 2000;15:93.

58. *Washington Legal Foundation v Henney*, 202 F3d 331 (D.C. Cir 2000).

59. *Perez v Wyeth Laboratories*, 734 A2d 1245 (NJ 1999).

60. Levy SB. The Antibiotic Paradox. New York: Plenum, 1992:1–12, 67–103, 157–182.

61. Harrison JW, Svec TA. The beginning of the end of the antibiotic era? I. The problem: Abuse of the "miracle drugs." Quintessence Int 1998;29:151–162.

62. Zucchelli G, Sforza NM, Clauser C, Cesari C, De Sanctis M. Topical and systemic antimicrobial therapy in guided tissue regeneration. J Periodontol 1999;70:239–247.

63. Minneman DC. Annotation, medical malpractice: Drug manufacturer's package insert recommendations as evidence of standard of care. 82 ALR 4th 166, sect 4.

64. *Newman v United States*, 938 F2d 1258 (11th Cir 1991).

65. *Morlino v Medical Center of Ocean County*, 152 NJ 563, 706 A2d 721 (1998).

66. *Spensieri v. Lasky*, No. 177 (N.Y. Ct. App. Dec. 2, 1999).

67. Strom BL, Abrutyn E, Berlin JA, Kinman JL, Feldman RS, Stolley PD, et al. Dental and cardiac risk factors for infective endocarditis. A population-based, case-control study. Ann Intern Med 1998;129:761–769.

68. Tong DC and Rothwell BR. Antibiotic prophylaxis in dentistry: A review and practice recommendations. J Am Dent Assoc 2000;131:366–374.

Appendixes

Appendix 1 Typical course of odontogenic infection management.

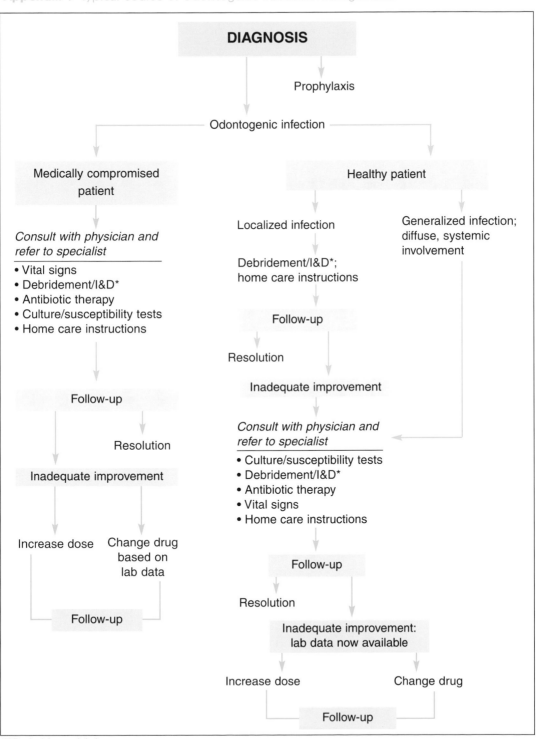

*I&D—Incision and drainage.

Appendix 2 Minimum inhibitory concentrations for 90% of anaerobic isolates.*

Antimicrobial agents	Minimum inhibitory concentrations†											
	Black-pigmented anaerobic rods (40)‡		Fusobacterium (3)		Other gram-negative bacilli (13)§		Veillonella (8)		Gram-positive cocci (11)		Eubacterium (7)	
	Range	90%	Range	90%	Range	90%	Range	90%	Range	90%	Range	90%
Penicillin G	≤0.06–64	0.5	≤0.06–8	0.5	≤0.06–32	4	0.25–0.5	0.5	≤0.06–0.5	0.25	≤0.06–0.5	0.5
Cefadroxil	≤0.06–128	4	0.25–16	8	0.25–64	64	≤0.06–1	0.5	≤0.06–64	16	0.13–64	4
Cephalexin	0.5–32	2	0.5–8	8	0.5–16	16	0.25–1	0.5	0.13–32	8	0.25–64	4
Cephradine	0.25–32	2	0.5–8	8	0.5–32	32	0.13–0.5	0.25	0.5–128	32	0.5–64	16
Cefoperazone	0.13–>128	1	≤0.06–8	1	0.25–128	32	0.25–2	2	≤0.06–1	1	≤0.06–2	1
Moxalactam	≤0.06–32	1	0.25–16	16	≤0.06–16	8	≤0.06–2	1	≤0.06–4	2	≤0.06–8	0.5
Sch 29.482	≤0.06–2	0.13	≤0.06–1	1	≤0.06–1	0.5	.013–0.5	0.25	≤0.06–1	0.5	≤0.06–0.25	0.25
Clindamycin	≤0.06–0.5	0.13	≤0.06–0.25	0.25	≤0.06–2	1	≤0.06–0.25	0.25	≤0.06–0.5	0.5	≤0.06–2	1
Erythromycin	0.13–>128	1	0.5–128	128	≤0.06–2	2	16–64	64	≤0.06–2	2	≤0.06–0.25	0.25
Metronidazole	≤0.06–32	1	≤0.06–0.25	0.25	≤0.06–2	2	0.5–1	1	≤0.06–2	2	≤0.06–64	64
Tetracycline	≤0.06–16	2	≤0.06–16	1	≤0.06–16	1	0.5–2	2	≤0.06–2	1	≤0.06–4	1
Colistin	0.5–>128	>128	0.25–2	1	≤0.06–>128	>128	1–2	1	32–>128	>128	4–>128	>128
Kanamycin	8–>128	>128	0.5–>128	128	0.5–>128	>128	32–>128	64	0.5–>128	128	4–>128	>128
Vancomycin	4–>128	128	16–>128	>128	1–>128	>128	32–>128	>128	0.13–1	1	0.5–2	1

*Source: Sutter VL, Jones JM, Ghoniem ATM. Antimicrobial susceptibilities of bacteria associated with periodontal disease. Antimicrob Agents Chemother 1983;23:483–486. Reprinted by permission of the American Society for Microbiology.

†Minimal inhibitory concentrations are expressed in micrograms per milliliter, except penicillin G, which is expressed in units per milliliter. Numbers in parentheses indicate number of strains tested. 90%, MIC inhibiting 90% of isolates.

‡Includes *Prevotella melaninogenicus, Prevotella loescheii, Prevotella denticola, Prevotella intermedia, Prevotella corporis, Porphyromonas asaccharolyticus, Porphyromonas gingivalis,* and the type of strain of *Bacteroides macacae.*

§Includes *Prevotella oralis, Bacteroides ureolyticus,* other *Bacteroides* spp, *Selenomonas* spp, and *Wolinella* spp.

Appendix 3 Minimum inhibitory concentrations for 90% of selected oral isolates (microaerophilic and facultative isolates only).*

Minimum inhibitory concentrations†

Antimicrobial agents	Capnocytophaga (17)		Eikenella and Haemophilus (2)‡		Actinomyces (22)§		Arachnia and Propionibacterium (6)§		Lactobacillus (16)§		Streptococcus (39)	
	Range	90%	Range	90%	Range	90%	Range	90%	Range	90%	Range	90%
Penicillin G	0.25–1	1	0.25–0.5	0.5	≤0.6–8	1	≤0.6–0.13	0.13	≤0.06–0.5	0.25	≤0.06–0.5	0.25
Cefadroxil	2–>128	128	8–32	32	≤0.06–2	1	0.13–8	8	≤0.06–1	0.5	0.25–32	16
Cephalexin	1–128	64	4–16	16	≤0.06–2	1	0.25–32	32	≤0.06–2	0.5	0.5–32	16
Cephradine	2–>128	128	8–16	16	0.25–8	4	0.25–64	64	≤0.06–1	1	0.25–32	16
Cefoperazone	0.25–32	8	≤0.06–0.13	0.13	0.13–4	4	0.13–8	8	≤0.06–1	1	≤0.06–4	2
Moxalactam	0.13–16	4	≤0.06	≤0.06	≤0.06–8	4	≤0.06–8	8	0.13–1	0.5	≤0.06–32	8
Sch 29,482	0.25–2	1	0.25–1	1	≤0.06–1	0.5	≤0.06–4	4	≤0.06–0.25	0.25	≤0.06–2	1
Clindamycin	≤0.06–0.13	0.13	16–32	32	≤0.06–4	1	≤0.06–16	16	≤0.06–2	1	≤0.06–128	0.13
Erythromycin	0.13–4	2	1	1	≤0.06–1	0.25	≤0.06–2	2	≤0.06–1	0.5	≤0.06–>128	0.13
Metronidazole	1–32	16	128–>128	>128	0.25–>128	>128	0.5–>128	>128	0.5–>128	>128	128–>128	>128
Tetracycline	0.25–2	2	1	1	0.25–64	4	0.13–2	2	≤0.06–16	1	0.5–128	64
Colistin	128–>128	>128	0.5–1	1	16–>128	>128	128–>128	>128	8–>128	>128	128–>128	>128
Kanamycin	128–>128	>128	1–2	2	8–>128	>128	16–>128	>128	2–128	128	0.5–>128	>128
Vancomycin	1.5–64	32	16–128	128	0.5–8	1	0.25–64	64	0.13–2	1	0.5–2	2

*Source: Sutter VL, Jones JM, Ghoniem ATM. Antimicrobial susceptibilities of bacteria associated with periodontal disease. Antimicrob Agents Chemother 1983;23:483–486. Reprinted by permission of the American Society for Microbiology.

†Concentrations are expressed in micrograms per milliliter, except penicillin G, which is expressed in units per milliliter. Numbers in parentheses indicate number of strains tested. 90%, MIC inhibiting 90% of isolates.

‡One strain each of Eikenella corrodens and Haemophilus aphrophilus.

§A few strains grew under anaerobic conditions only.

Index